Nursing Leadership and Management: Working in Canadian Health Care Organizations

Alice Gaudine
Memorial University of Newfoundland

Marianne Lamb
Queen's University

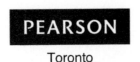

Toronto

Vice-President, Editorial Director: Gary Bennett
Senior Acquisitions Editor: Lisa Rahn
Marketing Manager: Jenna Wulff
Project Manager: Rachel Thompson
Developmental Editor: Mary Wat
Production Services: Cenveo® Publisher Services
Permissions Project Manager: Marnie Lamb
Photo Permissions Research: Luke Malone
Text Permissions Research: Khalid Shakhshir
Art Director: Zena Denchik
Cover Designer: Miguel Acevedo
Cover Image: Image Source/Gettyimages (Top Left); Sam Edwards/OJO Images/Gettyimages (Top Right); Justin Horrocks/E+/Gettyimages (Bottom Left); asiseelt/ E+/Gettyimages (Bottom Right)

5   18

Library and Archives Canada Cataloguing in Publication

Gaudine, Alice, 1955-, author Nursing leadership and management : working with Canadian healthcare organizations / Alice Gaudine, Memorial University, Marianne Lamb, Queen's University. – First edition.

Includes bibliographical references and index.
ISBN 978-0-13-273597-1 (pbk.)

    1. Nursing services–Canada–Administration. 2. Leadership.

I. Lamb, Marianne, 1948-, author II. Title.

RT89.G39 2013   362.17'3068   C2013-907063-X

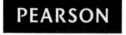

ISBN 978-0-13-273597-1

Brief Table of Contents

Detailed Table of Contents

14 Ethical Leadership and the Context for Ethical Practice in Health Care Organizations 410

Preface

Nursing Leadership and Management: Working in Canadian Healthcare Organizations provides a truly Canadian introduction to theory and practice while emphasizing key skills employed by highly successful nurse leaders and managers. Drawing on our experience as Canadian nurses and as instructors, we wrote this text with the goal of equipping our students with the knowledge to excel as nurse leaders. Our practical experience in nursing is grounded in Alice Gaudine's background in administration and Marianne Lamb's experience as a leader in organizations such as the Canadian Association of Schools of Nursing.

Written primarily as a resource for nursing students in a bachelor's program who are learning about nursing leadership, nursing management, and working in today's health care organizations, the book coaches readers in thinking critically, improving quality, communicating effectively, building teams, delegating successfully, handling conflict, leading change, and more. Throughout the book, we identify challenges nurses and health care organizations face and encourage the next generation of nurses to find positive solutions. Accordingly, the book is of interest to not only undergraduate nursing students but also practising nurses and graduate students. Practising nurses can use the book to help them prepare for a management or leadership position, to develop leadership skills in any position, and to learn about the responsibilities of their managers. Graduate students will find the book useful as a clear overview of key leadership and management topics.

We focused the book on issues for those working in the Canadian health care system. We drew on a wide range of research, but incorporated Canadian research and leading health care examples from different regions of Canada and from health care settings including hospitals, long-term care settings, nursing homes, and the community. Note that while we tried to be as inclusive as possible, some regions in Canada conduct more research on leadership, management, and nurses' work life than others. Additionally, more research in leadership, management, and quality of work life is carried out in hospitals than in other health care settings, possibly because the number of nurses employed by hospitals facilitates research at these sites. These two factors did constrain our ability to devote equal space to research from all regions of Canada and from a variety of health care sites.

HIGHLIGHTS OF THE FIRST EDITION

Four themes frame the contents of this book:

1. *Patient safety*
2. *Communication* in leadership and management
3. *Critical thinking* appears throughout the narrative and is exemplified in the cases and critical thinking questions and activities.
4. *Research* supports the content; we believe that nurse leaders and managers should use evidence-based practice.

We tried to engage the reader by using the active voice (first person) rather than exclusive use of passive voice (third person). Years ago, scientific writing did not allow the use of active voice but today active voice is encouraged for clear, concise writing (APA, 2010). "We" appears throughout to not only personalize the reading experience for students, but also to clarify when an idea is our own versus when an idea is widely known and accepted or when we are citing another author(s) (in which case we provide a reference).

PEDAGOGICAL FEATURES

A variety of features help students navigate this text.

- Chapter opening *learning objectives* and a *summary* allow students to confirm that they have absorbed key ideas.
- A chapter case study followed by questions encourages the application of concepts to a realistic scenario.
- *Critical thinking questions and activities* not only promote discussion and critical thinking, but also help the next generation of nurses to start thinking about innovations to improve our health care system.
- *Self-quizzes* assist with self-assessment of selected chapter content.
- Links to *useful websites* help the reader find further information or examples from organizations as these relate to the book's content.

In addition to this, the text includes **four types of boxed features**:

1. *At-a-glance* boxes: highlight key concepts
2. *Leading Healthcare Example* boxes: portray good practices in Canadian nursing and health care organizations
3. *Interview* boxes: a Canadian nurse leader provides examples and knowledge from his or her practice
4. *Related Research* boxes: showcase ongoing research in areas referred to in the chapter

INSTRUCTOR RESOURCES

The following instructor resources can be downloaded from Pearson's Instructor's Resource Centre. Please ask your Pearson Sales Representative for access information.

- **Instructor's Manual:** The Instructor's Manual helps prepare for lecture with its inclusion of topics for class discussion, solutions to questions, and more.
- **PowerPoint Slides:** PowerPoint slides provide visual talking points. Instructors can customize the decks if desired.
- **MyTest and Test Item File:** MyTest from Pearson Education Canada is a powerful assessment generation program that helps instructors easily create and print quizzes, tests, and exams, as well as homework or practice handouts. Questions and tests can all

be authored online, allowing instructors ultimate flexibility and the ability to efficiently manage assessments at anytime, from anywhere. MyTest for the first edition of *Nursing Leadership and Management: Working in Canadian Healthcare Organizations* is also available in Microsoft Word format (referred to as the Test Item File) on the Instructor's Resource Centre.

PEARSON CUSTOM LIBRARY

For enrollments of at least 25 students, you can create your own textbook by choosing the chapters that best suit your own course needs. To begin building your custom text, visit www.pearsoncustomlibrary.com. You can also work with a Pearson Sales Representative to create your ideal text—publishing your own original content or mixing and matching Pearson content. Contact your local Pearson Representative to get started.

COURSESMART FOR INSTRUCTORS

CourseSmart goes beyond traditional expectations—providing instant, online access to the textbooks and course materials. You can save time and hassle with a digital eTextbook that allows you to search for the most relevant content at the very moment you need it. Whether it's evaluating textbooks or creating lecture notes to help students with difficult concepts, CourseSmart can make life a little easier. See how when you visit www.coursesmart.com/instructors.

Acknowledgements

We want to acknowledge the assistance of Kate Edgar in the early phase of work on this book and the many reviewers of this textbook for their detailed, helpful comments. We appreciate the time and care that they put into their reviewing.

The reviewers include B. Maura MacPhee (University of British Columbia), C. Barbara Campbell (University of Prince Edward Island), D. Lillian Alexus (Langara College, School of Nursing), E. Kathleen Miller (Grant MacEwan University), F. Judith Wells (Western Regional School of Nursing, Memorial University of Newfoundland), G. Sandra MacDonald (Memorial University of Newfoundland), H. Willena Nemeth (Cape Breton University), J. Valerie Fiset (Algonquin College), D. Sharon Paton (Ryerson University), E. Kileen Tucker Scott (Ryerson University), F. Linda Brazier (BCIT), G. Kathleen Brophy (Centre for Nursing Studies), A. Ruth Chen (McMaster University), B. Beth Perry (Athabasca University), D. Eva Beattie (St. Clair College), B. Tanya Johnson (York University), D. Yolanda Babenko-Mould (UWO), E. Selma Kerr-Wilson (BCIT), and F. Denise Newton-Mathur (Laurentian University).

We would like to thank the tireless efforts of Pearson's editorial and production staff for all their work. In particular, we thank Lisa Rahn (Senior Acquisitions Editor), Mary Wat (Developmental Editor), Rachel Thompson (Project Manager), and Marnie Lamb (Permissions Project Manager) for their guidance and their hard work on our behalf.

About the Authors

Alice Gaudine, RN, is a professor at Memorial University of Newfoundland School of Nursing in St. John's, Newfoundland and Labrador. Prior to starting at Memorial University, Alice had approximately 15 years of experience in various nursing management positions as well as experience as a direct care nurse. Her masters degree is in Nursing (MScA, McGill) and her doctoral degree is in administration (organizational behaviour) (PhD, Concordia). She has published a number of journal articles on topics such as the ethical conflicts of nurses (and nurse managers) with organizations, and issues related to nurses' absenteeism and turnover. Alice has also held administrative positions in nursing education, as the Associate Director Graduate Programs and Research at Memorial University of Newfoundland School of Nursing, and the Associate Dean Academic at the University of Calgary-Qatar.

Marianne Lamb, RN, is a Professor Emerita at Queen's University in Kingston, Ontario. She has worked as a nurse in small and large hospitals in Ontario and Quebec, and completed graduate studies in acute care nursing (MSc, Alberta) and health policy/ health administration (PhD, Toronto). Marianne's leadership and management experiences include positions as Director of Professional Services with the Canadian Nurses Association, Director of the School of Nursing at Memorial University of Newfoundland, and Associate Dean (Health Sciences) and Director of the School of Nursing, Queen's University. Her most research work has focused on knowledge translation, patient safety, and clinical ethics. She is a past President of the Canadian Bioethics Society and the Canadian Association of Schools of Nursing.

Chapter 1
Leadership in Health Care

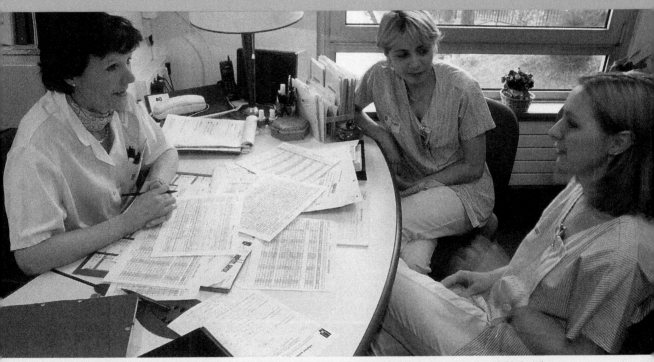

BSIP SA/Alamy

Learning Objectives

After reading, studying and reflecting on this chapter's content, you will be able to:

1. Distinguish between leadership and management
2. Discuss the evolution of theories of leadership
3. Describe the role and behaviour of followers in an organization
4. Debate the strengths and weaknesses of different styles of leadership in various health care settings
5. Analyze the components of emotional intelligence
6. Identify leadership behaviours in the various communities in which you participate (clinical work, educational institution, student organizations) and identify characteristics of leadership styles
7. Discuss the potential effects of leadership behaviour on nurses and on patient outcomes

INTRODUCTION

What is **leadership** and how is it different from **management**? We will briefly discuss how these two concepts differ, and then focus on leadership. We will discuss the concept of leadership, providing an overview of several theories of leadership. We will explore **leadership styles** and examine such concepts as **emotional intelligence** and **followership**. Finally, we will discuss the theories and research on nursing leadership and how nursing leadership and emotional intelligence in nurse leaders can affect outcomes for nurses, patients, and work environments.

THE CONCEPTS OF LEADERSHIP AND MANAGEMENT

Much has been written about the similarities and differences between the concepts of leadership and management, although you will find that many authors use the terms interchangeably. Management is a process that involves directing activities within an organization and managers carry formal authority with respect to the work of others in that organization. Kouzes and Posner (1995) wrote that management referred to "handling" things, whereas leadership referred to "going places." Leadership is a process that involves influencing the thinking and actions of others with respect to achieving a goal, and a person can be a leader without having the formal authority of a management position (Grossman & Valiga, 2013). Leadership is therefore relationship-based and vision-focused, whereas management is focused on orderly steps and coordination of details to implement a plan. Despite this distinction, leaders can manage projects and managers have a leadership role in an organization. Leadership is considered to be a skill, a behaviour, or a role that can emerge and be demonstrated by all practising nurses in some aspect of their professional work, even those who don't occupy a formal management position. Leaders influence others to achieve goals; they may be informal or formal leaders. Formal leaders are those in a position within an organization that confers authority on the individual, as well as a position description that sets out the responsibilities of the job.

Definitions of leadership vary, based on one's theoretical perspective. For the introductory purposes of this chapter, we will begin with Bass's (1990, p. 19) definition of leadership as:

> ...an interaction between two or more members of a group that often involves structuring or restructuring of the situation and the perceptions and expectations of the members. Leaders are agents of change—persons whose acts affect other people more than other people's acts affect them. Leadership occurs when one group member modifies the motivation or competencies of others in the group. (p. 19).

The above definition reflects a somewhat leader-centric view; as we will see later in this chapter, later approaches have shifted the perspective to a more interaction-based theory that focuses on followers as well as leaders. However, the key messages about leadership are these: it involves change and it is about influencing the actions of, and motivating followers towards goals.

Leadership and management do not begin with one's first formal promotion in nursing. As nursing students, you have had opportunities to demonstrate your leadership skills through class activities and student government, sports teams, or other extra-curricular activities. You may also have exhibited management skills in your role as class treasurer, planning events as social convener, and organizing fund-raising or other volunteer activities. We believe that new graduates in their first professional position in health care have opportunities to exhibit the characteristics of a leader in their workplace and beyond. For example, by teaching, coaching, and motivating patients and families with regard to self-care or illness management, you can inspire others to achieve goals that are important to them. If you are already an experienced registered nurse, you have had the opportunity to demonstrate leadership, for example, by volunteering to lead or participate in special work projects or to represent your unit in organization-wide projects; by volunteering for local, provincial/state, national, or international nursing organizations.

Box 1.1

Examples of Staff Nurse and Student Leadership

The College of Registered Nurses of British Columbia (CRNBC), formerly the Registered Nurses Association of British Columbia (RNABC) initiated a system of workplace representatives at hospitals and other agencies around the province (Priest, 2005). Nurses volunteered to take on nurse leader roles as "front-line supports" for registered nurses and acted as "role models, mentors and excellent communicators" (p. 8).

An example of such a nurse was Edie Pletzer, who several years after graduation became a workplace representative and a key person in the development of a new practice council for acute psychiatry at her workplace. She developed role descriptions and a competencies checklist for nurses as ways of improving the practice environment, and took on leadership roles in the community in an After-hours Response program related to mental health and addictions.

Santhi Lechimanan, a staff nurse and workplace representative for a senior's residential care home, set out to work with colleagues to make improvements in workplace support and education. She initiated monthly roundtables with colleagues on quality practice environments, at which participating nurses rotated the duty of chairing meetings. Santhi also joined the organization's nursing committee that embarked on setting up a mentorship program.

In 2004, a group of students launched a new organization called the New Health Professionals Network (NHPN) and advocated for a publicly funded and sustainable health care system in Canada. They engaged in the debate about public policy and the future of health care, making recommendations on ensuring appropriate training for new generations of health care professionals. The former student leaders came from the Ontario Association of Social Workers, the Canadian Association of Pharmacy Students and Interns, the Canadian Nursing Students' Association, and the Professional Association of Interns and Residents of Ontario.

Sources: Based on Priest, A. (February, 2005). Born leaders. *Nursing BC.* Diamond, Somers, Garreau & Martin (2005). New health professionals network: The future face of medicine, *Nursing Leadership, 18(4),* 44–46.

THEORIES OF LEADERSHIP

Theories of leadership have developed out of management theories, although leadership has been discussed since biblical times and was considered by philosophers in ancient Greece. Those interested in management science and organizational theory, especially those from the human relations school, which emphasized participative decision-making and manager treatment of employees, became particularly interested in leadership behaviour in organizations and sought to examine the nature of leadership. In much of the writing and discussion about leadership, the focus is clearly on "leaders" rather than "leadership." Many disciplines, including political science, psychology, sociology, history, philosophy, and management, have studied leadership. Each discipline contributes a different perspective on leadership. You will find that much, but not all, of the nursing and health care literature that focuses on leadership is really interested in its application to those with management or executive roles in organizations.

Great Man Theories and Trait Theories

Historic views and conceptions of leaders, if not leadership, included cultural and societal views of traditional leadership based on lineage and inherited headship. Societies often viewed members of a royal or distinguished family as having the qualities of "born" or "natural" leaders. Great Man theories were based on the study of famous or historic leaders to identify qualities and personal traits that could be said to characterize leaders, but this focus on individual leaders has provided little definitive knowledge about leadership (Bones, 2011; Roussel & Swansburg, 2009). There seems to be no universal and enduring sets of qualities or traits that one can attribute to leaders. Leaders are individuals who act in different time and social contexts (Ladkin, 2010). Therefore, whether or not anyone's behaviour is perceived as that of a leader will vary with the historical and cultural context. Researchers abandoned the trait approach as it did little to predict who would turn out to be a leader. Subsequent research began to focus on the activities of leaders (Glynn & DeJordy, 2010).

Behavioural Theories

Behavioural theories of leadership developed during the human relations period in management science (beginning around the 1920s). The focus of researchers was on the style of leadership exhibited by leaders. Leaders were divided into those with a "task orientation," focused on goals and structures, or those with a "people orientation," focused on relationships and interaction with followers (Glynn & DeJordy). The early work of behavioural theorists identified three styles: autocratic, democratic, and laissez-faire based on the behaviour of leaders in organizations and therefore focused on manager behaviour rather than on the concept of leadership (White & Lippitt, 1960; Bass, 1990; Stewart & Manz, 1997). Some of the characteristics of these styles are described in Table 1.1. Again, these lines of research found that no one style was more effective than all of the others or that the effectiveness of any one style varied depending on the setting.

While behavioural theories viewed the style of leadership as relatively fixed in an individual, situational or contingency theories examined behaviour in relation to the situation or aspects of the environment.

Table 1.1 Leader Styles and Behaviours

Team Leader Style	Behaviours
Autocratic	Authoritarian
	Directive
	Focused on task or production
	Focused on performance
	Control authority, power, and decision-making
Participative	Democratic
	Consultative
	People oriented/employee centred
	Group decision-making
	Share authority, power, and control with followers
Laissez-faire	Uninvolved in day to day activities
	Passive
	Not visible

Contingency Theories

Contingency theories were based on the assumption that there was variation in leadership depending on situations and that context can determine what is effective. Therefore factors such as the environment, readiness for change, the task at hand, and the expertise of followers influenced leadership. Contingency theorists proposed that a leader's style can and should vary depending on the situation and ranges from directive to supportive to participative to achievement-oriented (Glynn & DeJordy, 2010). These theories went beyond the notion of leadership as inherent qualities in the leader or a "one size fits all" leadership style that is suitable for all situations and that is always effective.

In current nursing literature on leadership and management, authors have emphasized two aspects of the context of health care: the pace of change and technological developments. **Innovation leadership** is a term used with respect to these contextual changes. Innovation leadership refers to "the process of creating the context for innovation to occur" (Malloch, 2010, p. 2) in organizations, given current and anticipated changes in work location, work media (digital), work time in a global and modern context, and altered lines of communication. This kind of leadership is seen as necessary in the future as the tasks of the leader shift from a focus on operations to include innovation planning and management, and transition to new operational work.

Interactional Theories

Interactional theories build on the earlier ones. From the 1970s to the present, there has been a greater focus on the leader's ability or style in bringing about change, and the influence on and interaction of leaders and followers. For example, Leader-Member Exchange theory (LMX) focuses on how leaders vary their behaviour depending on characteristics of their followers and the situation (Glynn & DeJordy, 2010). Here are some terms used in some of these theoretical approaches:

Transactional Leadership

Burns (1978) described transactional leadership as the traditional type of relationship between leaders and followers. Transactional leaders have a conventional approach in that they establish an exchange relationship with those who report to them, providing rewards in exchange for meeting objectives. They correct or punish when their employees fail to meet objectives, relying on reward and punishment as motivators. Rather than seeking shared goals or engaging employees, they use these extrinsic factors (rewards and punishment) and tend to focus on tasks. An exaggerated depiction of transactional leadership is shown in the cartoon of the traditional boss who uses a carrot (reward) approach.

Transformational Leadership

This style of leadership is inspirational and based on motivating followers to achieve a high level of performance. First described by Burns (1978), who focused on political leadership, this style has been of great interest to those seeking to improve organizational and management leadership. The leader creates and provides a vision and influences followers to achieve the goals that flow from that vision, exhibiting enthusiasm and optimism. Burns thought that transformational leaders engages the "full person" of the follower and satisfies their "higher needs." He therefore emphasized moral leadership, values, and responsibilities and focused on the wants, aspirations, and needs of followers. Transformational leadership is exhibited by leaders who inspire employees to achieve goals, collaborate, act as role models, mentor, and encourage questioning and creativity (Eagly & Carli, 2003; Rowold & Heinitz, 2007).

Full-range Leadership

This theory builds on Burns's earlier theory of transactional and transformational leadership, and proposes three types of leadership behaviour: transformational, transactional, and nontransactional laissez-faire leadership. Antonakis, Avolio, and Sivasubramaniam (2003) describe nine behavioural factors that go beyond earlier theories that focus on

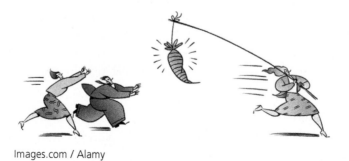

Images.com / Alamy

Creating and sustaining dementia special care units in rural nursing homes: The critical role of nursing leadership, 2005. Morgan, Stewart, D'Arcy, and Cammer (2005) describe the development of nursing home Special Care Units (SCUs) for residents with dementia in eight small, rural nursing homes in Saskatchewan. These units developed in recognition of the challenges of providing high quality and appropriate care to individuals with dementia, particularly in small facilities (fewer than 100 beds). The research study was conducted to examine how the units developed and how well they succeeded in achieving their planned purpose. A key finding of the study was the "critical role of nursing leadership and supervision in creating and sustaining the unit" (p. 75). To be effective, the SCU leaders required vision, passionate commitment, and a strong belief that the program would make a difference so they could inspire others to deal with the challenges in maintaining the program. Leadership behaviours described included support, guidance, and mentoring; daily role-modelling; and staff empowerment through increased staff decision-making and autonomy. Those nursing directors who were considered to be most successful used behaviours that were consistent with transformational leadership. The benefits for residents were related to living in a "smaller and more homelike scale, reduced stimulation and lessening of conflict with other residents" (p. 97).

Source: Morgan, D. G., Stewart, N. J., D'Arcy, C., & Cammer, A. L. (2005). Creating and sustaining dementia special care units in rural nursing homes: The critical role of nursing leadership, *Nursing Leadership, 18*(2), 74–99.

goals or role clarification exchanges and they emphasize how leaders influence followers. These factors are listed in Table 1.2: the first five are transformational, the next three are transactional and the final factor is laissez-faire leadership.

The transactional factors are contingent reward (reward for task completion), active management by exception (monitoring and active search for work standards with correction as needed), or passive management by exception (intervening only once errors are made or standards not met).

Resonant/Dissonant Leadership

According to Goleman, Boyatzis, and McKee (2002), a resonant leader skilfully moves between six styles of leadership according to the situation at hand. The four resonant styles are: visionary, coaching, affiliative, and democratic leadership. Resonant styles build the energy in a group, while dissonant styles may create more conflict. Two additional styles that are apt to create dissonance in an organization, unless used in a measured or limited way, are pace setting and commanding styles. The differences in these styles are identified in Table 1.3. The resonant styles build positive work environments, while the two dissonant styles result in leaders out of touch with staff, unless the styles are used with care in specific situations.

Table 1.2 Behavioural Factors of Leadership Types

Factor	Description
1. Transformational: Idealized influence (attributed)	Leader perceived by followers as charismatic, confident, powerful, and focused on ideals and ethics
2. Transformational: Idealized influence (behaviour)	Leaders actions are charismatic and centred on values, beliefs, and sense of mission
3. Transformational: Inspirational motivation	Leader energizes followers, views future optimistically, has ambitious goals, projects vision, communicates successful achievement of goals
4. Transformational: Intellectual stimulation	Leader appeals to followers' sense of logic, accepts new ideas, challenges followers to think critically and creatively to find solutions
5. Transformational: Individualized consideration	Leader shows empathy; advises, supports, and gives attention to individual needs of followers; supports their development and self-actualization
6. Transactional: Contingent reward	Leader clarifies goal, role, and task requirements; provides material or psychological rewards when contractual obligations met
7. Transactional: Management-by-exception active	Leader is vigilant to ensure standards are being met, searches for mistakes, and takes corrective action
8. Transactional: Management by-exception passive	Leader intervenes only if noncompliance or if mistakes have occurred
9. Nontransactional laissez-faire	Absence of leadership. Leader avoids decisions and responsibility and doesn't use his or her authority.

Sources: Data from Antonakis, J., Avolio, B. J. & Sivasubramaniam, N. (2003). Context and leadership : An examination of the nine-factor full-range leadership theory using the Multifactor Leadership Questionnaire. *Leadership Quarterly, 14,* 261–295; Kanste, O. Kääriäinen, M. & Kyngäs, H. 2009. Statistical testing of the full-range leadership theory in. nursing. *Scandinavian Caring Sciences 23 (4),* 775–782.

Charismatic Leadership

This kind of leadership is similar to transformational leadership in that it stems from the personal ability of the leader to inspire others to achieve a mission infused with values and meaning. Although similar to transformational and sometimes used interchangeably, charismatic leadership seems to be more focused on the leader than follower. Charismatic leadership involves the leader exhibiting personal risk and confidence in the outcome of the vision as well as unconventional behaviour that builds trust and commitment (Glynn & DeJordy, 2010; Rowold & Heinitz, 2007).

Values-focused Theories

Although many of the interactional theories emphasize the importance of integrity and values in leadership, notably Burns (1978) in his development of the idea of transformational leadership, a number of theorists have developed theories or models of leadership in which

Table 1.3 Emotionally Intelligent Leadership Styles

Style	Description
Visionary	Used when change requires a new vision or clear direction
	Articulates the big picture, but employees/team have freedom to innovate on how to reach goals
	Visionary, transformational style, improving climate and commitment
Coaching	Used to help an employee improve performance and build long-term abilities
	Focus is on personal development rather than tasks
	Helps employees identify their talents and areas to develop in relation to career goals
	Involves delegating, giving challenges, mentoring, tolerating failure
Affiliative	Used to bolster and heal a team and to strengthen connections
	When needed, the focus is on emotional needs of team over work goals, boosting morale in difficult or stressful times
	Exhibits empathy, but also deals with conflicts to create harmony
Democratic	Used to get employee input and ideas when direction is unclear and to build consensus or support for directions
	Useful for getting ideas about how to implement vision
	Needs to be open to feedback, to listen
Pacesetting	Used to get good results from a team that is already motivated and competent
	Sets and models high standards, expects employees to rise to challenges and perform
	Should be used sparingly, for example when a deadline must be met. Continual use can lead to a dissonant work place
Commanding	Used in a crisis, to get a change in a situation, and with problem employees
	May be useful in short term to turns things around, by being forceful and clear about changing the old culture
	Commanding tone, but done well in a limited time frame, without out-of-control behaviour
	Least effective style in most cases as it leads to dissonance if it sets an intimidating tone.

Source: Based on Goleman, Boyatzis & McKee (2002). *Primal leadership: Realizing the power of emotional intelligence.* Boston: Harvard Business School Press (p. 55).

values seem even more central. Curtin (1997) noted that integrity in leadership was receiving increased attention, which she considered to be a revival of the interest in "traits" of good leaders. Some of these theoretical approaches are:

Authentic Leadership

According to Avolio et al. (2004, p. 806), "Authentic leaders act in accordance with deep personal values and convictions, to build credibility and win the respect and trust of followers by encouraging diverse viewpoints and building networks of collaborative relationships with followers and thereby lead in a manner that followers recognize as authentic." The core idea is that authentic leaders know themselves; are aware of their beliefs and values and act in accordance with these; and have a positive influence on the attitudes, motivation, engagement, and performance of followers. Wong and Cummings (2009) describe this emerging theory as particularly relevant to nursing leadership because of four elements: the focus on leader-follower relationships, emphasis on moral/ethical aspects along with character and integrity, a positive leadership orientation that focuses on hope and strengths, and an emphasis on leader-follower development and learning.

Servant Leadership

This term was introduced in the 1970s and is a leadership style that involves a "servant-leader" who is focused on followers and who supports and encourages them to do their best (van Dierendonck & Patterson, 2010). The focus of the servant-leader is on others and he or she emphasizes the goals of an organization and what that organization contributes to society.

Spiritual Leadership

Spiritual leadership is defined by Fry (2003, p. 694–695) as "...comprising the values, attitudes, and behaviors that are necessary to intrinsically motivate one's self and others so that they have a sense of spiritual survival through calling and membership." This theory views spiritual leadership as exhibiting three qualities with related behaviours: vision (reflects high ideals, encouraging hope and so on), altruistic love (forgiveness, kindness, honest, etc.), hope and faith (endurance, perseverance, etc.). Spirituality is seen as an aspect of the workplace in that there is a need for a sense of meaning in work as well as a sense of having a calling through your work. Spirituality is viewed in terms of a relationship with a higher power rather than any specific formal religion.

Ethical Leadership

High profile examples of unethical behaviour by business leaders, such as those at Enron in the United States, prompted a great deal of interest in the ethical dimension of leadership and the study of this aspect of behaviour in leaders. Unlike transformative, authentic, servant, and spiritual leadership, the ethical leadership studies do not propose and study a particular leadership style, but rather an aspect of leadership. The term ethical leadership has been defined as "the demonstration of normatively appropriate conduct through personal actions and interpersonal relationships, and the promotion of such conduct to followers through two-way communication, reinforcement, and decision-making" (Brown & Treviño, 2006, p. 595–596). Normatively appropriate conduct refers to conduct that meets expected ethical standards in society. For example, for a nurse, normative behaviour would be conduct that conforms to the ethics of the profession.

FOLLOWERSHIP

As we have seen in the foregoing description of leadership, many models, frameworks, or theories of leadership are leader-centric ones, with the focus mostly on the leader and scant or little attention to followers. These theories emphasize leader responsibility for performance, often to the exclusion of followers. In response, theories and studies of **followership** developed as many in the field would note there can be no leaders without followers and vice versa (Grossman & Valiga, 2013). Burns (1978) challenged the focus on leaders and advocated greater attention to followers, the interaction between the two, and a focus on the process of leadership as opposed to a focus on individual leaders. Some of the lack of attention to followers has been attributed to both a negative view of followers as passive and relatively unimportant and a Western culture that idealizes and romanticizes leaders (Hoption, 2010). In 1985, Meindel, Ehrlich, and Dukerich wrote about the "romance of leadership" and accurately predicted that "the obsessions with and celebrations of it [leadership] will persist (p. 78).

What is meant by followers and followership? Kellerman (2008), in her book on followership, makes a distinction between rank and behaviour and defines followership in terms of rank: "Followers are subordinates who have less power, authority, and influence than do their superiors and who therefore usually, but not invariably, fall into line" (p. xix).

Kellerman notes that followers may be of three types; of these, the ones most commonly described are those in organizations who have less formal authority and whose positions are subordinate in the hierarchy. However, there are also followers who are not formally designated as such, as for example, a member of a professional association in relation to the president of that group. For example, many of us are members of the Canadian Nurses Association, but we would not be described as followers. In rare situations, followers may actually become more powerful than the designated leader, without gaining any formal authority. For example, a well-respected nurse in a clinical unit may have a powerful influence on nurses in that unit, influence beyond that of the nurse manager, without having a formal position. In this latter situation, rank remains, but behaviour is unusual. According to Kellerman (2008, p. xx), "…followership is the response of those in subordinate positions (followers) to those in superior ones (leaders).

Types of Followers

The study of followership is important, as very little is achieved without the efforts and contributions of followers in an organization or group. Followers and leaders interact to achieve results. Just as leaders are commonly described in terms of their characteristics and behaviours, followers are also, and one cannot assume that all followers are alike. While followers support the ideas and views of another, followers think about these in a critical way, not blindly, and they give feedback, working to accomplish group goals and make the achievement of those goals possible (Grossman & Valiga. 2013).

Those who study organizations, management, and political science have developed classification systems for followers. Zalenznik (1965) classified followers along two dimensions: active-passive and dominance-submission to yield four types of "subordinates": impulsive, compulsive, masochistic, and withdrawn.

A subsequent scheme by Kelley (1992) reflected his goal of promoting "good" followers and was based on degree of independent thinking and level of action. The dimensions of active-passive and critical/independent-dependent/uncritical thinking yielded four types of followers: alienated (independent and passive), exemplary (independent and active), conformist (dependent and active), and passive (dependent and passive).

Chaleff (2003) focused on courage in followers and promoted empowered or emboldened followers in their relationships with leaders. He classified followers in terms of how supportive they were of leaders and the degree to which they challenged the leader. The combinations along the two dimensions yielded four followership styles: implementer (high support and low challenge), partner (high support and high challenge), resource (low support and low challenge), and individualist (low support and high challenge).

Kellerman (2008), while noting that context makes a difference in the behaviour of followers, devised a classification scheme based on one dimension—the level of engagement. She identified five types that fall along a continuum of little or no feeling and acting to followers who were deeply committed and involved. These five types are:

1. Isolates: detached from and indifferent to leaders, do not know them or respond to them

2. Bystanders: decide not to participate and disengage from leader and group; a declaration of neutrality

3. Participants: engaged and either favourable or opposed to leader, group or organization, so they are invested in trying to have an effect

4. Activists: feel strongly about leaders and act accordingly; eager, energized, engaged, and heavily invested; working hard to either support or undermine the leader

5. Diehards: deeply devoted to leaders or ready to remove them from power/influence by any means; ready to sacrifice themselves for a person, an idea, or both

Kellerman notes that at some point we are all followers, although sometimes we lead. She uses two criteria to distinguish "good" followers from "bad" followers, and although she is primarily interested in political science, her work is applicable to the workplace, including the organizations in which nurses work. One criterion is level of engagement—she argues that some level of engagement is better than none. The second criterion is being motivated by the public interest rather than self-interest. Kellerman would therefore assert that to do nothing or to be uninvolved is bad, to support a good leader is good, to support a bad leader is to be a bad follower, to oppose a good leader is to be a bad follower, and to oppose a bad leader is to be a good follower. Kellerman also emphasizes that followers are very important to other followers, and good followership depends on this relationship.

THE CHANGING VIEW OF LEADERSHIP AND FOLLOWERSHIP

In the workplace, superior-subordinate relationships have changed over time, becoming more equal, and the literature has reflected this change. For the most part, the term "subordinate" has been replaced by "follower" and "superior" has been replaced by "leader." At times, work now seems to take place in groups with no designated leader. Ladkin (2010) describes how members of a group working on a hydrogen-powered car in Europe interacted without one person in a leader role; in fact, a group participant said he considered the purpose of producing a sustainable product as "the leader," guiding all of their decisions. According to Ladkin, leadership emerges from a collective process and she describes her view of leadership as "the leadership moment." This idea of the leadership moment suggests that, at times, the actions of a leader may underpin the phenomenon of leadership, while at other times followers may drive the moment. At still other times, the goal or purpose itself can create leadership. As mentioned, some work groups today are "leaderless," and while this is not the norm in most health care organizations, hierarchies have fewer levels (are likely flatter) than they used to have.

Despite the sporadic interest in followers and followership and some study of these concepts, most research has focused on leaders and leadership, and little research has been done on the connection and relationship between the two. What attention was given to followers within the leadership literature was not due to an interest in followers themselves, but rather an interest in searching for ways of improving managers' leadership. There is growing recognition that theories should combine leadership and followership because these two are conceptualized as forming a partnership with the partners affecting the views and actions of each other. In other words, leadership theory and followership theory need to merge to understand how leaders influence followers as well as how followers influence leaders—leaders are not all-powerful beings. In order to learn about effective organizations, we need to understand how both leaders and followers interact and what makes them effective in their roles. In a review of the theoretical developments on followership, Baker (2007, p. 58) summarizes the "basic tenets of active followership theory":

(a) followers and leaders are roles, not people with inherent characteristics;

(b) followers are active, not passive;

(c) followers and leaders share a common purpose; and

(d) followers and leaders must be studied in the context of their relationship. (pp. 50–60).

As you begin or develop your nursing career, you can consider when and how you take on follower and leader roles and the extent to which the various frameworks, styles, and classifications fit with your experiences in health care.

EMOTIONAL INTELLIGENCE

Emotional intelligence (EI) refers to abilities, skills, and personality traits and/or competencies that enable you to recognize your own feelings and emotions and those of others, and to manage those emotions in your decisions, relationships, and adaptation to daily work and life. Although the term **emotional intelligence** was first coined within academia by Salovey and Mayer (1990), the concept was popularized by Goleman (1995) in a book on the topic and subsequently became of great interest to businesspeople, management consultants, and health administrators (Freshman & Rubino, 2002). The proposition that emotional intelligence predicts success and is an important factor in effective leadership led to interest in measuring EI for the purposes both of testing propositions about and developing theories of EI through research and applying the concepts in management practice. The burgeoning interest in the relationship of EI to leadership was reflected in a dramatic increase in theoretical and research articles on the topic. In a review of the literature, Akerjordet and Severinsson (2008) found that while there were no such articles in health care and psychology literature in 1997, these articles began appearing, and by 2005 there were 28. During this period, discussion of the importance of EI for nurse leaders began to appear in nurse management journals (Vitello-Cicciu, 2002; Amendolair, 2003).

The Concept of Emotional Intelligence

The concept of emotional intelligence has evolved since the term was first coined in 1990, as a number of theorists and researchers have expanded on the original work on the topic. Smith, Profetto-McGrath, & Cummings (2009) summarized three theories that authors have pursued: those who see EI as an ability to process emotional information and use core abilities related to emotion; those who view EI as a set of personality traits and abilities that predict emotional and social adaptation; or, those who view EI as a set of learned skills and competencies enabling one to understand self and others and manage emotions (see Table 1.4).

Goleman, Boyatzis, and McKee (2002) see the key task of a leader is to "drive" emotion positively so that everyone's performance is enhanced. They identify the four domains of emotional intelligence that add up to emotional intelligence. They are self-awareness (knowing one's own emotions), self-management (knowing how to handle one's emotions constructively), social awareness (being empathetic and attuned to the emotions of others), and relationship management (handling the emotions of others appropriately).

Criticism of Concept of Emotional Intelligence

The concept of emotional intelligence has been the subject of considerable debate and there have been numerous critiques of EI in the literature (Freshman & Rubino, 2002; Feather, 2009; Smith, Profetto-McGrath & Cummings, 2009; Akerjordet & Severinsson, 2010). One criticism is that EI is not a new concept, but an aspect of existing ideas or a repackaging of the concepts of intelligence, empathy, coping, and adaptation. Since there is no consensus on the definition of EI and the concept has not been clearly delineated, measurement of EI is suspect and it is questioned whether the various methods of measurement being used are really examining the same concept. Given the measurement problems, it is argued that EI research cannot explain and predict human behaviour, as proposed, and the rush to market programs and training in EI for managers or to use measures of EI in the workplace is premature and ill-advised and even "unconscionable" (Antonakis, Ashkanasy, & Dasoborough, 2009). As work progresses on measuring EI and the theory underpinning those measures develops, research on the role of emotional intelligence in leadership will likely continue to grow and the interest in EI and nursing leadership will continue.

Emotionally Intelligent Nurse Leadership

As noted earlier, the fields of business and health care became interested in the developing research related to emotional intelligence because it is thought to improve human performance. EI fits with the view that human relations are central to management,

Table 1.4 Concepts and Models of Emotional Intelligence

Author/Sources	View of EI and Features
Mayer and Salovey (1993; 1997)	Ability to perceive, appraise, and express emotion
Salovey and Mayer (1990)	Ability to process emotional information and use it
	Ability to understand and regulate emotions
	Can be learned
	Increases with age
	Contributes to success in life
Bar-On (2013)	A set of competencies, skills and behaviours that make up emotional-social intelligence
	Enables individual to adapt in work and other environments
	Key components in the model include ability to understand and express emotions and those of others, to manage and control emotions, ability to deal with change and solve interpersonal problems, ability to motivate self and general a positive mood.
	Can be learned, predicts success in human performance
Goleman (1995, 1998, 2005)	Set of learned skills and competencies
	Capacity to recognize own feelings and that of others
	Able to manage own emotions well and control responses. Manages emotions in relationships and motivates self and others
	Skills can be taught, and EI is predictive of emotional competency in the workplace

Source: Based on Emotional intelligence and nursing: An integrative literature review, by K.B. Smith et al. International Journal of Nursing Studies, 46(12), 1624–1636.

and transformational leaders as ones who inspire others to achieve goals within organizations.

It is not surprising that EI has been examined in relation to nursing and nursing leadership. Smith, Profetto-McGrath, and Cummings (2009) conducted a review of articles on emotional intelligence and nursing, drawing on the literature published in English between 1995 and 2007. Their final sample consisted of 39 articles, 9 of which were research-based, 21 theoretical articles, and the remainder editorials or opinion pieces. They summarized the findings in terms of four areas or themes, namely EI and the nature of nursing, nursing education, nursing leadership, and nursing research:

■ Because nursing is a profession that deals with human emotion and understanding humans, it is believed that nurses should be emotionally intelligent. Empathy and emotional understanding of others is seen as a nursing competency or core skill.

- Nursing students must be prepared for emotional competence, something required for practice and successful outcomes despite difficult working environments. Experiences that enable students to learn about their own emotions and that of others, mentoring and coaching through self-reflection, and emotionally intense experiences while thinking critically and balancing emotions are necessary aspects of nursing education.

- Emotional intelligence in nurse leaders is considered to be critically important, as this skill or ability is required to inspire others to be successful in achieving goals and providing high level care, even in difficult circumstances. These leaders understand the emotions of others with whom they work and enable them to manage their emotions, even in stressful environments.

- Nursing research related to emotional intelligence is growing, and both qualitative and qualitative studies have been conducted. There is some evidence that leaders with emotional intelligence have a positive influence on the workplace environment and employee stress (Cummings, Hayduk, & Estabrooks, 2005), and that the EI of leaders is positively related to nurse job performance and satisfaction (Wong & Law, 2002). Young-Ritchie, Laschinger, and Wong (2009) in a study of 300 emergency staff nurses in Ontario found that nurses who thought their front-line leader showed emotionally intelligent behaviour reported that they had greater access to power in their organization—in other words, they felt empowered by the leader's behaviour.

NURSING THEORY AND NURSING LEADERSHIP

In the past several decades, the profession has experienced hospital downsizing and restructuring (Cummings, Hayduk, & Estabrooks, 2005), nursing shortages (Baumann et al., 2001), concerns about healthy work environments (Shamian & El-Jardali, 2007), and a growing concern about safety (Cummings, Midodzi, Wong, & Estabrooks, 2010). These conditions have challenged the profession and increased interest in nursing leadership. Nurses are often poorly prepared for leadership, and an increasing number of research studies have explored how leadership styles affect staff nurses and patient care outcomes (Carney, 2009). Many of the leadership theories we have just described have been examined for their fit and application to nursing contexts. For example, Wong and Cummings (2009) examined the emerging theory of authentic leadership and noted that a number of its features meant that it was "…closely aligned with current and future nursing leadership practice and research priorities for the creation of sustainable changes in nursing work environments" (p. 534).

In addition to examining how theories of leadership apply to nursing, some nurses have proposed models of nursing leadership that stem from theories of nursing or that meld nursing theories with leadership theories. Some nurses have proposed that a theory of nursing leadership is needed, one that specifically addresses the science and art of nursing. Laurent (2000) proposed that Ida Jean Orlando's model for nursing practice, developed in the 1960s, provided a framework for nursing leadership in that Orlando's model does not manage or control patient care, but sees the nurse as leading the patients into active participation in care by validating needs and plans with them. Similarly, Laurent thinks this kind of a leadership model would see managers releasing control to the employees, in a dynamic leader–follower relationship. She distinguishes between management and leadership, seeing management as focused on control, stability, and status quo, whereas leadership involves release of control, risk-taking, and providing direction.

Jackson, Clements, Averill, and Zimbro (2009) note many calls in the nursing leadership literature for adopting a transformational leadership approach as opposed to the traditional "command and control" approach. They propose that this approach is too general for the discipline of nursing and not necessarily appropriate for health care settings. They propose a theory for nursing leadership based on Carper's (1978) four *Fundamental Patterns of Knowing in Nursing*, because they believe that it would address the issues addressed by managers and administrators who now confront a chaotic health care environment. The patterns of knowing and associated qualities and examples are presented in Table 1.5.

Another nursing model that is focused less on nurse administrators than the previous ones is proposed by Parse (2008). This model relates to her "humanbecoming school of

Table 1.5 Patterns of Knowing in Nursing Leadership Theory: Description, Qualities, and Examples

Pattern of Knowing	Nursing Leadership Knowing	Description and Qualities	Examples
Empirics	Empiric Leadership Knowing.	Evidence-based nursing leadership. Factual, objective.	Annual report card. Empiric research, outcome-based practice. EBM.
Aesthetics	Aesthetic Leadership knowing	Art of nursing leadership. Empathetic subjective, visionary.	What is significant for nursing staff? Perceptive leadership.
Personal	Personal Leadership Knowing	Relationship-based nursing leadership. Listening, being authentic, empowering. Mutual respect.	Interpersonal relationship between leader and staff. Validate staff concerns. Maximize individual potential.
Ethics	Ethical Leadership Knowing	Ethical nursing leadership. Values, standards, morality.	Code of ethics, professional organizations, accountability, justice.
Sociopolitical	Sociopolitical Leadership knowing	Politics of nursing leadership. Strategic, cultural, diversity, gender-based.	Laws, regulations, external and internal health care environment.
Unknowing	Unknowing Leadership	Openness in nursing leadership. Humility, awareness, flexibility.	Leaders do not know all the answers. Open-minded, adaptable leadership.
Emancipatory	Emancipatory Leadership Knowing	Motivational nursing leadership. Consciousness raising. Transformative workplaces.	Governance partnerships. Policy changes.

Source: Jackson et al. Proposing a theory for nursing leadership. *Nursing Economics, 27*(3), 149–159. Reprinted by permission of Janetti Publishing.

Effects of Leadership and Span of Control on Nurses' Job Satisfaction and Patient Satisfaction (2009)

This study by McCutcheon et al. (2009) was undertaken following a period in which widespread hospital restructuring had resulted in the loss of nursing management positions, a flatter organizational structure, and a wider span of control (meaning an increase in the number of individuals reporting to a single manager). The purpose of the study was to examine the relationship between leadership style, span of control, and two outcomes: nurses' job satisfaction and patient satisfaction. The researchers were also interested in how span of control affected the relationship between leadership style and the two outcomes. The intent was to learn if one could see better outcomes with different leadership styles and spans of control.

This study involved a convenience sample of seven hospitals that had a total of four levels of management: president,

vice-president, program director, and manager. Participants were nurse managers of units, staff registered nurses and registered practical nurses (or licensed practical nurses), and adult patients on the unit who were to be discharged within 24 hours. The final sample consisted of 41 managers from 51 units, 717 nurses, and 680 patients. Staff nurses completed a questionnaire that included a leadership scale that asked about the manager's behaviour and a satisfaction scale. This scale was based on full-range leadership theory and thus included items on transformational, transactional, management by exception, and laissez-faire behaviours. Patients completed a scale on satisfaction with nursing care, and nurse managers completed a questionnaire on span of control as well as a demographic questionnaire.

The study found that nurses' job satisfaction scores varied according to lead-

thought" about nursing. She conceptualizes leadership as residing within the "constituents of a situation" rather than with a designated leader or executive/manager (p. 369). She believes that three essentials in leading are commitment of a vision, willingness to risk, and a reverence for others. She views leading-following as deliberate pursuit of innovation to seek excellence. She discusses the process as requiring the ability to live with ambiguity and vagueness as well as carefully watching ideas emerge and situations unfold.

WHAT DOES THE RESEARCH INTO NURSING LEADERSHIP TEACH US?

Theories of nursing leadership are still relatively new and little has been done to test these theories through research. Most research in this field has been about applying or testing more general theories of leadership and examining their applicability to nursing. Vance and Larson (2002) examined the health care and business literature on leadership between 1970 and 1999 and found that there was little research into the results of leadership on individuals, groups, or organizations, the focus of their review. What little ership style, with transformational and transactional styles having a positive effect and management by exception having a negative effect. Span of control was not a predictor of nurses' job satisfaction, but the positive effects of transformational and transactional leadership styles on job satisfaction were reduced in units where managers had wide spans of control. Patients were more satisfied on those units with lower span of control and a leader with a transactional leadership style.

These authors noted that while the positive effect of transformational style on staff has been demonstrated in previous research, the finding that patient satisfaction is higher with a transactional style was new. One possible explanation for this finding is that transactional leaders provide direction and clarification of duties, which may facilitate patient care. As managers with wide spans of control

may have less time to plan and implement systems that enhance patient care, that situation might explain the effect of span of control on patient satisfaction. A wide span of control might also reduce the time a manager has to interact with staff on an individual level to develop such systems. The authors conclude that organizations should support leaders in developing leadership styles that facilitate staff and caution that no leadership style can overcome the effects of a wide span of control, so organizations need to ensure a reasonable number of reporting relationships.

Source: McCutcheon, A. S., Doran, D., Evans, M., McGillis Hall, L. & Pringle, D. (2009). Effects of leadership and span of control on nurses' job satisfaction and patient satisfaction. *Nursing Leadership, 22* (3), 48-67.

research had been published to that point was descriptive in nature. They located only a few studies that provided some support for the view that leadership had a substantial effect on people and organizations. They concluded that leadership was one of a number of factors that exert influence on outcomes and that all of these influences must be examined together to try and sort out the impact of the leadership factor. Since that time, more research focused on nursing leadership has been reported in the literature. In the following sections we have summarized some of the findings from research on nursing leadership.

What Factors Contribute to Leadership?

Cummings et al. (2008) completed a systematic review of the literature on factors that contributed to nursing leadership and the effectiveness of educational interventions for developing leadership in nurses. They identified 24 quantitative studies that met their inclusion criteria, and the 20 factors that were identified were grouped into four themes: behaviours and practices of individual leaders, traits and characteristics of individual leaders, influences of context and practice settings, and leader participation in educational activities related to leadership development. Factors that contributed to leadership behaviour included:

1. older age and experience (but not length of time in a position),
2. previous leadership experience,
3. relational competencies and style,
4. practising and modelling leadership behaviour,
5. transformational leadership style,
6. openness and extroversion,
7. contact between leader and staff nurse,
8. facilitative leadership style rather than control, and
9. participation in formal and informal leadership education.

Educational activities, such as leadership development programs, were a significant factor in increased leadership practices.

How Do Staff Nurses Perceive Nurse Leaders and Their Leadership Style, and How Is Style Related to Outcomes for Nurses?

Stordeur, Vandenberghe, & D'hoore (2000) examined leadership styles across management levels of 464 nurses in 41 units in eight Belgian hospitals to test the hypothesis that there is a cascading effect of leadership. Theory and some previous research had indicated that leadership styles used at higher levels cascade and are replicated at lower levels of the hierarchy. Their study did not support this hypothesis, and analysis suggested that leadership patterns are related to hospital culture and structure rather than hierarchical level. The researchers did find that transformational leadership was related to several positive outcomes: satisfaction with the leader, willingness to exert extra effort, and perception of unit effectiveness. This relationship also was found for transactional leadership style, but not as strongly as for transformational style. As has been found in previous research, the style of management-by-exception that was passive was negatively related to these outcomes.

Cummings (2004) tested a model of the effects of hospital restructuring on nurses in Alberta through a 1998 survey, following a period of nurse layoffs in the province. Nurses working in dissonant leadership environments reported the highest scores on the negative effects, while those in resonant leadership environments reported the lowest scores on the negative effects. In a study testing a model of authentic leadership and staff nurse trust in their manager, work engagement, voice behaviour, and perceived unit care-quality, researchers found a significant and positive relationship between trust and work engagement that, in turn, predicted voice behaviour (speaking up) and perceived quality (Wong, Laschinger, & Cummings, 2010).

Pearson et al. (2007) conducted a systematic review of evidence that examined nursing leadership and healthy work environment in health care. They found 48 papers, most of which examined relationships between leadership style and characteristics and specific outcomes, such as satisfaction. Based on 11 studies, they found a positive relationship between staff empowerment and positive staff outcomes, such as job satisfaction, accountability, decreased job tension, organizational commitment, and trust. Transformational leadership was associated with job satisfaction and extra effort. Particular leader behaviours, such as consideration, provision of opportunity, and quality mindedness were also shown to be related to positive staff outcomes such as intent to stay in an organization, productivity, and higher levels of motivation.

Cummings et al. (2010) conducted a systematic review on leadership styles and outcomes for nurses and the work environment. They found 53 studies and examined these using content analysis. Outcomes were grouped into four categories: staff satisfaction with work, role, and pay; staff relationships with work; staff health and wellbeing; work environment factors; and productivity and effectiveness. Key findings of the review were that leadership styles that focused on people and relationships were associated with higher nurse job satisfaction whereas styles focused on tasks were associated with lower satisfaction by nurses; staff health was better, and anxiety, emotional exhaustion, and stress were lower with transformational leadership whereas management by exception or dissonant leadership were associated with emotional exhaustion and lower emotional health. In most of the reviewed studies that addressed productivity and effectiveness, these outcomes were higher in settings with charismatic, transformational, and change-oriented leadership, but reduced with management by exception, transactional, laissez-faire, and peer leadership.

What Are the Outcomes of Leadership Style for Patients?

Wong and Cummings (2007) conducted a systematic review of the literature to examine the relationship between nursing leadership and patient outcomes. They identified seven quantitative studies that addressed the relationship between these two variables, and although the findings on mortality outcomes were mixed and not conclusive, they did find a relationship between positive leadership behaviours and patient satisfaction in two of three studies, a relationship between leadership and reduced patient adverse events in three studies, and reduced complications in two studies. The authors conclude that organizations would benefit from developing transformational nursing leadership as a way to improve patient outcomes.

Cummings et al. (2010) studied nursing leadership styles in relation to 30-day patient mortality in 90 acute-care hospitals in Alberta. Using data from a nurse survey from 1998, patient data from the provincial health insurance plan from 1 April 1998 to 31 March 1999, and institutional data for the study hospitals from 1998, a secondary analysis was conducted that examined leadership styles and 30-day mortality. The leadership style of each hospital was determined by examining the responses to 13 survey questions. These reflected emotional leadership competencies and styles and were grouped into three types: resonant—visionary, coaching, affiliative, and democratic styles; dissonant—pacesetting and commanding style; and mixed—neither completely one or the other. Hospitals were then grouped into five categories: high resonant, moderately resonant, mixed, moderately dissonant, and high dissonant based on the scores of nurses' responses to the 13 survey

Interview with Greta Cummings, RN, PhD

Dr. Greta Cummings has more than 15 years of senior administrative leadership experience in hospital, regional, and provincial health services and is currently a faculty member at the Faculty of Nursing, University of Alberta. She holds two investigator awards and has received a number of awards for research excellence. She established the CLEAR Outcomes research program in leadership science in health services, which focuses on the leadership practices of health care decision-makers and managers to achieve better outcomes for providers and patients.

Q: There are many theories of leadership and types of leadership styles described in the literature. Which of these resonate with you, based on your leadership experience and your research into nursing leadership?

A. There are numerous theories of leadership and each one of them focuses on a somewhat different approach. The one that I particularly use that resonates with me and that I really like in both my leadership research and in my everyday life, is an approach of looking at emotional intelligence (EI) as a core requirement of good, strong leadership. And within the EI approach, I particularly gravitate to the work of Goleman, Boyatzis, and McKee who look at EI from the perspective of how well people are aware of their own emotions right at the time that they have them. So they know if they are angry, they know if they are sad, they know if they are anxious. And then, they can manage these emotions appropriately. They are also very aware of the relationships that are going on around them—the kind of socio-political relationships that are around them. They can manage relationships with other people in a way that is effective, everybody grows, and they are able together, to develop a preferred future. So why that works for me or resonates for me is that in fact there are four different leadership styles that are resonant leadership styles because they build energy, they build the harmony in relationships to actually jointly create a preferred future to develop something new, to change the current situation. Two styles are known as dissonant leadership styles that actually lead to more conflict, stress and strain, and anxiety, and don't necessarily lead to the achievement of something together. Most people who are in leadership positions have analytical smarts, so they do have IQ, but what studies and my research has shown is that IQ is not enough. You need EI or other forms of intelligence to complement that. So, EI, just by itself, is not necessarily the most important thing, but it strengthens leadership in someone who has analytical ability as well.

Q: How does the idea of followership fit in?

A: I wouldn't say there is real consensus around followership in the literature. There are a number of people who talk about the real importance of followers and that you are not a leader if you don't have followers. And I'm not totally comfortable with that approach because I think that dichotomizes people too much into those who are always followers and could never lead, when in fact, people can lead in a variety of situations. They might work with a leader in one situation and have the role of follower, and in another situation, they are the leader. So they take turns. It is almost like the analogy of the geese flying and they form a V and they always take turns being the leader because being out front they have to buffer the wind for the others. It's tiring and the rest of the team is with them, so they take turns and they rotate through that leadership. And that's a common kind of approach to leadership that is very real. Now, I think that the role of leader is actually not to develop better followers. I think that the role of leader is to develop more leaders—my approach to leadership is that you are always trying to do yourself out of a job.

Q: How would you advise new nurses to develop their leadership skills and experiences?

A: The EI approach includes being visionary, being a coach, being affiliative, being concerned for emotion in the setting and stakeholder involvement, getting the right people involved, and [having] democratic leadership styles, which requires ensuring that people affected by a decision are involved in the decision. To become a resonant leader like that, you need self-awareness. You've got to have an awareness of your emotions, of your passions, of your values, of your mission for your own life, how you are going to achieve that, and how you relate to other people. So, you need to be clear on that before you can try and lead a group of people. And the approach that I use with students or young people is to have them identify what their values and their vision and mission are for their life. Their values are where they spend their time and their money. And if you don't know what your values are, you just need to look at that and your time and your money will tell you what they are. And then, if in order to determine what their mission and vision is for their own life, in terms of what they want to achieve or what kind of legacy they would like to leave behind, to think ahead what they would like to have written on their tombstone about their life.

When it comes to actually how nurses can see opportunities for leadership in practice, whether it's a community hospital or hospice or family care—they can start to look at opportunities and be aware of opportunities where they feel uncomfortable. So, if they feel somewhat uncomfortable about a situation or they feel there are some inequities happening or that a patient's not getting safe and appropriate care, then that gives them an opportunity to identify a gap in the quality of care for this one patient. How could I improve the quality of care tomorrow? That is being able to turn a current reality into what could be a preferred future. And then of course, being able to look at the situation and say "what's the problem here?" So the problem might be lack of education, or their own education, lack of attention to standards and guidelines, an unwillingness to actually apply evidence, or there might actually be something sinister going on that needs to be attended to. So, depending on what's at the root cause of this situation, let's say in this case, unsafe or poor quality care that is being provided to a patient, then the next step is to be able to declare that this isn't good enough—things have to change. And the next step after that one would be figuring out who they could talk to about this. Because you need to get some allies, especially as a student or new graduate, be able to talk to the appropriate nursing manager, nursing support, other staff, and to engage others and to see that maybe things could be done differently. Then together, they could start taking some action to change the situation so that these patients would get care in a different way with different outcomes. So that's the beginning of leadership and that's an opportunity.

Source: Interview with Greta Cummings, RN, PhD. Reprinted by permission.

questions. Hospitals with high resonant leadership styles had the lowest 30-day mortality after controlling for patient demographics, co-morbidities, and characteristics of hospitals and nurses. However, those hospitals with dissonant styles were the next in lower mortality rates, followed by mixed types of leadership styles, suggesting that clarity of leadership may be better than a mixed type. The authors concluded that hospital leadership styles may contribute to 30-day mortality of patients.

Squires et al. (2010) examined the link between leadership and safety outcomes in hospitals. They were interested in examining patient and nurse safety outcomes in relation to resonant leadership, interactional justice (fairness), quality of the nursing work environment, and safety climate of the hospital. Based on survey responses from 266 acute care hospital nurses, they found that resonant leadership and fairness enhanced nurse leader–nurse relationships and that these relationships were associated with a positive safety climate. While the work environment was also important in a safety climate, trusting and high quality relationships between nurses and nurse leaders improved both patient and nurse outcomes, such as medication errors, nurse emotional exhaustion, and intentions to leave.

A CRITIQUE OF THE FOCUS AND RESEARCH ON LEADERSHIP

As mentioned earlier, there has been criticism of the rush to develop emotional intelligence training by management consultants who may overemphasize this aspect of leadership. There is also a current critique of the "leadership movement" itself and the emphasis on leaders in general, particularly the top leaders of organizations. In his book *The Cult of the Leader*, Christopher Bones (2011) is primarily taking aim at large corporations, big business, and "celebrity leaders" in his argument that leadership has to become organization-centric rather than leader-centric. Similarly, Barker (2001) criticized leadership studies that examine leadership as a discrete event rather than a continuous process, as well as studies that assume the actions of one person, such as a president or CEO, are the cause of outcomes of an organization.

SUMMARY

In this chapter we have distinguished between leadership and management in health care, focusing primarily on leadership. The idea of leadership has changed over time—once viewed as specific qualities or fixed traits of "born" leaders, the concept of leadership has evolved through study of aspects beyond personal characteristics. The examination of leadership expanded to consider the focus of leaders, their behavioural styles, how behaviour does and ought to vary depending on the context, the values exhibited by leaders, and the way in which leaders interact with followers. Most of the nursing literature defines leadership in terms of influencing and inspiring followers to achieve goals; however a developing view is that followership should be incorporated into the concept of leadership. There are no leaders without followers and no followers without leaders—both participate and interact in the achievement of goals and the accomplishment of enterprises. In nursing, there is growing evidence of how important the interaction of leaders and followers is in achieving desired goals, such as patient safety, high quality care, and healthy workplaces.

Glossary of Terms

Emotional intelligence (EI) refers to the abilities and skills of an individual to identify, recognize, and manage the emotions of oneself and others. EI is considered key in leader effectiveness.

Followership is the response of followers to leaders (Kellerman, 2008). The notion of followership refers to the process of interaction and relationship with leaders.

Innovation Leadership refers to leader behaviour that creates the conditions for innovation to occur.

Leadership is a process whereby one person influences others to achieve goals. Definitions vary in detail with different theoretical perspectives on leadership.

Leadership style refers to the pattern of behaviour of leaders as they engage in the process of leadership and interact with followers.

Management is a process whereby one or more persons with formal authority in an organization directs the activities of others to achieve goals.

CASE

Pierre Tremblay is a nurse manager in community health organization and is responsible for the day-to-day operations of client care programs in the home and in other community settings. He is responsible for supporting, supervising, and managing front-line service providers including registered nurses and licensed practical nurses. He is also responsible for planning the training of nursing staff and has several ideas about what important topics to address in the coming year. He decides to raise the issue of education sessions at the next staff meeting, identify some of the topics he thinks are important, and ask the nurses to suggest other topics.

Questions:

1. What style of leadership do you think Pierre exhibits? Contrast his style with that of others and identify what behaviour you would expect with those other styles.

2. What do you see as the role of the staff nurses as followers in this situation? What is the range of ways in which followers may respond?

3. Pierre convenes the meeting and nurses identify five topics that they think are more important than the ones that he has identified. They also take the opportunity to discuss their complaints about their work schedules and problems with the new documentation requirements for home visits. His initial impulse is to argue for the topics he has identified, as he believes they are more important to ensure quality care. However, he is aware that he is feeling anger as an initial response and decides to just listen to the responses. He tells the staff that he will bring back a final list to the next meeting for further discussion. What do you think of Pierre's response?

4. How do you think that Pierre could empower nurses through continuing education? What nurse outcomes of such empowerment would you look for in the organization?

5. What would Pierre need to do to make you consider him to be a resonant leader? A transformational leader? A transactional leader?

Critical Thinking Questions and Activities

1. Describe two leaders you have encountered in your personal life or nursing practice who reflect at least two leadership styles. What behaviours did you observe that led you to choose those styles?

2. What leadership styles do you consider to be most appropriate for leading practising nurses and why did you choose those?

3. Have you had the opportunity to take on a leadership role in your personal or nursing experience? How did you interact with followers? Would you do anything differently now that you have read about leadership theory?

4. Think about clinical, professional, and school-related situations in which you accepted the role of follower. How would you describe your role as a follower and how has your behaviour fit with that role?

5. Reflect on the concept of emotional intelligence. How would you assess yourself in terms of the following abilities?

- Awareness of the emotions of others in a situation.
- Recognizing your own emotions in a situation.
- Regulating your own emotions in a situation.
- Ability to express your emotion in a situation.
- Deal with the emotions of another in a situation.

6. Interview a nurse in a practice setting about her or his experience of clinical leadership. Ask the interviewee to talk about his or her views and beliefs about leadership and how leadership skills were developed.

Self-Quiz

1. One difference between leadership and management is that leadership:
- **a.** Is focused on directing and organizing the work of others
- **b.** Requires a position of formal authority
- **c.** Involves inspiring others to achieve goals
- **d.** Has been shown to require specific personal qualities

2. A leadership style that is based on reward or punishment for accomplishing goals is known as:
- **a.** Transformational
- **b.** Authentic
- **c.** Transactional
- **d.** Spiritual

3. A core idea of authentic leadership is that a leader:
- **a.** Knows self
- **b.** Inspires others
- **c.** Handles emotions well
- **d.** Creates a vision

4. Laissez-faire leadership refers to:
- **a.** A casual approach to supervision
- **b.** Intermittent feedback to followers
- **c.** Management by exception
- **d.** Absence of leadership

Useful Websites

Canadian Nurses Association
www.cnanurses.ca/CNA/documents/pdf/
publications/Nursing_Leadership_Development_
Canada_e.pdf
www.cna-aiic.ca/CNA/practice/leadership/
default_e.aspx
www.nanb.nb.ca/PDF/CNA_Nursing_
Leadership_2009_E.pdf

The Academy of Canadian Executive Nurses
www.acen.ca

Registered Nurses Association of Ontario
www.rnao.org

Winnipeg Regional Health Authority
www.wrha.mb.ca/osd/leadership.php

Nursing Leadership Network of Ontario
www.nln.on.ca/index.php?option=com_
content&view=article&id=13&Itemid=28

Association of Registered Nurses of Newfoundland and Labrador
www.arnnl.ca

Canadian Association of Schools of Nursing
casn.ca/en/Nursing_Leadership_47/items/1.html

ANDSOOHA – Public Health Nursing Management
www.andsooha.org/

Dorothy Wylie Leadership Institute
dwnli.ca/about/dorothy-wylie/

Canadian Health Leadership Network
www.chlnet.ca/front_page

Harvard Business Review
hbr.org/

American Organization of Nursing Executives
www.aone.org/

The Future of Nursing
www.thefutureofnursing.org/topics/
leadership?page=2

American Association of Critical Care Nurses
www.aacn.org/wd/volunteers/content/
frameworkforgovernanceleadershippositions.
pcms?mid=2890&menu=

International Council of Nurses
www.icn.ch/
www.icn.ch/pillarsprograms/global-nursing-
leadership-institute/
www.icn.ch/pillarsprograms/leadership-for-
change/

The Foundation of Nursing Leadership
www.nursingleadership.org.uk/

Current Nursing
currentnursing.com/nursing_management/

References

Akerjordet, K., & Severinsson, E. (2008). Emotionally intelligent nurse leadership: A literature review study. *Journal of Nursing Management*, 16(5), 565–577.

Akerjordet, K., & Severinsson, E. (2010). The state of the science of emotional intelligence related to nursing leadership: An integrative review. *Journal of Nursing Management*, 18(4), 363–382.

Amendolair, D. (2003). Emotional intelligence: Essential for developing nurse leaders. *Nurse Leader*, 1(6), 25–27.

Antonakis, J., Ashkanasy, N.M., & Dasborough, M.T. (2009). Does leadership need emotional intelligence? *The Leadership Quarterly*, 20, 247–261.

Antonakis, J., Avolio, B.J., & Sivasubramaniam, N. (2003). Context and leadership : An examination of the nine-factor full-range leadership theory using the Multifactor Leadership Questionnaire. *Leadership Quarterly*, 14, 261–295.

Avolio, B.J., Gardner, W.L., Walumbwa, F.O., Luthans, F., & May, D.R. (2004). Unlocking the mast: A look at the process by which authentic leaders impact follower attitudes and behaviors. *The Leadership Quarterly*, 15, 801–823.

Baker, S. D. (2007). Followership: The theoretical foundation of a contemporary construct. *Journal of Leadership and Organizational Studies, 14*(1), 50–60.

Bar-On, R. (2013). *The Bar-On model.* Retrieved from http://reuvenbaron.org/wp/?page_id=14 June 14, 2013.

Barker, R.A. (2001). The nature of leadership. *Human Relations, 54*(4), 469–494.

Bass, B.M. (1990). *Bass & Stodgill's handbook of leadership* (3rd ed.). New York: Free Press.

Baumann, A., O'Brien-Pallas, L., Armstrong-Stassen, M., Blythe, J., Bourbonnais, R., Cameron, S., et al. (2001). *Commitment and care: The benefits of a healthy workplace for nurses, their patients and the system.* Ottawa, Ontario, Canada: Canadian Health Services Research Foundation.

Bones, C. (2011). *The cult of the leader. A manifesto for more authentic business.* Chichester, UK: Wiley.

Brown, M.E. & Treviño, L.K., (2006). Ethical leadership: A review and future directions. *Leadership Quarterly, 17*(6), 595–616.

Burns, M.M. (1978). *Leadership.* New York: Harper & Row.

Carney, M. (2009). Leadership in nursing: Current and future perspectives and challenges. *Journal of Nursing Management, 17*(4), 411–414.

Carper, B. (1978). Fundamental patterns of knowing in nursing. *Advances in Nursing Science, 1*(1), 13–23.

Chaleff, I. (2003). The courageous follower: Standing up to and for our leaders. 2nd ed. San Francisco: Berrett-Koehler.

Cummings, G. (2004). Investing relational energy: The hallmark of resonant leadership. *Nursing Leadership, 17*(4), 76–87.

Cummings, G., Hayduk, L., & Estabrooks, C. (2005). Mitigating the impact of hospital restricting on nurses. The responsibility of emotionally intelligent leadership. *Nursing Research, 54*(1), 2–9.

Cummings, G., Lee, H., MacGregor, T., Davey, M., Wong, C., Paul, L., & Stafford, E. (2008). Factors contributing to nursing leadership: A systematic review. *Journal of Health Services Research & Policy, 13*(4), 240–248.

Cummings, G.G., MacGregor, T., Davey, M., Lee, H., Wong, C.A., Lo, E., & Stafford, E. (2010). Leadership styles and outcome patterns for the nursing workforce and work environment: A systematic review. *International Journal of Nursing Studies, 47*(3), 363–385.

Cummings, G.G., Midodzi, W.K., Wong, C.A., & Estabrooks, C.A. (2010). The contribution of hospital nursing leadership styles to 30-day patient mortality. *Nursing Research, 59*(5), 331–339.

Curtin, L.L. (1997). How—and how not—to be a transformational leader. *Nursing Management, 28*(2), 7–8.

Diamond, J., Somers, A., Garreau, M., & Martin, D. (2005). New health professionals network: The future face of medicine. *Nursing Leadership, 18*(4), 44–46.

Eagly, A.H., & Carli, L.L. (2003). The female leadership advantage: An evaluation of the evidence. *The Leadership Quarterly, 14,* 807–834.

Feather, R. (2009). Emotional intelligence in relation to nursing leadership: Does it matter? *Journal of Nursing Management, 17,* 376–382.

Freshman, B., & Rubino, L. (2002). Emotional intelligence: A core competency for health care administrators. *Health Care Manager, 20*(4), 1–9.

Fry, L. W. (2003). Toward a theory of spiritual leadership. *The Leadership Quarterly, 14,* 693–727.

Glynn, M.A., & DeJordy, R. (2010). Leadership through an organization behaviour lens. A look at the last half-century of research. In: Nohria, N. & Khurana, R. (Eds.) *Handbook of leadership theory and practice.* Boston: Harvard Business Press, pp. 119–157.

Goleman, D. (1995). *Emotional intelligence.* New York: Bantam.

Goleman, D. (1998). *Working with emotional intelligence.* New York: Bantam.

Goleman, D., Boyatzis, R., & McKee, A. (2002). *Primal leadership. Realizing the power of emotional intelligence.* Boston, Massachusetts: Harvard Business School Press.

Grossman, S.C., & Valiga, T. M. (2013). *The new leadership challenge. Creating the future of nursing.* 4th ed. Philadelphia: F.A. Davis.

Hoption, C.B. (2010). Towards a relational and dynamic perspective of leadership. (Unpublished doctoral dissertation). Queen's University, Kingston, Ontario. Retrieved from http://hdl.handle.net/1974/5430

Jackson, J.R., Clements, P.T., Averill, J.B., & Zimbro, K. (2009). Patterns of knowing: Proposing a theory for nursing leadership. *Nursing Economics, 27*(3), 149–159.

Kanste, O., Kaariainen, M., & Kyngas, H. (2009). Statistical testing of the full-range leadership theory in nursing. *Scandinavian Journal of Caring Sciences, 23,* 775–582.

Kellerman, B. (2008). *Followership. How followers are creating change and changing leaders.* Boston: Harvard Business Press.

Kelley, R. E. (1992). *The power of followership: How to create leaders people want to follow and followers who lead themselves.* New York: Doubleday).

Kouzes, J.M., & Posner, B.Z. (1995). *The leadership challenge. how to keep getting extraordinary things done in organizations.* San Francisco: Jossey-Bass Publishers.

Ladkin, D. (2010). *Rethinking leadership. A new look at old leadership questions.* Northampton, MA: Edward Elgar.

Laurent, C.L. (2000). A nursing theory for nursing leadership. *Journal of Nursing Management, 8*(2), 83–87.

Lorsch, J. (2010). A contingency theory of leadership. In: Nohria, N. & Khurana, R. (Eds.) *Handbook of leadership theory and practice.* Boston: Harvard Business Press, pp. 411–429.

Malloch, K. (2010). Innovation leadership: New perspectives for new work. *Nursing Clinics of North America, 45*(1), 1–9.

McCutcheon, A.S., Doran, D., Evans, M., McGillis Hall, L., & Pringle, D. (2009). Effects of leadership and span of control on nurses' job satisfaction and patient satisfaction. *Nursing Leadership, 22*(3), 48–67.

McGregor, D. (1966). *The human side of enterprise.* New York: McGraw-Hill.

Morgan, D.G., Stewart, N.J., D'Arcy, C., & Cammer, A.L. (2005). Creating and sustaining dementia special care units in rural nursing homes: The critical role of nursing leadership. *Nursing Leadership, 18*(2), 74–99.

Parse, R.R. (2008). The Humanbecoming leading-following model. *Nursing Science Quarterly, 21*(4), 369–375.

Pearson, A., Laschinger, H., Porritt, K., Jordan, Z., Tucker, D., & Long, L. (2007). Comprehensive systematic review of evidence on developing and sustaining nursing leadership that fosters a healthy work environment in healthcare. *JBI Library of Systematic Reviews, 5*(5), 279–343.

Priest, A. (2005). Born leaders. *Nursing BC, 37*(1), 8–11.

Roussel, L., & Swansburg, R.C. (2009). *Management and leadership for nurse administrators.* 5th Ed. Sudbury, MA: Jones and Bartlett Publishers.

Rowold, J., & Heinitz, K. (2007). Transformational and charismatic leadership: Assessing the convergent, divergent and criterion validity of the MLQ and the CKS. *The Leadership Quarterly, 18,* 121–133.

Salovey, P., & Mayer, J. (1990). Emotional intelligence. *Imagination, Cognition, and Personality, 9,* 185–211.

Shamian, J., & El-Jardali, F. (2007). Healthy workplaces for health workers in Canada: Knowledge transfer and uptake in policy and practice. *HealthcarePapers, 7,* Special Issue, 6–25.

Smith, K.B., Profetto-McGrath, J., & Cummings, G.G. (2009). Emotional intelligence and nursing: An integrative literature review. *International Journal of Nursing Studies, 46*(12), 1624–1636.

Squires, M., Tourangeau, A., Laschinger, H., & Doran, D. (2010). The link between leadership and safety outcomes in hospitals. *Journal of Nursing Management, 18*(8), 914–925.

Stewart, G.L., & Manz, C.C. (1997). Leadership for self-managing work teams: A typology and integrative model. In: Vecchio, R.P. (Ed.). *Leadership. Understanding the dynamics of power and influence in organizations.* Notre Dame, Indiana: University of Notre Dame Press, pp. 396–410.

Stordeur, S., Vandenberghe, C., & D'horre, W. (2000). Leadership styles across hierarchical levels in nursing departments. *Nursing Research, 49*(1), 37–43.

van Dierendonck, D. & Patterson, K. (2010). Servant leadership: An introduction. In: K. Patterson & D. van Dierendonck (Eds.) *Servant leadership. Developments in theory and research.* New York: Palgrave Macmillan, pp. 3–10.

Vance, C., & Larson, E. (2002). Leadership research in business and health care. *Journal of Nursing Scholarship, 34*(2), 165–171.

Vitello-Cicciu, J. M. (2003). Innovative leadership through emotional intelligence. *Nursing Management, 34*(10), 28–32.

White, R.K., & Lippitt, R. (1960). *Autocracy and democracy. An experimental inquiry.* New York: Harper & Brothers.

Wong, C.A., & Cummings, G. G. (2007). The relationship between nursing leadership and patient outcomes: A systematic review. *Journal of Nursing Management, 15*(5), 508–521.

Wong, C., & Cummings, G. (2009). Authentic leadership: a new theory for nursing or back to basics? *Journal of Health Organization and Management, 23*(5), 522–538.

Wong, C.A., Laschinger, H., Cummings, G. G., Vincent, L., & O'Connor, P. (2010). Decisional involvement of senior nurse leaders in Canadian acute care hospitals. *Journal of Nursing Management, 18*, 122–133.

Wong, C., & Law, K.S. (2002). The effects of leader and follower emotional intelligence on performance and attitude: an exploratory study. *Leadership Quarterly, 13*, 243–274.

Young-Ritchie, C., Laschinger, H., & Wong, C. (2009). The effects of emotionally intelligent leadership behaviour on emergency staff nurses' workplace empowerment and organizational commitment. *Canadian Journal of Nursing Leadership, 22*(1), 70–85.

Zaleznik, A. (May-June, 1965). The dynamics of subordinacy. *Harvard Business Review*, 119–131.

Chapter 2
Health Care Management and the Canadian Context

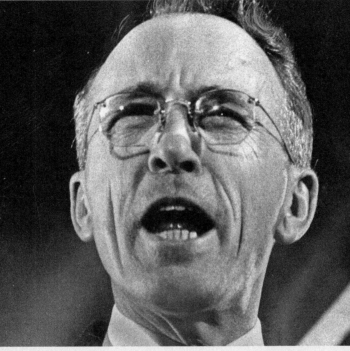

Barry Philp/Toronto Star/ZUMA Press/Newscom

Learning Objectives

After reading, studying and reflecting on this chapter's content, you will be able to:

1. Discuss the evolution of theories of management and how they are reflected in current health care organizations
2. Compare the focus and activities of leaders and managers
3. Identify the components of health systems and the factors influencing the organization of health services
4. Distinguish among municipal, provincial/territorial, and federal levels of responsibility and jurisdiction with respect to health care services and the legislative framework governing health care and health care professionals
5. Describe the levels of health care and the range and types of health care services in Canada
6. Discuss the range and types of regulated and unregulated health workers and professionals in Canada
7. Identify trends and issues in health systems in Canada and how performance of health systems might be evaluated

INTRODUCTION

In the first part of this chapter we focus on the concept of management and discuss the evolution of management theories over time. We discuss the key functions of management and compare management activities with those of leadership, which were highlighted in Chapter 1. We discuss health care management, noting particularly nurses' roles in the management of health care. In the second part of this chapter, we provide a "macro" view of the health care system in Canada and the many factors that shape and change health care over time. Although many of you may begin your early nursing career in a staff nurse position within a health care organization or have had such positions in your career to date, we would like you to consider the system within which you work. We aim to help you develop an understanding of the wide-ranging forces that influence your workplace and the management of those organizations in which you work, be they large or small.

THEORIES OF MANAGEMENT

In Chapter 1, we distinguished between leadership and management, noting that management focuses on organizing and directing activities within an organization and is done by individuals who have a role that carries formal authority and responsibility for such activities. Management theories predate the more recent development of leadership theories, so most of the organizations we have dealt with during our lives have been shaped more by ideas of management than ideas of leadership. These theories aimed at explaining how organizations work, while leadership theories tend to focus on individuals and their interaction with groups.

Ideas about how to accomplish goals can be traced back to the earliest human efforts to undertake group projects, but over time, management theories developed as people began to question and examine the best way to accomplish tasks. These theories have been categorized in terms of their major focus or approach and we present them here because, although there have been changes in how organizations and managers function, you will see elements of these theories today in many of the organizations in which nurses work, and these theories will be reflected in the practice of many managers. The categories of theories presented here are: classical management, human relations, open systems/contingency theories, and decision-making theories. You will see parallels between management theories and leadership theories, but theorists in each category provide a differing perspective on management and organizations.

Classical Management Theories

The development of machines at the time of the industrial revolution stimulated a trend of mechanizing work to more efficiently accomplish goals (Morgan, 2006). **Classical management theory** and **scientific management** gained currency at a time when the focus was on production using machinery. Scientific management theorists, such as Frederick Winslow Taylor, were interested in the design of individual jobs or tasks to increase the output of workers and to increase the efficiency of management through the "scientific" analysis of jobs and the training of workers to use scientific principles and managers to carry out their management functions. Taylor broke production into minute tasks and hierarchical managerial roles were established to oversee the standardized steps carried out by the workers (Dunbar & Statler, 2010). Morgan (2006) sees the approach of McDonald's in the prescribed steps to prepare and serve hamburgers efficiently as stemming from the task analysis approach of scientific management.

Other classical management theorists were interested in the design of organizations as a whole. Henri Fayol developed principles of management that touched on administration, human relations, and production efficiency (Morgan, 2006). He and other theorists in this period viewed management as a process consisting of activities of planning, organization, command, coordination, and control. Included in Fayol's principles are ideas about management that continue today, particularly in large organizations (Fayol, 1949). Some of these principles are:

- Division of work—the idea of specialization in work that increases efficiency.
- Authority—a person in a position should have authority to give orders and be responsible for executing the work.
- Unity of command—an employee takes orders from only one person.
- Scalar chain—there is a line of authority that runs from the bottom to the top of an organization and it is also the line of communication and decision-making.
- Subordination of interest—the individual's interests are subordinate to those of the general interest, so there must be fair agreements.
- Centralization—some degree of centralization of authority is required.
- Discipline—obedience to authority and behaviour in accord with agreed rules.

Classical management theory, either scientific management or management processes for efficiency, views organizations as mechanisms or like mechanisms in the way they should operate.

Management Functions

Although initially identified by Henri Fayol in the 1920s, others have created variations in the categories of management activities (Koontz & Weihrich, 1990). These categories describe the overall functions of managers and management:

- Planning: involves the selection of goals and objectives as well as the means to achieve objectives. This activity involves the consideration of alternatives and the selection of means, so decision-making is required, followed by the mapping of details.
- Organizing: involves establishing structure to achieve the plan, including the roles of individuals and the task assigned to roles. Such activity involves grouping activity and establishing appropriate levels of authority for those involved.
- Staffing: involves recruitment, hiring, and retention of people for positions in the organizational structure. This activity involves human resource activities, such as interviewing, staff development, career planning, compensation, and promotion.
- Leading: involves influencing others to contribute to goals. The more traditional title for this activity was directing, but both terms refer to an interpersonal aspect of the

role of managers, including motivating others, managing conflict, delegating, coaching, and communicating.

■ Controlling: involves measuring achievement in terms of performance and taking corrective action as required. Such activity includes measurement of productivity; budget reviews and fiscal outcomes; quality control measures; and ethical, legal, or other reviews.

You will note that "leading" is included here as a management function, but is similar to the earlier discussion of the concept of leadership. Chapter 1 was devoted to what is listed here as one of several functions of management, as thinking currently emphasizes leadership as a behaviour or activity that is not exclusive to management roles. Although leadership behaviour is required of managers, nurses exhibit it in all nursing roles. Many of the subsequent chapters in this book will relate to the foregoing categories of management functions. For example, Chapters 6 and 8 discuss aspects of staffing and Chapter 13 discusses fiscal control, part of the controlling function. As you work in organizations, you will observe and experience the management functions as they operate in your workplace.

Human Relations Theories

Due in part to worker unrest in the era of scientific management, some rejected the hard science approach to management theory and became interested in what motivated workers and how cooperation of workers could enhance performance. Studies of the effects of lighting, coffee breaks, and so on, on the productivity of factory workers (known as the Hawthorne studies) led to the realization that almost anything that was tried as an experiment improved production, a result that initially puzzled researchers. The researchers eventually realized that the attention given to the workers improved attitudes and social relationships, which enhanced cooperation and reduced worker alienation (Dunbar & Statler, 2010).

The human relations school began to examine not only motivation, but also the role of hierarchy in organizations and democratic approaches to management as an alternative to autocratic or authoritarian approaches that had been traditional in most organizations. Organizational psychologists began to examine employee satisfaction and how to alter structures and enrich jobs and leadership styles that promoted employee autonomy, creativity, and decision-making (Morgan, 2006). The emphasis on managerial-command approaches changed to one of leader support of employees who participated in workplace decision-making (Dunbar & Statler, 2010). McGregor's work in the 1960s focused on manager behaviour and worker motivation (1966). His Theory X and Theory Y contrasted a managerial view that people must be rewarded, punished, persuaded, or supervised to ensure things get done, a view that saw workers as passive at best and lazy at worst (Theory X). In contrast, managers who perceive workers as having a willingness to meet organizational goals and the potential to develop and to direct their own work (Theory Y) are less controlling and more democratic in their approach to making decisions.

Such work by those interested in human relations research formed the basis for human resource management, which became an important focus in organizations as a way to improve working life and employee satisfaction while reducing absenteeism and turnover. This focus ensured that the human aspect of organizations was considered, not just the technical aspect or design of a job or organization, because they were interdependent in a social system like the workplace.

Open Systems and Contingency Theories

Open systems theory was a general one that, when applied to organizations, proposed that organizations were not closed systems, but open to the environment in which they existed. Therefore, the design of an organization and its activities should reflect sensitivity to the environment. In the case of health care organizations, this means that they must consider and respond to other organizations in their environment such as government agencies, unions, other health agencies, and businesses with which they share responsibilities and on which they depend. For example, in the past decade, hospitals have had to respond to what is going on in the wider environment with the development of antibiotic-resistant infections, pandemic planning, or shortages of vaccines or isotopes. Managers must think about the relations between their subsystem and the whole organization and between their subsystem and the environment, an approach that views organizations as organisms, rather than as mechanisms (Morgan, 2006).

Contingency theory emphasizes that there is no one best way to organize and that organizational forms vary depending on the nature of the environment. Classical management principles are not appropriate in certain kinds of firms, like high technology firms that must quickly adjust to new developments in the field. Units and organizations as whole may require different degrees of hierarchy, contingent on the nature of the work or the environment. For example, research and development units in industry have goals that are less specified than production departments, and finance departments require more guidelines and controls than public relations units.

Decision Theories

Theorists who viewed organizations as information processing machines initially used theory and research to focus on efficiency (Dunbar & Statler, 2010). Morgan (2006) likened this approach to viewing organizations as "institutionalized brains" in that these theorists focused on organizations as decision-making systems. While these theorists acknowledged that organizations and managers could not be perfectly rational, given that humans have limited abilities to process information and must make decisions based on limited information, the approach did give emphasis to rationality, routinizing decision-making where possible, and enhancing rationality in practice. These theories led to operations research, goal-setting and management by objectives, management information systems, detailed examination of process, total quality management (TQM), and other widespread management approaches.

While these theorists recognized that there were limits to rationality in decision-making within organizations, the thrust of this approach was to examine not only how managers might optimize decisions and reduce uncertainty, but also propose how to deal with the reality of uncertainty by transcending the rational model. Development of the computer, information technology, the internet and "networked intelligence" have transformed many industries and organizations, speeding information processing, changing how humans can interact and expanding capacities and possibilities. Morgan (2006) writes that the challenge now is that of constant learning and describes how **cybernetics**, the scientific study of information, communication, and control, arose from the challenge of designing machines that had adaptive capacity. Notions and principles from cybernetics have influenced many ideas about management of organizations, including learning to learn, developing feedback mechanisms to become self-correcting, and the development of a culture that focuses on team learning.

ROLES IN NURSING MANAGEMENT AND LEADERSHIP

What kinds of nursing management and leadership roles are there? Organizations engaged in the provision of health care are concerned with how to best organize and deliver care. Health care organizations range in size and structure from small health centres with one manager or administrator to large multi-hospital systems with several layers of management. Administrative roles in nursing are usually described in terms of two levels: nurse managers and nurse executives (Jones, 2010; Kleinman, 2003). At one time, a distinction was made between a front-line nurse manager and a middle manager. The latter category is less evident now in health care organizations as the trend has moved away from more layers of management. Where there are middle layers, they are usually considered under the broader category of nurse manager, but with fewer layers in organizations, the responsibilities of both nurse managers and nurse executives have expanded (Kleinman). Nurse managers are often responsible for one or more specific clinical services or unit while nurse executives are the top level of nursing administration, often responsible for more than nursing care services. Nurse manager titles differ and may range widely, depending on the kind of organization and level of responsibility, for example, Nurse Manger, Rapid Response Team; Clinical Manager, Surgical Services; or Director, Home Care Services. Nurse executives are typically members of the senior management team in a health care organization. The senior nurse may carry the title of Chief Nursing Officer because he or she is the designated leader for professional nursing, but he or she may also carry other titles, such as Vice-President, Patient Care, because the position's scope of responsibilities extends beyond nursing activities. Position titles within these levels vary from organization to organization and from time period to time period, as titles come in and out of fashion and as management and leadership theory evolves. Many argue that the word "nurse" has disappeared from senior management levels, as such titles as Vice-President, Patient Care, have replaced those responsibilities with the broadening of the scope beyond nursing care.

There are other kinds of management and leadership roles in nursing that do not deal with the provision of health care services, but rather focus on nurses and the profession. For example, there are such positions in institutions that educate nurses and that focus on the socio-economic welfare of nurses (nurses' unions) and on the profession (regulatory bodies and professional associations). Examples of these roles include dean of a school or faculty of nursing, president and chief executive officer of a union or professional association, and executive director of a regulatory college of nurses in a province.

As mentioned earlier, because the concept of leadership differs from that of management, organizations often seek individuals who have strength in both leadership (vision-

Table 2.1 A Comparison of Management and Leadership

Management	Leadership
Dealing with complexity, producing results	Dealing with change, producing change
Order and consistency	Anticipating, preparing for and responding to a changing environment
Quality	
Planning by setting targets and goals, budgeting and allocating resources	Developing a vision and setting a direction as well as strategies to make needed changes
Organizing by establishing organizational structure and staffing positions with qualified people. Focus on structuring positions to fit together	Aligning people to vision and securing commitment. Focus on communication with those at various levels to understand vision and who can help or hinder
Controlling and problem-solving by comparing results to the plan, identifying deviations from plan and solving problems. Focus on system norms, standards, and processes.	Motivating, inspiring, and empowering people to pursue change and overcome barriers by coaching, role modelling. Emphasis on needs for achievement, values, emotions

ing, inspiring, and motivating) and management (planning, organizing, coordinating, and directing) aspects of a role. Indeed, as mentioned in the section on management functions, leadership is considered a function of anyone in a management position. Kotter (2001, p. 103) described these as "two distinctive and complementary systems of action" that are required by managers in organizations. Although not everyone excels at both the ability to lead and to manage, there is value in seeking to develop the skills and abilities of both dimensions. Table 2.1 illustrates the strengths and abilities of a leader-manager who demonstrates a balance in these abilities.

As you work in health care organizations, you will become increasingly aware of leadership and management in action and likely begin to identify the strengths and weaknesses of the workplaces you encounter. You will take on leadership roles, and perhaps formal management roles, as your career develops, and you will learn more about the broader context of your work and the larger forces that influence what happens in your workplace. Health care management requires you to deal with the complexity of providing health care as well as having the leadership skills to manage a dynamic and changing environment. We now turn to discuss the larger external environment of health care management.

THE HEALTH SYSTEM—THE CONTEXT FOR HEALTH CARE

We begin this section with a model that provides a broad overview of the organization of health care systems and an indication of how these may differ around the world. We will then focus on health care systems in Canada and discuss some of the basics of the health care context, exploring the forces that affect health care services and organizations. This overview will illustrate the complexity of health care and health care organizations, and therefore, some of the challenges inherent in health care management. We believe that an appreciation of the many factors influencing health care and the dynamic nature of the system within which you work will help you to identify trends that will influence your practice and working life.

A Model of the Health System

For the purposes of learning about the health care system, a model of a health system is presented in Figure 2.1. We will use this model to provide a big picture of the health care system in Canada and to guide the discussion of key elements of the system.

As depicted in the model, the values and goals of a culture and society have an effect on the political system of a country that in turn shapes policy on education, health, health care, and research. These policy areas or fields are ones that influence the way in which health services are organized to address health needs in an attempt to influence the health status of individuals, families, groups, and communities. While health services are designed to influence the health status of citizens, there are other determinants of

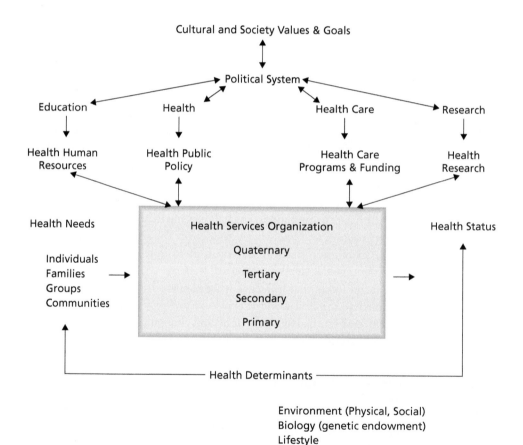

Figure 2.1 Model of Health System

Source: Based on Y. Bergevin and N. Mahamed, Challenge of policy formulation for growth promotion. In *Growth promotion for child development.* Proceedings of a colloquium, Nyeri, Kenya, 12–13 May, 1992.

health, such as the environment, biology, and lifestyle. We will discuss each of these elements, especially as they relate to Canada, in the following sections.

CULTURAL AND SOCIETAL VALUES AND THE POLITICAL SYSTEM

This model of the health system indicates that societal and cultural values shape, and are shaped by, the political system. Canada's political system addresses **public policy** on education, health, health care, and research, all of which have an influence on the way in which we plan, organize, and provide health care.

As cultural and societal values around the world vary, political systems and political values develop differently and influence the way in which national health care systems are developed and structured in various ways. You should not be surprised to find differences in the way in which countries organize health care for their citizens, given differences in resources, priorities, and values. The last major review of health care in Canada was carried out by the *Commission on the Future of Health Care in Canada*. Often referred to as the Romanow Report, after its commissioner, it contains a key message, based on substantial public consultation, which is the importance that Canadians placed on the values that shaped medicare and health care and access based on need rather than ability to pay. According to Romanow (2002, p. 6), "Canadians view medicare as a moral enterprise, not a business venture," and he underscored the values of equity, fairness, and solidarity as ones that formed the basis for health care in the country. He noted that Canadians viewed the system as "a national program, delivered locally" and that they wanted their governments to work together to ensure the system adhered to these values.

Variations in National Health Care Systems

National health care systems are designed and structured in a variety of ways. Roemer (1993) classified systems into four types, based on the degree to which a government was involved in the funding, planning, and management of the system. These range from systems in which the national government provides all of the funding for health services and governs all of the health care facilities in the country, and is thus the employer of health care professionals to systems that are mostly privately funded with services delivered by private enterprise. Table 2.2 provides examples of countries that would illustrate the different types of systems. It must be acknowledged that with time and changes in

Table 2.2 Examples of Types of Health Systems

Classification	Example
Entrepreneurial and permissive	United States
Welfare-oriented	Canada, Japan
Universal and comprehensive	Sweden, United Kingdom
Socialistic and centrally planned	China, Cuba

governments, policy changes in systems may alter the way a particular country would be classified. For example, Canada is considered a welfare-oriented system because our federal legislation with respect to insured services only addresses a portion of services—hospitals and physicians. Countries such as Sweden and the United Kingdom have traditionally addressed a full range of services under national health legislation.

In entrepreneurial systems, individuals purchase health insurance or work for employers that purchase such insurance for employees under private insurance schemes, and most health care services are paid for in this way. In countries with such systems, there is often a mix of publicly funded services for the poor and/or the elderly, with most services being provided and paid for privately. Welfare-oriented systems are publicly funded to a great extent, at least for the expensive components of health care, such as acute care hospital and physician services. Therefore, while citizens may pay for some services, these are typically for less catastrophic services, such as dental care or drugs, for which private insurance may be purchased. Universal and comprehensive services are publicly funded ones that provide a full range of services for all citizens, although there may be access to a private, parallel service in addition to that guaranteed by the government. Socialistic and centrally planned services are the ones available to all citizens and they are designed and delivered by government-funded organizations.

The type of system does not necessarily reflect the economic conditions of the country, and each of the four systems can be found in very poor countries or in affluent and industrialized countries. In entrepreneurial and permissive systems, the private market is very evident, and the government does not intervene to a great extent—people pay for health care through private insurance or private means, and those who provide health services, be they physicians, hospitals, or others, operate as private businesses. In these countries, only a relatively small portion of services and programs are provided by the government through public funding (that is, supported by taxes). In countries with welfare-oriented health systems, governments do take on a larger role, often by financing personal medical care and providing some direct services, especially in rural areas. In comprehensive-type systems, almost all of a country's health services are universally available through a publicly funded system. In socialist health systems, the government centrally plans and delivers health services with almost total elimination of private health care—government not only finances the services, but also hires almost all those who provide the services, educates all health professionals, and produces pharmaceuticals.

Even among Western, industrialized countries, different decisions are made about the degree to which governments will be involved in health care, the extent to which it will publicly finance health care, and how involved it will be in delivering it. In part, these decisions are influenced by cultural and political beliefs about the appropriate role of governments and the responsibilities of the individual vis-à-vis the collective. Furthermore, government policy changes over time, bringing about changes in the health care system. For example, the United States has differed from Canada in health care policy in that it has not had universal health care under a publicly funded scheme. Although health policy reform under the Obama administration has brought some changes in the United States, the majority of Americans must purchase private insurance for health care (to consult a physician or to get a hospital stay covered) in the same way that we, in Canada, may purchase private insurance for services that are not insured through provincial plans, such as dental care or prescription drugs. The publicly funded plans in the United States are "medicare," a special plan for seniors and others with special needs, and "medicaid" for the poor.

Political values drive the kind of health care system that is and can be adopted in a country. In Canada, society has come to value health care services available to all equally when needed, rather than being based on the ability to pay, and a belief that government ought to be involved in ensuring this kind of system is in place. In countries in which there might be distrust of government involvement and more emphasis on the responsibility of the individual for health care rather than the collective, or a greater emphasis on the role of the free market, there will be marked differences in the context in which health care operates. While it is clear that most Canadians support a publicly funded system, there is a recurring debate about the extent to which there should be more or less privatization of health care funding and delivery. This debate is evident in the numerous federal and provincial reports over the past few decades that have come down on different sides of the private versus public debate in their recommendations (Bryant, 2009).

CANADIAN POLITICAL SYSTEM, GOVERNING AUTHORITY, AND POLICIES AFFECTING HEALTH CARE IN CANADA

In Canada, jurisdiction for various aspects of public life were divided among federal and provincial levels of government in the original British North America Act of 1867 (Vayda & Deber, 1984) and for the most part, matters considered to be of local concern and at that time, matters that were not costly, came under the authority of provincial governments. Therefore, education, asylums, hospitals, and charities came under provincial jurisdiction, while only some aspects of health care were considered matters of national concern and were governed by the federal government, which had a broader tax base and "spending power." Municipal levels of government have also taken on roles in providing physician and hospital services as these services developed in the country, but the nature and specific responsibilities of all three levels of government with respect to health care have evolved over time. Both the federal and provincial governments have had some involvement in the four **policy fields** identified in the model: education, health, health care, and research, but in general, authority for education and health care lies with the provinces and territories.

Federal Government

Under the Constitution Act of 1982, the federal government carries responsibilities for a limited range of health services, such as services for members of the military and for Aboriginals on reserves, while most responsibilities for health care are given to the provinces. However, following the Second World War, the federal government became involved in health policy related to services by virtue of its spending power and the offer to cost share services with the provinces. Following Saskatchewan's lead, the federal government introduced legislation to enable universal insurance for hospital care and diagnostic services in 1957. Once again, Saskatchewan led the way by introducing **medicare** in 1962, a program to provide physician services under a universal, publicly funded program. (Tommy Douglas, the then Premier of Saskatchewan, is often called the Father of Medicare and his photograph appears at the beginning of this chapter.) Following a Royal Commission on Health Services report, federal legislation was introduced that enabled universal insurance for physician services in 1966. Known in popular terminology as "medicare," the funding of hospitalization and physician services represented a major aspect of federal health policy, perhaps the most popular and politicized program in Canada. As noted by O'Neill, McGuinty, and Teskey (2011) in a review of six decades of political science literature on Canadian medicare, the scholarly community has a "...near-consensus on medicare as a defining characteristic of the country and its people" (p. 49).

Initially, the federal government provided half of the funding for hospitalization and medical care that was spent by a province or territory; however, this arrangement changed in 1977 as the federal government sought to limit the mounting costs of such programs. In changing the basis on which funds were transferred to the provinces, the federal government softened the blow somewhat by providing the provinces with some greater flexibility to use funds for other types of health services. The new funding system moved from 50–50 cost-sharing to block grants, tax point transfers, growth rates, cash transfers, and per capita cash contributions for some extended services such as nursing homes, and ambulatory and home care. Further changes in funding and cost-sharing have occurred since that date, the latest occurring in a 2004 agreement that extends until 2013–14 (Health Canada, 2011).

Over time, concerns began to be expressed about user fees applied in some provinces for emergency room visits or "extra-billing" charges by physicians, requiring people to pay a fee "out-of-pocket" when they received a service that was supposedly paid for through taxes. Following a review of medicare, user fees and extra-billing for insured services were essentially outlawed, and the federal acts for hospital care and physician care were consolidated in 1984 under the Canada Health Act (Department of Justice, 2011). This act also enshrined the principles for the publicly funded system detailing the criteria that must be met for provinces to receive a cash contribution from the federal government (see Table 2.3).

Provincial/Territorial Governments

Provincial/territorial governments play a major role in financing and organizing health services within their jurisdictions and thus reference is often made to Canada's 13 health systems, as there is some variation across provincial and territorial borders. Even if Canadians, as noted earlier, consider health care to be a national system, the provincial government has the jurisdiction and authority to govern health care within a province. While there are transfers of funding to provincial/territorial governments from the federal government that contribute to health care, provincial governments contribute a substantial proportion of their resources to a range of services that extend beyond the original focus on hospitals and physician services. Per capita spending on health by provincial/territorial governments varies with higher per capita spending in the more remote and less populated province/territories. See Table 2.4 for health expenditures by province/territory.

Table 2.3 Program Criteria for Federal Funding to Provinces under the Canada Health Act

Program Criteria	Explanation
Public Administration	Provincial health insurance plan must be administered and operated on a non-profit basis by a public authority
Comprehensiveness	Provincial health insurance plan must insure all insured health services provided by hospitals, medical practitioners, or dentists, and where the law of the province so permits, similar or additional services rendered by other health care practitioners
Universality	Provincial health insurance plan must entitle 100 percent of the insured persons of the province to the insured health services provided for by the plan on uniform terms and conditions
Portability	Provincial health insurance plan must not impose any minimum period of residence in the province, or waiting period, in excess of three months before residents are eligible for insured services
	During a waiting period of three months or less in a "new" province, the previous province of residence pays for the insured service
	Where the insured health services are provided in Canada, payment for health services is at the rate that is approved by the health care insurance plan of the province in which the services are provided (unless the two provinces involved agree to a different apportioning)
	Where the insured health services are provided out of Canada, payment is made on the basis of the amount that would have been paid by the province for similar services rendered in the province
Accessibility	Provincial health insurance plan must provide for insured health services on uniform terms and conditions and on a basis that does not impede or preclude, either directly or indirectly whether by charges made to insured persons or otherwise, reasonable access to those services by insured persons

A major area of provincial/territorial health policy relates to the health insurance plan for hospital and physician services, which must be consistent with the principles of the Canada Health Act to receive full federal funding. A substantial portion of provincial/territorial expenditures (34.9% on average in 2010) is devoted to health care spending (CIHI, 2011a). Not surprisingly, health care spending is closely examined for reductions when there are economic downturns. Given the public support for health care however, politicians are reluctant to reduce funding, and generally, must maintain or increase funding to this sector every year.

Beyond administration of the health insurance plans, the provincial and territorial governments have overall responsibility to allocate funding for hospitals and other health

Table 2.4 Per Capita Health Expenditure by Provincial/Territorial Government, 2010

Province/Territory	Per capita Expenditure in Dollars by Provincial/Territorial Government
Newfoundland	4,564
Prince Edward Island	3,988
Nova Scotia	3,944
New Brunswick	3,789
Quebec	3,341
Ontario	3,548
Manitoba	4,155
Saskatchewan	4,077
Alberta	4,295
British Columbia	3,544
Yukon Territory	5,234
Northwest Territory	5,954
Nunavut	8,862

Source: Canadian Institute for Health Information (CIHI), 2011a. Reprinted with permission.

care facilities, negotiate fee schedules for physicians, plan and implement health promotion campaigns and public health services, and address other health policies and services that are not part of the Canada Health Act. For example, nursing homes, workers' compensation, ambulance services, mental health and human resources planning, and regulation of professions all fall within provincial and territorial jurisdiction. Each jurisdiction has legislation that addresses the full range of matters pertaining to health care, such as health insurance, regulated health professionals, health institutions, public health, mental health, etc. Therefore, this level of government has a great influence on the organizations within which most health professionals work and the professions to which they belong.

Municipal Government

The municipal level of government, that level responsible for local matters in cities, towns, and smaller communities, operate under provincial legislation that sets out the framework for local government. Depending on the province, this level of government may have some responsibilities with respect to health care, for example, in Ontario where public health units across the province have local health boards with regional municipal representatives. The costs are shared with the provincial government (Ontario Ministry of Health and Long-term Care, 2011). To a great extent however, the provision of health services by local government has diminished since the early days of Canada's history.

Regionalization of Health Services

Although provincial governments have jurisdiction for health care services within a province, in recent decades all of them have established regional bodies, based on geographic areas, and delegated some degree of responsibility for decision-making about health services to them. This development represents one of the major changes in the governance and organization of health services during the 1990s and the first decade of the twenty-first century. **Regionalization** meant that, in many provinces, individual hospital and agency boards were replaced by regional ones, and decision-making for planning and implementation shifted from central provincial authorities in departments of health to more local ones. The benefits of regionalization were thought to be increasing citizen participation in decision-making, better planning that met more local needs, **horizontal integration** and **vertical integration** of services that improved services, and efficiencies that created economies of scale and better expenditure control (Church & Barker, 1998; Lewis & Kouri, 2004). Horizontal integration refers to an organization becoming larger by joining with a similar organization(s). Vertical integration refers to an organization becoming larger by joining with another organization(s) that is a supplier or purchaser of products or services of the organization. The responsibilities of regional authorities vary across the county—some incorporate a wide range of health services such as home care, public health, acute care, and long-term care while others have a narrower focus. In some provinces, but not all, regional authorities are responsible for allocating budgets to the services within their region while in other provinces they are responsible for planning and implementation of services. Provinces continue to adjust policy on regional health authorities and thus there have been changes over time in the degree to which authority is centralized or decentralized. For example, Alberta abolished its health regions in 2008 and moved to the creation of one health authority or "super board," Alberta Health Services (Duckett, 2011). In Ontario, Local Health Integration Networks (LHINs) were established in 2006 and have engaged in planning and priority-setting in the regions, but without replacing hospital boards or the authority for managing the system as has occurred in some other provinces (Falk, 2011).

Intergovernmental Agreements

As discussed in the previous section, provincial/territorial governments have major responsibilities for policy about how health care is organized within their jurisdictions. Provincial/territorial governments, through their ministries of health, determine the overall structure of the health system, how the system is organized and regulated, the major policies governing system functioning, and the major priorities within the jurisdiction with respect to health and health policy. Given that the federal government has been involved in developing and funding aspects of the health system and health policy, there have been periods of time during which there was considerable conflict between the two levels of government. The tensions over health care funding and jurisdiction that existed between the 1960s and the 1980s gave way by the mid-1990s to what has been described as collaborative federalism (Bryant, 2009), leading to the Social Union Framework Agreement (SUFA) between the two levels of government in 1999. All jurisdictions except Quebec signed this agreement that aimed to clarify responsibilities and obligations in the area of social policy (that is, health, social services, post-secondary education, social assistance, and training policy). Subsequent to that agreement, the federal minister of health and provincial and territorial counterparts met to come to an agreement known as the Health Accord Agreement. These accords (in 2000, 2003, and 2004) addressed health care issues and established funding for early childhood development, improved medical equipment, primary care reform, and Canada Health Infoway, a not-for-profit corporation established by federal and provincial/territorial first ministers in 2001. This corporation works with governments to develop and adopt electronic health record (EHR) systems in Canada and promote sharing of such development across regions. The 2004 Health Accord set out a 10-year plan to renew the health care system.

Policies Affecting Health Care

As illustrated in the health system model, the political system generates policies in several fields that have an effect on the health system. Education policies affect the training of people who will work in the health field and more attention is given to health human resources later in this chapter. A second set of policies can have a positive or negative effect on the health status of the population. Factors that contribute to one's health include the physical and social environment (for example, war, pollution, natural disasters), biology (your genetic makeup or endowment), and lifestyle (for example, use of tobacco or alcohol, exercise, and eating habits). Public policy that is considered **healthy public policy** refers to those measures that promote health, for example tax incentives for engaging in regular exercise, nutrition labelling that might improve dietary habits, taxes on tobacco products, non-smoking policies in public places, and fines on industries that pollute the environment. It is also well known that housing, income, nutrition, and other factors are important determinants of health. A wide range of public policy can be considered from the perspective of its impact on the health of the population.

A third area of health public policy relates to funding. Most people think of health services as having the greatest impact on the health status of the population, but as noted earlier, it is only one factor, and many challenge the traditional assumption that it is a key one (Evans, Barer, & Marmor, 1994). In Canada, public policy relevant to health services includes both federal policy such as the Canada Health Act and the transfer of funds to provincial governments in support of health care services, as well as an array of programs and funding that fall within provincial jurisdiction, for example legislation regulating hospitals, health regions, health professionals, and diagnostic services. Legislation and regulations governing every kind of health care facility constitute policies that affect how the health system is structured and operates.

A fourth area is research policy. Health research is one aspect of the health system that garners a relatively small share of the spending on health. According to the Canadian Institute of Health Information (2009), in Canada we spent approximately 1.4 percent of the $84 billion in health expenditures in 1997–1998 on health research, while this percentage increased to 1.8 percent of the $172 billion in health spending in 2007–2008. A major agency funding health research is the Canadian Institutes of Health Research (CIHR), an organization that was established in 2000 out of the former Medical Research Council of Canada. CIHR (2012) funds the training of researchers through scholarships and awards as well as research projects and programs in four areas: 1) biomedical, 2) clinical, 3) health system services, and 4) social, cultural, environment, and population health. Researchers (usually organized into teams) submit funding applications to CIHR, and there are always many more applications than there are funds available, so the process is highly competitive and many strong applications are not successful. CIHR has 13 Institutes that are organized around particular areas of research and these networks bring together researchers (including nurse researchers) ranging from basic scientists to clinical scientists to population health scientists together with voluntary agencies and policy-makers to focus on topics and goals in the following areas:

- Aboriginal Peoples' Health
- Aging
- Cancer Research
- Circulatory and Respiratory Health
- Gender and Health
- Genetics
- Health Services and Policy Research
- Human Development, Child and Youth Health
- Infection and Immunity
- Musculoskeletal Health and Arthritis
- Neurosciences, Mental Health, and Addiction
- Nutrition, Metabolism, and Diabetes
- Population and Public Health

Many provinces also have agencies that fund health research and these are also important organizations for the development and training of researchers and the funding of studies and programs of health research.

Another important research agency is the Canadian Foundation for Healthcare Improvement (CFHI), formerly the Canadian Health Services Research Foundation (CHSRF). Established in early 1997, CHSRF received an initial endowment in 1997 from the federal government, followed by a second endowment of $60 million that included "$25 million that was earmarked for the development and support of nursing research" (CHSRF, 2007). This organization was an important one in the development of research focused on nursing in health care and it supported health services research and the development of researchers. CFHI no longer provides research grant funding for health policy, but does undertake research and analysis to advance improvements in health care, usually by commissioning research on health services topics (CFHI, 2013).

THE ORGANIZATION OF HEALTH SERVICES IN CANADA

The organization of health services varies from one country to another, but in general, there are four levels that are used to describe the kinds of services that are provided in many countries: primary, secondary, tertiary, and quaternary. These levels are depicted in the centre of the health system model and these levels are intended to address the health needs of citizens to achieve optimum health status of the population as an outcome.

Primary Health Care

Primary health care (PHC) is "a comprehensive system of essential health care that is focused on preventing illness and promoting health" (CNA, 2002, p 1). PHC refers to the first level of care, that level sought by individuals requiring health information or assistance for health issues, disease prevention, common health problems, and injuries. This is the level at which people have first contact with the health system, where people can obtain direct service that meets their needs without the requirement of being referred elsewhere. As this level is the most basic and fundamental one in meeting health care needs, the World Health Organization (WHO) made an effort to promote the development of PHC as a priority in the 1970s, particularly in countries with very few resources. At WHO's International Conference on Primary Health Care in Alma-Ata in what was then the USSR, the Declaration of Alma-Ata was adopted by members of the World Health Assembly who supported the principles embodied in the Declaration and expressed in the theme "Health for All by the Year 2000" (WHO, 1978). These principles are identified and described in Table 2.5.

As PHC encompasses the level at which individuals, families, and communities enter the health system and access health services, there is a wide range of organization of services at this level. Perhaps the kind of service that is most familiar to generations of Canadians is the provision of **primary care** by a physician in a solo, private practice. Primary care is the provision of health care to an individual (often called personal health services), typically to assess, diagnose, and treat a common health problem, but also to promote health through advice and teaching or to prevent disease through immunization or education. This kind of health service is also found in group practices, nurse practitioner clinics, urgent care centres and clinics, and a wide variety of community-based clinics and programs aimed at specific services and client groups. All of these fall within the umbrella level of care referred to as primary health care.

Although the terms "primary care" and "primary health care" are often used interchangeably, in Canada, **primary care** is usually one component of a loosely integrated system of primary health care services available in a community that does not usually embody all of the principles of primary health care. There are some organizations that aim to incorporate principles such as public participation, health promotion, and intersectoral cooperation. Some community health centres provide a range of health and social services that are designed for the group of clients they serve. Examples include community health centres in a geographic area with a high number of recent immigrant families, or Quebec's network of more than 140 centre local de services communautaires (CLSCs) or local community health centres.

Table 2.5 Principles of Primary Health Care

Principle	Explanation
Accessibility	Essential health care (promotive, preventive, curative, rehabilitative/palliative services) that address the main health problems in the community
	Universally available to individuals and families in the community
	Integral part and central function and main focus of country's health system
	Brings health care as close as possible to where people live and work
	First element of a continuing health care process
Public participation	Full participation of individuals, families and communities in PHC and services designed at a cost that the community and country can afford to maintain
	Spirit of self-reliance and self-determination
	Participation in planning, organization, operation, and control of PHC
	Appropriate education to develop the ability of communities to participate
Health promotion	Includes at least education on prevailing health problems, prevention and control methods, promotion of food supply, nutrition, supply of safe water, basic sanitation, maternal and child health care, including family planning, immunization
Appropriate skills and technology	Care based on practical, scientifically sound, and socially acceptable methods and technology
	Modes of care adapted to community's society, economy, and culture.
	Application of results of social, biomedical, and health services research and public health experience
Intersectoral cooperation	Recognizing the determinants of health and role of agriculture, food, industry, education, housing, public works, and communications in health
	Ensure collaboration between disciplines and sectors and the coordinated efforts of all sectors in government policy and service delivery

Sources: Data from CNA (2002). *Effective health care equals primary health care* (PHC); CNA (2000). The primary health care approach; WHO (1978). *Declaration of Alma–Ata: International conference on primary health care, Alma-Ata, USSR, 612* September 1978. Geneva: WHO.

Primary care has been the focus of reform in many provinces as governments have introduced incentives to encourage more accessibility to services (24/7 access), team models of care that focus on disease prevention and health promotion, improved management of chronic illnesses, and better coordination of a range of available services. Many younger physicians seek practices other than solo fee-for-service ones because they prefer the more balanced working life group practices provide and the collegial, collaborative working relationships that such centres and interdisciplinary settings can offer them as well as the quality of care that they can provide to patients.

There are a number of settings in which nurses work that are components of the primary health care system, although some would argue that "system" is too strong a word for these somewhat fragmented services. These positions include occupational health nurse in businesses and industrial firms where nurses provide first contact care in the workplace to promote health, prevent disease or injury, and to treat and monitor common health problems or injuries. Public health nurses in geographic communities provide direct services to individuals through immunization clinics, sexual health and other programs, and health promotion strategies to reduce smoking or prevent falls in the elderly. These services, focused on health promotion and disease prevention, are provided in the community through home visits and clinics or in easily accessible locations, such as schools and shopping malls.

Data for 2009 from the Canadian Institute for Health Information (2010) on registered nurses indicates that approximately 14.2 percent of RNs work in the community, a small increase from 2005 when the percentage was 13.5 percent. However, this report includes nurses working in home care, which is not part of primary health care, in addition to those who work at the level of primary health care, such as public health nurses and nurses in community health centres, nursing stations, clinics, and outposts.

Secondary Health Care

The **secondary health care** refers to a more specialized level of care in a variety of settings, such as community hospitals, home care, and long-term and chronic care settings. Individuals are normally referred to this level of health care by someone in the primary health care level, such as a family physician, community agency, or sometimes a family member or the individual themselves. There is a wide variety of services provided in these secondary settings, including medical and surgical treatment, rehabilitation, continuing, and palliative care.

Most community hospitals are governed by community boards of trustees, voluntary organizations, or regional health authorities and are funded by provincial or territorial governments. Most of the hospitals in Canada are of this type and they offer a wide range of services in rural, small, and large communities. In addition to acute inpatient care for an episode of illness and treatment, hospitals may offer emergency and ambulatory care services on an outpatient basis.

Hospitals receive most of their funding from provincial governments. An annual budget is prepared by the hospital, normally based on the previous level of activity, any approved planned changes in services, and any guidelines set by the body that negotiates funding with the hospital, be it a ministry of health or a regional health authority. Hospitals are a major component of health care spending and fall within the Canada Health Act provisions and what many refer to as the five principles of medicare mentioned earlier.

Continuing care is provided in settings that may be termed rehabilitation hospitals, or chronic care, extended care, or complex continuing care institutions. Because acute care hospitals are designed for illness that is typically severe, episodic, and of limited duration, continuing care institutions are designed to care for those who no longer need acute care services, but who require ongoing care to deal with complex health problems.

Two types of secondary services that are not part of the Canada Health Act are home care and long-term care (called nursing homes in some places). Home care is a service that enables individuals with a physical or mental health issue to live at home and receive professional care (nursing, physiotherapy, and so on), personal care (bathing, toileting, and so on) and homemaking services (house cleaning, laundry, and so on) or some combination of these services through home visits by personnel. Although all provincial governments have provided some level of home care, the Romanow Commission found a wide variation in service availability between and within provinces, criteria for eligibility and budgets devoted to this kind of alternative to institutional care. For that reason, the Commission recommended that home care be covered by the Canada Health Act, beginning with three areas of priority: mental health, post-acute care, and palliative care (Romanow, 2002). However, despite an expansion of such services, they have not yet become an insured service in the way that hospitals and physician services are recognized as an essential service under the Canada Health Act. There has been little appetite by governments to expand any health service in this way.

Long-term care refers to residential care facilities for those requiring continuing, 24-hour care that includes nursing care and personal support. These facilities are partly subsidized by provincial governments, but they are not an insured service under the Canada Health Act—residents or their families normally pay a monthly fee for long-term care. As with home care, access to, availability of, and funding for long-term care varies across the country. In addition to issues of access, concerns have been expressed about the quality of care in these institutions (Jansen, 2011; Samuleson, 2011). Many residents in such facilities are elderly, and the number of beds has increased as the population ages, but the numbers have not kept pace with demand and there are waiting lists for admission across the country.

Tertiary Health Care

Tertiary health care includes more specialized services than one would find in a general or community hospital. These services are usually found in larger centres that can bring together the equipment and personnel required. While tertiary level hospitals offer the range of services of community hospitals, they are typically associated with an academic setting, are known as academic health centres, and offer services that are unavailable in community hospitals. For example, kidney transplants and cardiac surgery are available in tertiary care settings. Some specialty hospitals, such as those designed for the care of children, are included within this level of care.

Quaternary Health Care

Quaternary health care refers to yet more specialized services that are only available in limited locations due to the highly specialized equipment and personnel involved. These services may only be available in a few cities in a country and poorer countries may not provide any of these services. For example, some experimental therapies and heart-lung transplantation would be done in a hospital designated as a quaternary level centre for that service. These services are located in the largest Canadian cities.

HEALTH HUMAN RESOURCES IN CANADA

A major component of the model of the health system is health human resources—the people who carry out the work of the health care system. There is a broad range of workers: regulated health professionals; other professionals in finance, management, law, technology, skilled trades, and services personnel; unregulated health workers; administrative and secretarial personnel, and so on. Federal and provincial public policy on education and training has an impact on the planning for and availability of the appropriate numbers and kinds of workers in the health care system. As with health care, the federal government in Canada has played a role in funding post-secondary education, the level at which many health professionals are educated, although education policy is primarily within the jurisdiction of provincial governments.

Major changes in the demand for or supply of health workers can cause problems in the delivery of health care to citizens unless there is planning at some level. For example, the building of a new hospital requires consideration of the requirement for additional nurses and other types of workers. In the past, periods of shortages followed by an oversupply of nurses has resulted in a roller coaster of employment problems. Layoffs of nurses in the 1990s due to health care spending cuts were followed by shortages of nurses. Other shortages will occur as the "baby boomer" nurses retire. Similar concerns arose about a shortage of physicians when many Canadians were unable to find a doctor when their long-term family physician retired. Consequently, more research attention has been given to understanding the factors that need to be considered in planning human resources in the health sector. Educational preparation is one of these factors, as is licensing requirements for some professions. Requirements for some of the health occupations are presented in Table 2.6 as an illustration of the complexity of health human resources.

Please note that data are not available for unregulated health workers, such as physician assistants or health care aides/personal care workers. The minimum education required for any health care group varies over time, as groups seek change in the nature and length of their education programs. For example, the nursing profession at the national level and in many provinces set a goal in the 1980s for establishing a bachelor's degree as the new educational requirement for registered nurses and they set the year 2000 as a target date. At the time of writing, all jurisdictions in Canada require a baccalaureate degree for entry to practice except the province of Quebec, where a diploma in nursing is the minimal requirement.

Health Care Occupations

Specialized preparation is required for health care professions and occupations. Individuals who pursue education in these fields make a considerable investment in time and funds. Many, but not all, occupations in health care are regulated ones, and fairly accurate numbers are available for professional colleges that have members who are registered or licensed, as an active membership is required each year in order to practice. In Table 2.7 we present numbers for selected health occupations over a five-year period to give you a

Table 2.6 Educational Programs and Licensing Requirements for Health Occupations in Canada

Occupation	Minimum Education Required*	Internship/ Practicum Required	National Exam
Audiologists	master's	√	√
Chiropractors	professional doctorate	√	√
Dental Hygienists	diploma	√	√
Dentists	professional doctorate	√	√
Dieticians	bachelor's	√	√
Environmental Public Health Professionals	diploma or bachelor's	√	√
Licensed Practical Nurses	diploma	√	√
Medical Laboratory Technologists	diploma	√	√
Medical Physicists	master's or doctorate	√	√
Medical Radiation Technologists	diploma	√	√
Midwives	bachelor's	√	√
Nurse Practitioners	post-baccalaureate certificate or master's	√	√
Occupational Therapists	master's	√	√
Optometrists	professional doctorate	√	√
Pharmacists	bachelor's	√	√
Physicians	md plus residency	√	√
Physiotherapists	master's	√	√
Psychologists	doctorate	√	√
Registered Nurses	diploma or bachelor's	√	√
Registered Psychiatric Nurses	diploma or bachelor's	√	√
Respiratory Therapists	diploma	√	√
Social Workers	diploma, bachelor's or master's	√	√
Speech-Language Pathologists	master's	√	√
Health Information Management Professionals	diploma or bachelor's	√	√

* The minimum requirements are reported here, but they vary by province/territory.

Source: Canadian Institute of Health Information (2011b). Reprinted with permission.

Table 2.7 Numbers in Selected Health Occupations in Canada, 2005 to 2009

Category	2005	2006	2007	2008	2009
Chiropractors	7,108	7,318	7,434	7,615	7,796
Dental Hygienists	18,403	19,389	20,928	22,365	23,902
Dentists	18,688	18,925	19,201	19,433	19,655
Dietitians	8.135	8,422	8,797	9,027	9,369
Environmental Public Health	1,220	1,375	1,420	1,245	1,288
Medical Laboratory Technologists	20,103	19,873	19,813	19,300	19,238
Midwives	520	626	639	738	826
Occupational Therapists	11,378	11,782	12,297	12,649	13,122
Optometrists	3,999	4,141	4,255	4,507	4,581
Pharmacists	29,471	27,094	28,495	29,010	30,333
Physicians	61,622	62,307	63,682	65,440	68,101
Physiotherapists	15,772	16,108	16,419	16,889	17,312
Psychologists	14,715	15,751	16,097	15,780	16,156
Respiratory Therapists	7,636	7,886	8,211	8,796	9,611
Speech-Language Pathologists	6,331	6,661	6,992	7,316	7,611

Source: Canadian Institute of Health Information. (2011b). Reprinted with permission.

sense of the relative size of some of these groups in Canada. Information on nursing groups is presented in a subsequent table. Normally, one would expect regular growth in the numbers of health care workers that reflects the growth in Canada's population over time. However, as the baby boomers represent a large group within the Canadian population and they have now started to reach retirement age, one can expect that larger replacement numbers will be needed over the next few decades.

Regulated Nursing Personnel

There are four kinds of regulated nursing personnel in Canada: registered nurses (RN), nurse practitioners (NP) (who are also registered nurses), registered psychiatric nurses (RPN) in the four Western provinces and Yukon Territory only, and licensed practical nurses (LPN/RPN) who are called registered practical nurses in Ontario. Table 2.8 indicates the first year in which each group became regulated.

As you can see in Table 2.9, the category of registered nurse is a major one among nursing groups and the largest group of all the health professions. All categories of regulated nursing personnel have increased in number during the past decade, but between 2005 and 2009, percentage growth has varied, 18.5% for licensed practical nurses, 6% for

Table 2.8 First Year of Regulation of Regulated Nursing Personnel by Province/ Territory as of 2010

Category	N.L.	P.E.I.	N.S.	N.B.	Que.	Ont.	Man	Sask.	Alta.	B.C.	Y.T.	N.W.T.	Nun.
RN	1954	1949	1910	1916	1946	1922	1913	1967	1916	1918	1994	1973	1999
NP	1997	2006	2002	2002	2003	1997	2005	2003	2002	2005	NR	2004	2004
RPN	-	-	-	-	-	-	1960	1948	1955	1951	2009	-	-
LPN	1983	1959	1957	1960	1974	1947	1946	1956	1986	1988	1987	1988	2011

Source: Canadian Institute of Health Information. (2011b). Reprinted with permission.

registered nurses and 5% for registered psychiatric nurses. The percentage growth for nurse practitioners was not reported by CIHI (2010) because of data variations and their relatively recent appearance as a regulated category.

The registered nurse workforce is a large one that participates in a wide variety of health care settings. Data from 2009 indicate that 62.6% of employed RNs work in hospitals, 14.2% work in community health (which includes community health centres, home care, and public health) while 9.9% work in nursing homes or long-term care. The remainder is self-employed or works in such settings as educational institutions, government, physician offices, and so on.

Unregulated Nursing Personnel

In many health care facilities and agencies in Canada, unregulated personnel assist in nursing care of individuals and families under the guidance of regulated nursing personnel (RNs, RPNs, and LPNs). The title of these unregulated workers varies by agency, region, or province/territory, and there is also variation in the kind and length of educational preparation that they may have received. They have been called nursing aides, health care aides, personal support workers, personal care workers, and so on. The Canadian Nurses Association (CNA) has referred to them as **unregulated health workers**

Table 2.9 Numbers of Regulated Nursing Personnel by Category in Canada, 2005–2009

	2005	2006	2007	2008	2009
Registered Nurses	251,242	253,819	257,961	261,889	266,341
Nurse Practitioners	976	1,162	1,393	1,669	2,048
Registered Psychiatric Nurses	4,964	5,051	5,124	5,162	5,214
Licensed Practical Nurses/ Registered Practical Nurses (Ontario)	64,953	67,300	69,709	74,380	76,944

Source: Canadian Institute of Health Information. (2011b). *Canada's health care providers 2000 to 2009—A reference guide.*

(UHW). CNA defines UHW as "an umbrella term used to describe care providers or assistant personnel who provide some form of health service and who are not licensed or regulated by a professional or regulatory body" (2009, p. 1). At one time, these workers may have received on-the-job training, but now they tend be prepared in short programs in high schools, private training organizations, community colleges, and other settings. They frequently work in nursing homes, but can be part of care teams in hospitals and community agencies, including home care settings. As they are unregulated and have various position titles, an accurate count of their numbers is difficult to maintain, but CNA (2009) cites a 2003 estimate from Statistics Canada of 188,800 people in such occupations.

As a nursing student or registered nurse, you may have worked with UHWs and can appreciate the contribution they can make to health care and the role of the registered nurse in working with people in this category of personnel. As a registered nurse, you are apt to be in a team leadership position and may work with UHWs who are members of the team. It is important that you develop your leadership knowledge and skills and understand your responsibilities and liabilities with respect to delegating and guiding the work of others. Because of inconsistencies from one workplace to another, it is important to seek clarity about the roles and abilities of UHWs you are working with. CNA and other national organizations have recommended more national discussion of how to integrate this group into the health care system and the need to clarify their roles and levels of education.

HEALTH SYSTEM OUTCOMES AND CURRENT ISSUES IN HEALTH CARE

From the earlier sections it is evident that a great deal of time and attention has been and continues to be given to the development and maintenance of a health system. Considerable amounts of public and private funding support the system, and large numbers of individuals bring a wealth of expertise and professional skill in pursuit of the goals of the health system. As you have already learned through your nursing education so far, the health care system is not the only determinant of the health of a population, and such factors as the physical and social environment, as well as biology and lifestyle, also play key roles in determining health.

There are many ways in which one could look at health outcomes. The Organization for Economic Co-operation and Development (OECD) has examined a number of factors that contribute to health status. The OECD (2012) is an international organization, currently composed of 34 countries, that is interested in sharing ideas on policies that range from economic to social. The member countries share an interest in democracy and market economies. They compile data and generate reports on health matters that provide useful comparisons, because many members of OECD have an economic status similar to Canada. As a member of OECD, Canada uses data and contributes data. This sharing is one of the ways that Canada can assess how well it is doing. How does Canada compare to other OECD countries in terms of health of the population? Figure 2.2 on life expectancy at birth and Figure 2.3 on infant mortality rates present

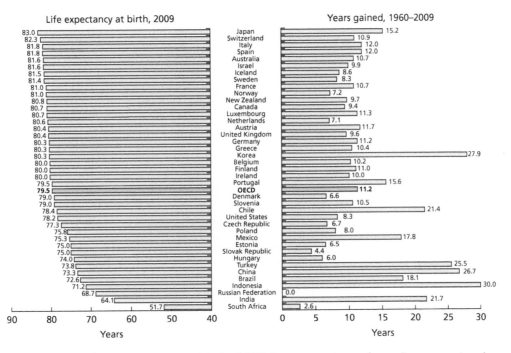

Life expectancy at birth, 2009   Years gained, 1960–2009

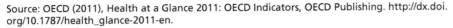

Figure 2.2 Life expectancy at birth, 2009 (or nearest year), and years gained since 1960

Source: OECD (2011), Health at a Glance 2011: OECD Indicators, OECD Publishing. http://dx.doi.org/10.1787/health_glance-2011-en.

measures that are considered to be two indicators of the relative health status of a population.

The OECD (2011) is interested in how a country's health systems perform and has identified three aspects that can be examined in greater detail: quality of care, access to care, and cost/expenditure. These three aspects are ones that many health authorities and health institutions examine when evaluating performance. A number of the current issues in health care in Canada relate to these three aspects of performance. For example, the 2004 Health Accord, mentioned earlier, focused on improving wait times for services, which is a concern related to access to care. Use of technology and development of electronic health records was another issue addressed in the accord and that issue is viewed as a factor in ensuring quality of care as well as efficiency, which can reduce health care costs. One of the solutions that many believe is key in addressing issues of quality, access to care, and costs is an integrated health system.

Integrated Health Care System

Canada shares the international concern about fragmentation of health care services. A common solution posed in response to those concerns is "integrated care" (Kodner, 2009). The range of concerns include problems in accessing services; lack of coordination of

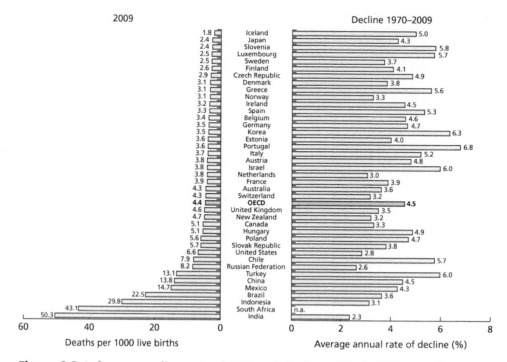

Figure 2.3 Infant mortality rates, 2009 and decline 1970-2009 (or nearest year)

Source: OECD (2011), Health at a Glance 2011: OECD Indicators, OECD Publishing. http://dx.doi. org/10.1787/health_glance-2011-en.

services for individuals, especially those with multiple and complex problems; a focus on acute care that fails to address the needs of those with chronic conditions; disjointed, inefficient, and low quality care; and out-of-control costs. Many examples can be given of patients who "fall between the cracks" in health care or who are "lost in the system," not obtaining the kind of care they require in a timely manner. Given the range of concerns, the meanings given to integrated care also range widely and encompass such phrases as case management, continuity of care, seamless care, patient-centred care, and vertical and horizontal integration of services.

One definition of integration in health care comes from a technical brief by the World Health Organization (WHO, 2008). It defines integrated service delivery as "the organization and management of health services so that people get the care they need, when they need it, in ways that are user-friendly, achieve the desired results and provide value for money." (p. 5). This kind of service delivery is a way of making navigation through the system easier and more seamless for clients; however, in addition, integration can be more extensive than just service delivery and can extend to include funding, administrative, organizational, and clinical integration. While there are examples of some types and levels of integration, full integration at all levels is an enormous challenge. Some of these challenges have been discussed in proposals in Ontario for integrated health care organizations that combine delivery of acute care, primary care, and homecare in one organization (McLellan, Egberts, & Ronson, 2011).

Thomas McKeown, meet Fidel Castro: Physicians, population health and the Cuban paradox, 2008.

Robert Evans (2008) discusses the "remarkable" Cuban achievement with regard to health status of the population. Although a poor country in terms of most measures of wealth, such as per capita Gross Domestic Product (GDP), based on data from the World Health Organization, Cuba is comparable to high-income countries on common measures of population health, such as life expectancy at birth and mortality before the age of five. Cuba is considered an "outlier," performing well above what one would expect of a poor country. Evans notes that there has been little examination of how Cuba has accomplished this result and suggests that further scholarly attention should be given to this question. He notes that one of the unusual characteristics of Cuba that can be found in health data is the doctor-to-population ratio in the country, which is the highest in the world. Evans considers those countries closest to Cuba's doctor-to-population ratio to see if they might suggest an answer. In general, poorer countries with a similar physician supply do not achieve the same outcomes as Cuba, while wealthy countries achieve comparable outcomes. The question remains—how does Cuba achieve these outcomes, given their GDP? Evans discusses the nature of primary health care in Cuba and physician training and speculates that these might be factors in Cuba's success:

The difference appears to be that in Cuba, primary care physician (and nurse) teams have responsibility for the health of geographically defined populations, not merely of those patients who come in the door. These teams are then linked to community- and higher-level political organizations that both hold them accountable for the health of their populations and provide them with channels through which to influence the relevant non-medical determinants. (p. 31)

This article illustrates how a focus on health outcomes leads one to examine what it is that improves health outcomes for a population other than a greater infusion of funds. The data that Evans examines do seem to suggest that an emphasis on primary health care principles, accountability systems, and population health approaches may well help explain improved health outcomes at the national level. The author, who is an eminent Canadian health care economist, has raised questions about health care policy approaches that are applicable to any country, even one like Canada, which would be considered wealthy compared to many other countries.

Source: Evans, R. G. (2008). Thomas McKeown, meet Fidel Castro: Physicians, population health and the Cuban paradox. Healthcare Policy, 3(4), 21–32.

SUMMARY

In this chapter we have focused on management theories and functions and the environment in which managers operate. The idea of management has evolved over time so that, while key management functions remain important, the leadership dimension has taken on equal importance as the pace of change in society increases. Managers and leaders with skills in both spheres are needed to organize and lead complex health care organizations amid constant and fast-paced change. Health care management occurs within an environ-ment that has great complexity; is affected by public policies and regulations in many sectors; is of great concern to individuals, their families, and communities; and must con-tinually change to ensure accessible, safe, high quality effective care that is provided in an efficient way at a cost the country care sustain.

Glossary of Terms

Classical management theory is a view of management as a process of planning, organizing, commanding, and controlling.

Cybernetics is an interdisciplinary science that studies information, communication, and control. It is considered a technique for designing self-regulating systems and is used in thinking about how organizations learn.

Healthy public policy refers to govern-ment policy that promotes health.

Horizontal integration refers to an orga-nization becoming larger by joining with a similar organization(s). In the case of hospi-tals, horizontal integration is when a hospital joins with another hospital(s).

Medicare is a term used by Canadians to refer to publicly funded health care services to which they have access in provincial and territorial health systems. It refers to insured health services and at a minimum includes hospital care and physician care.

Policy fields refer to areas of policy interest, such as health, transportation, agri-culture, education.

Primary care refers to the provision of per-sonal health services to individuals and fami-lies, normally on a continuing basis in their home community. This is usually first level of contact that individuals have with the health system, and the provider is the gateway to health services required beyond assessment, diagnosis and treatment of common illness or injuries, disease prevention, or individual health promotion.

Primary health care encompasses the level at which individuals, families and communi-ties enter the health system and access health services and includes the provision of individual

health services for injuries and illness, but extends beyond that to include disease preven-tion and health promotion. There is a range of organizations that provide PHC services.

Public policy refers to courses of action by governments. Public authorities, be they municipal, provincial, or federal, through policy may decide to take actions (or decide not to take action) with respect to problems within their respective jurisdiction or area of responsibility.

Quaternary health care refers to the most specialized services that are only avail-able in limited locations due to the highly specialized requirements for equipment and personnel. These services may only be avail-able in a few cities in a country, and poorer countries may not have any of these services available. Heart and lung transplantation is an example of such a service.

Regionalization refers to the decentraliza-tion of authority and responsibility for health services from a more central authority to a regional body. The trend in Canada has been for provincial governments to establish regional bodies based on geographic areas and delegate some degree of responsibility for decision-making about health services to them.

Scientific management refers to an approach to management from the early 1900s that emphasized designing work to maximize time, energy, and efficiency, and training or hiring workers so that skills matched the jobs. The role of managers was to plan and supervise workers.

Secondary health care is a specialized level of care in a variety of settings, such as community hospitals, home care, and long-term and chronic care settings. Individuals are normally referred to this level of health care by someone in the primary health care level, such as a family physician

Tertiary health care refers to the third level of care that provides more specialized services than one would find in a general or community hospital, so these services are usually found in larger centres that can bring the equipment and personnel together required. For example, cardiac surgery may be carried out in a tertiary health centre.

Unregulated health worker (UHW) refers to care providers or assistant personnel who provide some form of health service and who are not licensed or regulated by a professional or regulatory body. Those who assist with nursing care may have job titles like nursing aide, health care aide, or personal support worker.

Vertical integration refers to an organization becoming larger by joining with another organization(s) that is a supplier or purchaser of products or services of the organization. In the case of hospitals, vertical integration refers to a hospital becoming larger by joining with health care organizations where patients may be referred to the hospital, or go to after hospitalization, such as community health centres and long term care centres.

Critical Thinking Questions and Activities

1. Describe how your current clinical placement or workplace exhibits characteristics of classical management theory or human relations theory.

2. Choose one of the health care organizations in which you have had experience and describe how that organization would be "open to the environment." What has the organization had to respond to in the environment and how has it responded?

3. Interview a nurse in a managerial role in a clinical area and ask him or her to give examples of his or her experience in the five management functions described in this chapter.

4. Identify a nurse at a senior level of management in your organization and give examples of her or his skills and activities as a manager and as a leader.

5. Think about your own experiences as someone who has used and received health care services. At what level of the system were the services provided? What health occupations were involved in providing these services? Now answer the same questions about someone else that you know and that person's health care experiences.

6. Where does the funding come from for the health services you or someone you know received? Who was responsible for the costs of the health services required? Were there health care costs that were paid by the individual?

Self-Quiz

1. The management theory associated with designing positions for work flow and efficiency is known as:
   a. Cybernetics
   b. Human relations
   c. Theory X and Theory Y
   d. Scientific management

2. Leadership is distinguished from management in that:

    a. Leadership is focused on quality standards

    b. Management is concerned with coaching

    c. Leadership is dealing with change

    d. Management involves developing a vision

3. The Canada Health Act criteria require that:

    a. Out-of-country services are available to Canadians

    b. All citizens have access to drug therapy

    c. Provincial health insurance is publicly administered

    d. Long-term care is an insured service

4. Public health services would be considered what level of health care?

    a. Primary

    b. Secondary

    c. Tertiary

    d. Quaternary

Useful Websites

Academy of Chief Executive Nurses (ACEN)
http://acen.ca

Canadian Association of Schools of Nursing
www.casn.ca/en/

Canadian Institute for Health Information (CIHI)
www.cihi.ca/CIHI-ext-portal/internet/EN/Home/home/cihi000001

Canadian Nurses Association
www.cna-aiic.ca/CNA/default_e.aspx

Health Canada
www.hc-sc.gc.ca/index-eng.php

Health Council of Canada (HCC)
www.healthcouncilcanada.ca/en/

International Council of Nurses
www.icn.ch/

Parliament of Canada
www.parl.gc.ca/Default.aspx?Language=E

Public Health Agency of Canada
www.phac-aspc.gc.ca/index-eng.php

Registered Psychiatric Nurses of Canada
www.rpnc.ca/pages/about.php

Statistics Canada
www.statcan.gc.ca/start-debut-eng.html

Victorian Order of Nurses Caregiver Connect Portal
www.von.ca/en/caregiver-connect/home/default.aspx

World Health Organization
www.who.int/en/

References

Bergevin, Y., & Mohamed, N. (1993). Challenge of policy formulation for grown promotion. In. J. Cervinskas, N.M. Gerein, & S. George (Eds.). *Growth promotion for child development*. *Proceedings of a colloquium*, Nyeri, Kenya, 12–13 May, 1992. Ottawa: International Development Research Centre.

Bryant, T. (2009). *An introduction to health policy*. Toronto: Canadian Scholar's Press.

Canadian Foundation for Healthcare Improvement. (2013). *Frequently Asked Questions*. Retrieved from www.cfhi-fcass.ca/AboutUs/FAQs.aspx, May 31, 2013.

Canadian Health Services Research Foundation. (2007). *2007 Annual Report on the Nursing Research Fund*. Ottawa: CHSRF.

Canadian Institute for Health Information. (2009). *Health care in Canada 2009. A decade in review*. Ottawa: CIHI.

Canadian Institute for Health Information. (December, 2010). *Regulated nurses: Canadian trends, 2005 to 2009*. Ottawa: CIHI.

Canadian Institute for Health Information. (2011b). *Canada's health care providers 2000 to 2009—A reference guide*. Ottawa: CIHI.

Canadian Institute for Health Information. (2011a). *National health expenditure trends, 1975 to 2011*. Ottawa: CIHI.

Canadian Institutes of Health Research. (2012). CIHR Grants and Awards Guide. Retreived from www.cihr-irsc.gc.ca/e/22630.html#1-A

Canadian Nurses Association (2000). *The primary health care approach. Fact sheet*. Ottawa: CNA.

Canadian Nurses Association (2002). *Effective health care equals primary health care (PHC). Fact sheet*. Ottawa: CNA.

Canadian Nurses Association (2009). *Increasing use of unregulated health workers. Issues discussion at Annual Meeting 2009*. Ottawa: CNA.

Church, J. & Barker, P. (1998). Regionalization of health services in Canada: a critical perspective. *International Journal of Health Services, 28*(3), 467–486.

Department of Justice. (2011). Canada Health Act (R.S.C., 1985, c. C-6). Retrieved from: http://laws-lois.justice.gc.ca/eng/acts/C-6/

Duckett, S. (2011). Getting the foundations right: Alberta's approach to healthcare reform. *Healthcare Policy, 6*(3), 22–26.

Dunbar, R.-L.-M., & Statler, M. (2010). A historical perspective on organizational control. In S.B. Sitkin & Cardinal, L.B., & Bijilsma-Frankema, K.M. (Eds.), *Organizational control*. Cambridge: Cambridge University Press.

Evans, R.G. (2008). Thomas McKeown, meet Fidel Castro: Physicians, population health and the Cuban paradox. *Healthcare Policy, 3*(4), 21–32.

Evans, R.G., Barer, M.L., & Marmor, T.R. (1994). *Why are some people healthy and others not? The determinants of health of populations*. New York: de Gruyter Inc.

Falk, W. (2011). Will Falk comments on John Ronson's essay "LHINs at five years—What now?" Retrieved from www.longwoods.com/content/22529/print September 12, 2011.

Falk-Rafael, A., Fox, J., & Bewick, D. (2005). Report of a 1999 survey of public health nurses: is public health restructuring in Ontario, Canada moving toward primary health care? *Primary Health Care Research and Development, 6*, 172–183.

Fayol, H. (1949). *General and industrial management*. London: Pitman.

Health Canada. (2011, September 13). *Canada's health care system*. Retrieved from http://hc-sc.gc.ca/hcs-sss/publs/system-regime/2011-hcs-sss/index-eng.php

Jansen, I. (2011). Residential long-term care: Public solutions to access and quality problems. *Healthcare Papers, 10*(4), 8–22.

Jones, R.A. (2010). Preparing tomorrow's leaders. A review of the issues. *Journal of Nursing Administration, 40*(4), 154–157.

Kleinman, C.S. (2003). Leadership roles, competencies, and education. How prepared are our nurse managers? *Journal of Nursing Administration, 33*(9), 451–455.

Kodner, D. (2009). All together now: A conceptual exploration of integrated care. *Healthcare Quarterly, 13*(October Special Issue), 6–15.

Koontz, H. & Weihrich, H. (1990). *Essentials of management. 5th edition*. New York: McGraw-Hill.

Kotter, J.P. (2001). What leaders really do. *Harvard Business Review, 68*(3), 103–111.

Lewis, S. & Kouri, D. (2004). Regionalization: making sense of the Canadian experience. *Healthcare Papers, 5*(1), 12–31.

McGregor D. (1966). The human side of enterprise. In: Bennis, W.G. & Schein, E.H. *Leadership and motivation. Essays of Douglas McGregor* (pp. 3–29). Cambridge, Massachusetts: MIT Press.

McLellan, B., Egberts, M.C. & Ronson, J. (2011). Are integrated healthcare organizations right for Ontario? Retrieved October 20, 2011 from www.longwoods.com/content/22607.

Morgan, G. (2006). *Images of organization*. Thousand Oaks, California: Sage Publications.

O'Neill, M.A., McGuinty, D., & Teskey, B. (2011). Canadian political science and medicare: Six decades of inquiry. *Healthcare Policy*, 6(4), 49–61.

Ontario Ministry of Health and Long-term Care. (2011). Public health units. Retrieved from www.health.gov.on.ca/english/public/contact/phu/phu_mn.html

Organisation for Economic Cooperation and Development. (2011). Health at a glance. p2011. Retrieved from DOI : 10.1787/health_glance-2011-en

Organisation for Economic Cooperation and Development. (2012). About the Organisation for Economic cooperation and Development. Retrieved from www. oecd.org/pages/0,3417,en_36734052_36734103_1_1_1_1_1,00.html

Roemer, M.I. (1993). National health systems throughout the world. Lessons for health system reform in the United States. *American Behavioral Scientist*, 36(6), 694–708.

Romanow, R. (2002). *Building on values: The future of health care in Canada. Final report*. Commission on the Future of Health Care in Canada.

Samulelson, K. (2011). What does quality look like to the resident? *Healthcare Papers*, 10(4), 24–29.

Vayda, E., & Deber, R.B. (1984). The Canadian health care system: An overview. *Social Science & Medicine*, 18(3), 191–197.

World Health Organization. (1978). *Primary health care: Report on the International Conference on Primary Health Care, Alma-Ata, USSR, 6-12 September, 1978*. Geneva: Author.

World Health Organization. (2008). *Integrated health services—what and why? Technical brief no.1*. Geneva: Author, 1–10.

Chapter 3

Organizational Power and Politics

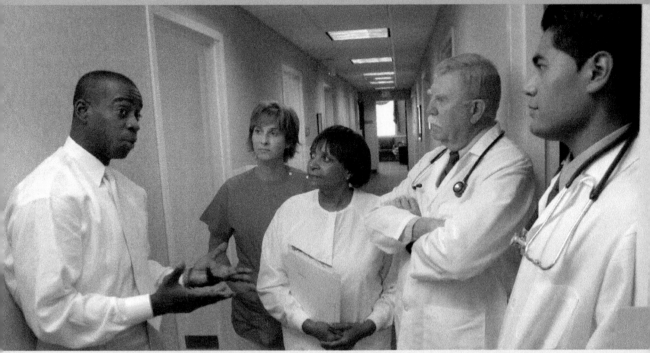

Thinkstock/Getty Images

Learning Objectives

After reading, studying, and reflecting on this chapter's content, you will be able to:

1. Define power and politics and describe differing perspectives on their use in organizations
2. Analyze power relationships in the workplace and the sources of power of the actors or units/departments of an organization
3. Debate the positive and negative perceptions of power and politics in the workplace
4. Discuss how an organization may be structured to empower employees
5. Describe the groups in organizations who can exert power and ways in which power can operate
6. Discuss how politics plays out in organizations and the strategies and games that can be used in health care organizations
7. Identify the types of situations in health care organizations that give rise to use of power and politics

INTRODUCTION

You have spent some time working in organizations, as a volunteer, an employee, or a student and you have therefore had the opportunity to observe and participate in organizational life. Have you ever been influenced by a preceptor, a teacher, a colleague, or a manager to think about your work in a different way and therefore, do it differently? Have you ever wondered how a decision that affected your work or somehow changed the workplace got made? Have you ever influenced others whom you have worked with, either intentionally or unintentionally? Why does one department's proposal for expansion get chosen over another? Why does one part of the institution get renovated or new equipment when another seems just as outdated? Is it all a matter of rational choice or evidence-based decision-making? One of the ways you can examine these questions is from the perspective of **power** and **politics**.

Many people have a negative reaction to the idea that power and politics may be key factors in the life of organizations—they believe that the use of power and politics is always destructive, unfair, subversive, and somehow, morally wrong. Some who work in organizations acknowledge that power and politics do play a role in their workplace, but they prefer to ignore that aspect of working life and stay out of "political games." Others view power and politics as normal in social contexts, and, therefore, a reality in organizations. They see the exercise of power as one way that goals are chosen and achieved and consider politics as a key way of integrating and resolving differing views in an organization, such as a hospital, health centre, public health unit, or nursing home.

As a member of an organization, you may consider your own role in power and politics from various viewpoints: as an observer, an analyst, or a participant. You can begin this study by learning more about the many views on what power is; where it comes from; when, where, and how it operates in organizations; and how it can affect individuals and organizations in positive and negative ways.

In this chapter, we begin with definitions of power and politics. We then discuss views of power and politics in organizations together, followed by subsections that focus first on the phenomenon of power and then on politics in organizations. The final section of this chapter will discuss power in health care organizations and nursing. We will highlight the types and sources of power that individuals, groups, or subunits of an organization might have, discuss how and when power and politics flow and play out in organizational life, and examine the consequences of power and politics. We believe that power and politics are a reality in organizational life and that those who work in organizations, no matter what the size, can benefit from an understanding of situations that give rise to power and politics. In your nursing roles, you will exercise power and participate in politics, either knowingly or unknowingly. We believe that you should do so knowingly. As you reflect on and understand your own behaviour and that of others, you can participate fully in an ethical and positive way to accomplish goals. We recognize that power and politics can be used in a destructive way, but you can contribute through thoughtful action to constructive, effective, and ethical health care. We will discuss ethical leadership more fully in Chapter 14.

DEFINITIONS OF POWER AND POLITICS

The concepts of power and politics both involve the idea of influence. We agree with Alexander and Morlock (2000) who define power as "the ability (or potential) to exert actions that either directly or indirectly cause change in the behavior and/or attitudes of another individual or group" (p. 216). Kanter (1997), who focused on power in organizations, defined it as "the ability to mobilize resources (human and material) to get things done" (p. 136). Power can be viewed as a positive or negative social force and many traditional views of power are negative, viewing it in terms of dominance over others or a holdover from pre-democratic periods where the leader was a cruel tyrant. Lammers & Galinsky (2009) believe that these conflicting perspectives on power stem from two Western philosophies, one that sees power differences in social organization as contributing to order and effectiveness, while the other sees power differences as leading to social inequality, abuse, and rule by elites. The international Occupy Movement, at home exemplified by the 2011 Occupy Bay Street, reflects current concerns about inequities in society between those with high incomes (the 1 percent) and those without (the 99 percent). Fundamentally, the movement is about the relationships between those perceived to have power and those who do not.

Politics refers to tactical activities or strategies a person takes to influence the decisions or actions of others. Definitions of politics vary in several respects. Some definitions embody the idea that the use of politics in organizations is inherently legitimate or illegitimate. A negative view is one that sees politics as "a domain of activity in which participants attempt to influence organizational decisions and activities in ways that are not sanctioned by either the formal authority system of the organization, its accepted ideology, or certified expertise" (Alexander & Morlock, 2000, p. 248). Other authors do not define politics in terms of legitimacy, but rather as competing interests and goals, jockeying for a favourable position, or approval of one over another. For example, Liu, Liu, and Wee (2010) define political behaviour as "the exercise of tactical influence by individuals intended to facilitate personal or organizational goals" (p. 1433). Buchanan and Badham (1999) define political behaviour as "the practical domain of power in action, worked out through the use of techniques of influence and other (more or less extreme) tactics" (p. 11). Butcher and Clarke (2002) argue that constructive politics "represent the logical processes by which diverse interests and stakeholders are reconciled in organizations" (p. 41). This definition casts politics in a positive light, provided that it is "constructive" politics, hinting that politics can be negative and destructive.

PERSPECTIVES ON ORGANIZATIONAL POWER AND POLITICS

Observations of power and politics have been made for a long time, but classical management theory and rational management theory have tended to ignore these features of organizational life. As discussed in earlier chapters (see Chapter 1 on theories of leadership), many theories developed from the 1920s to the current day that depict organizations as cohesive and logical entities in which decisions are made in a rational manner, based on known cause and effect relationships, accurate and timely information, formal leadership, and orderly processes. In the 1950s and 1960s, researchers interested in group dynamics and social psychology examined power and influence in groups (Cartwright & Zander, 1968), particularly as they functioned in organizations. In the 1970s and 1980s, power and politics was given greater attention by organizational theorists and researchers as they recognized that these were a reality, although not openly discussed (Kanter, 1979; Kotter, 1985; Pfeffer, 1992). Kanter (1979), in a book on new ways of managing in organizations, wrote:

> Power is one of the last dirty words. It is easier to talk about money—and much easier to talk about sex—than it is to talk about power. People who have it deny it; people who want it do not want to appear to hunger for it; and people who engage in its machinations do so secretly. (p. 135)

Many of us in Canada have a Western view of organizations, so our views on power and politics influence our view of how organizations operate. As mentioned earlier, there is a cultural component to how people view power that has been explored in behavioural studies (Lammers & Galinsky, 2009). The findings of these studies suggest that while Westerners showed a positive association between power and reward, the association between power and cooperation was negative. In contrast, East Asians associated the idea of power positively, with restraint and with cooperation. Differing cultural views of power may lead to differing psychological and behavioural consequences in the workplace.

Politics is even more likely than power to evoke a negative image, even among those who acknowledge its reality in organizational life. They describe politics as creating havoc in organizations and derailing efficient functioning. Mintzberg (1983) viewed political behaviour in organizations as essentially illegitimate and compared it to an illness— dangerous to healthy functioning, yet having value, in that it alerted the organization to the need to adapt. In his view, when politics became a dominant force in an organization, it affected legitimate power, that form of power that belongs to an official position with formal authority. Similarly, others have described politics as unsanctioned behaviour in terms of an organization's goals, formal authority, or accepted policies and procedures (Cavanagh, Moberg, & Velasquez, 1981; Alexander & Morlock, 2000). Others have a less negative view. Pfeffer (1992) argued that there is a great deal of ambivalence about power in organizations, and while we may acknowledge that politics exist in organizations, we think that it interferes with efficiency. He believes that power, influence, and politics are used to get things done. Butcher and Clarke (2002) take a positive view of politics in organizations, describing it as being "the constructive reconciliation of competing causes" (p. 40) by which diverse interests and views can be sorted out in a just way.

Bases of Power

How does one get or develop power? French and Raven's (1968) work from the 1950s and 1960s generated a theory of social influence and power in terms of two social agents, one having influence on the other. Influence was conceptualized as psychological change, including change in behaviour, opinion, attitude, goals, needs, values, or other psychological aspects. They examined the relationship between the influencer and the one influenced and the bases of the power in the relationship, all of which depend on the perceptions of the person being influenced. In this theory, the influencer might be a person, a particular role, a part of a group, or a whole group, while the influenced is an individual. French and Raven categorized five bases of power that they considered to be the most common and important:

- Reward power is based on the ability of the person in the senior position to provide rewards, such as pay increases, promotions, special privileges, and other benefits.

- Coercive power is the power to apply punishment or withhold rewards, for example the power to fire someone based on work performance.

- Legitimate power is based on the official or formal position of someone and the perception that that person has the right to exert influence and expect compliance. This power is based on a kind of internalized value held by the one being influenced, for example, a cultural value that an older person can give direction to a younger one or that a department head can give direction to someone lower in the organizational hierarchy.

- Referent power is based on personal attractive qualities. Those influenced by this power identify with the person and would like to be associated with him or her, even if those being influenced are not aware of the power. Sometimes this is referred to as charisma. When a group has referent power, the influenced individual would like to join that group and the stronger the identification, the greater the referent power of the group.

- Expert power is based on the perceived extent of a person's knowledge or expertise. For example, a health care professional or a lawyer might have expert power because a patient or client perceives that this professional has a more extensive knowledge of the relevant field.

You can see how all of these bases of power may play a role in many of your social relationships, but they are particularly worth noting in relation to your working life as a nurse in a health care organization. You will have greater knowledge of health care than most of those you care for, and you will therefore have expert power within that relationship. You will want to use that power in a responsible, thoughtful, and ethical way, but to do so, you need to first be aware of that power and the effect that it can have on others. You will also be in roles that could confer reward, coercive, referent, and legitimate power in relationships with clients, family, visitors, and colleagues.

French and Raven proposed that not all types of power are the same when used. For example, they proposed that coercion leads to high resistance and a decrease in attraction to the influencer, while reward power has the opposite result, that is, higher attraction and less resistance. They also proposed that the more legitimate the coercion, the less it is apt to lower attraction and generate resistance. Randolph & Kemery (2011) conducted a study of the use of different bases of power by managers in a wide variety of industries, including health organizations. They were interested in determining if the use of different kinds of bases of power by managers affected the management practices they used to empower employees and if indeed the employees felt psychologically empowered (a sense of meaning, competence, self-determination, and ability to have an impact). They surveyed 195 manager–employee pairs in the United States and found that there was a positive relationship between managerial **empowerment** practices and employee psychological empowerment, but the key predictors were use of expert, reward, and referent power bases, not coercive and legitimate power.

Sources of Power

Some theorists have focused on sources of power for those who work in organizations. According to Pfeffer (2009), sources of power include personal and structural ones. Some of these personal sources include:

- Personal attributes, for example, being articulate, self-confident and sensitive to others can be considered qualities that enable one to influence others.

- Personal behaviour can influence others and lead others to perceive an individual as powerful. For example, behaviour that expresses strong emotion, like anger, can convey the impression of power.

- Personal actions, such as transforming a function or activity into something enhanced or more valued and useful can enhance an individual's power. For example, successfully marketing a previously unprofitable product in a business can increase the power of the leader of the marketing unit.

Individual attributes, actions, and behaviour can enable people to become influential in an organization, beyond what would be expected based on their actual position.

Structural sources of power may be more important in organizations than personal ones. Structural sources of power include:

- Formal position in the hierarchy provides the occupier of the position with a sphere of influence and the right and responsibility to make decisions, give direction, and take action. This source of power comes from one's position in the **formal authority system**, meaning that the power to act and exert authority is legitimate (Alexander & Morlock, 2000). Figure 3.1 depicts the formal authority structure one might find in an acute care hospital, with three levels of management.

- Control over resources, such as money and budgets, provides a person with structural power. Often, representatives from finance departments have this kind of influence or power on decision-making, especially in periods of resource constraint. Other kinds of resources also provide power and influence to the person who controls them, for example individuals who control access to people (personal secretaries, for instance) or who allocate space and equipment. Resources are always limited, but the more limited, the more scarce they are and more important as a source of power.

- Control of decision processes has several aspects that confer power. According to Morgan (2006), those who can influence the premises, processes, issues, and objectives for a decision have the ability to control decisions. Setting the ground rules and shaping the discussion of issues provides considerable influence in decision-making. Senior administrators often have this power in organizations because they chair important committees and set agendas for them, so can control the timing and sequence of discussion and decision making.

- Control over or access to knowledge and information is identified by some as a structural source of power. The structure of an organization and the way in which the structure is designed is important because it influences the way in which information flows and determines who has access to and control of information. Often, financial

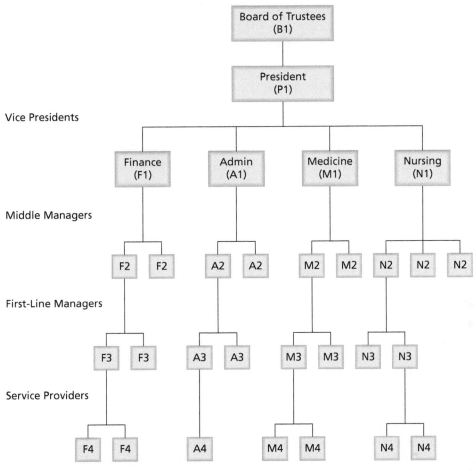

Figure 3.1 Formal Authority Structure: Acute Care General Hospital

Source: From Shortell. *Health Care Management*, 4th ed. © 2000 Delmar Learning, a part of Cengage Learning, Inc. Reproduced by permission. www.cengage.com/permissions.

departments are considered powerful in organizations, because they design and control information about budgets and spending, making them key in many organizational decisions.

- Ability to cope with uncertainty on behalf of the organization is another source of power. For example, individuals or departments with expertise in a critical area, such as infection control in a health care organization, can accrue power because of the critical nature of their knowledge in preventing and limiting the dangers of infection that can affect the whole organization. This is particularly true now when antibiotic-resistant infections are major problems in health care organizations.

- Being central in communication networks is related to access to knowledge critical to the organization and the ability to bring parties together to coordinate and accomplish results. The ability to bring together two parties who benefit from each other is a brokering role that can bring power and influence to an individual. Similarly, those who are networked with individuals and groups, can form alliances and accrue considerable informal power outside of the chain of command or formal system of authority.

Power-dependence Theory

Power-dependence theory focuses on social exchange and the relations between actors who might be individuals (like the director of care in a nursing home or a staff nurse) or a collective (like a maternal health team in a public health unit or a renal unit in a hospital). The actors in an interdependent relationship depend on one another for some results that they value and this provides the basis for power (Molm, 2009). Independent individuals have no power over each other, interdependent individuals are dependent on each other to some degree, and a dependent relationship is when one individual has substantial power over another. In any relationship however, it is not always the person you expect who has the power.

However nobody is all powerful in all relationships. Control of resources can serve as a source of power, and two parties in a relationship (however temporary, such as a customer in a restaurant and the waiter serving that customer) may have a power imbalance, with the one seeking the resource being dependent on the one with the resource. Even the CEO of an organization is interdependent—she or he must depend on others to accomplish the goals set for the organization. The basic idea of power-dependence theory is that power is usually asymmetrical between two agents, because of differences in influence and interdependence. We are primarily interested in more sustained relationships than that between the waiter and the customer, such as those we experience in a work setting. The idea of social exchange is that people seek results that they value and that individuals exchange valued goods or benefits with each other over time in a continuing relationship, so there is a mutual dependence that can lead to a balanced relationship or there can be inequalities in power. Understanding even the power relationship between two individuals in the workplace is difficult though, because it is embedded in larger power structures or networks that affect power balances. In organizations, you are dealing with a complex social system, with multiple relationships and dependencies. How an organization is structured can influence the power relationship between individuals and departments (Molm, 2009). Power relations can be examined at the individual level, as well as at the level of groups or units within organizations.

A Post-Structural View of Power

More recent views of power are those developed by a French philosopher, Michel Foucault, whose interest focused on prisons and the use of discipline and punishment (Foucault, 1977). Unlike prevailing notions of power, he viewed power in positive terms and saw it as diffused in society, not limited to a few individuals. Buchanan and Badham (1999) note that his writings are difficult to follow, but they identify two concepts that are central to Foucault's view of power: bio-power and disciplinary power. Bio-power is described by Perron, Fluet, and Holmes (2005) as intended to "manage and administer individuals and, by extension, communities and populations" (p. 537), so it is pervasive in society. It establishes what is normal and abnormal, socially deviant or acceptable, and this is judged by "competent" authorities. Bio-power applies to society as a whole and has a continuity that is unlike episodic uses of power. We come to view what is normal in a social sense, through bio-power. For example, Buchanan and Badham note that at one time society viewed a woman's aspiration for senior executive positions as unacceptable.

Disciplinary power is a second concept and it is aimed at individuals and groups. Using tools of control or disciplinary practices, such as surveillance and assessment, individual behaviour is controlled and one can see these practices in daily operation in schools, hospitals, and factories. Such power can be viewed as productive and beneficial to society, or negative. However, a third aspect of Foucault's ideas, related to knowledge, mean that power and practices change and the prevailing "web" of practices shifts over time. Developing knowledge opens opportunities for power—knowledge is continually changing and shifting. Some of the ways in which traditional ideas about power differ from those of Foucault are that traditional concepts see power as belonging to individuals, usually elites, as most of us are dominated by the more powerful among us; as typically destructive and negative, as something you are able to see when activated; and as something that can be overcome through knowledge of power sources. In contrast, Foucault viewed power as pervasive in social life; as a network of power that we build; as productive and constructive and everchanging; as operating as part of regular daily life; and as being maintained through knowledge (Buchanan & Badham, 1999).

While Foucault's ideas may not give guidance with respect to the use of power and politics in a specific organization, Buchanan and Badham (1999) believe that this perspective enables us to look at our ideas, practices, and behaviour in organizations in a more critical way. Nurses have done just that. For example, Perron, Fluet, and Holmes (2005) describe breastfeeding as an example of bio-political intervention in which nurses often participate. They believe that new mothers are pressured, given the scientific and authoritative support for breastfeeding, to only breastfeed. Through media, disciplinary practices, and advocacy, the current view is established that it is a mother's duty to do so. These authors use Foucault's ideas to analyze a number of nursing practices and illustrate the ways in which nursing power may be evident in organizations. Polifroni (2010) examines power in nursing using the ideas of Foucault, particularly those related to knowledge, to analyze the power of clinical nursing.

Kanter's Theory of Structural Power in Organizations

Kanter studied structural sources of power in organizations and makes the case that understanding these is important for managers as they are major factors in organizational success. She believes that the key source of power for productivity and accomplishment in the workplace is not the individual person, but the person's position and the power built into the position, or the structural sources of power. Table 3.1 illustrates organizational factors that contribute to power or powerlessness in a position.

Kanter's work has been used in numerous nursing studies to examine the relationship between structural factors and a sense of workplace empowerment. Empowerment refers to increases in the influence that employees have in an organization, through various organizational designs, approaches, and changes. Cho, Laschinger, and Wong (2006) reported

Table 3.1 **Ways Organizational Factors Contribute to Power of Powerlessness**

Factors	Generates Power when Factor is	Generates Powerlessness when Factor is
Rules inherent in the job	few	many
Predecessors in the job	few	many
Established routines	few	many
Task variety	high	low
Rewards for reliability/predictability	few	many
Rewards for unusual performance/innovation	many	few
Flexibility around use of people	high	low
Approvals needed for nonroutine decisions	few	many
Physical location	central	distant
Publicity about job activities	high	low
Relation of tasks to current problem areas	central	peripheral
Focus of tasks	outside work unit	inside work unit
Interpersonal contact in the job	high	low
Contact with senior officials	high	low
Participation in programs, conferences, meetings	high	low
Participation in problem-solving task forces	high	low
Advancement prospects of subordinates	high	low

Source: Kanter, R.M. *Frontiers of Management.* Copyright ©1997, Harvard Business Publishing. Reprinted with permission.

on a study of new graduate nurses in Ontario hospital settings to examine relationships between workplace empowerment, work engagement, and organizational commitment. In total, a sample of 226 nurses who had graduated within the previous three years was obtained. The researchers found support for the empowerment model based on Kanter's work, with a direct positive effect of structural empowerment on six areas of work life.

Kanter (1979) argues that leaner and flatter organizations with fewer levels of bureaucracy mean that formal position is less important as a source of power than it used to be when you always had to go through "the **chain of command**" to get things done. Now, there are more channels of communication within and across organizations that organization members are expected to develop and use. Being at the centre of numerous networks now enables people or units to get things done and this centrality is a structural source of power. At one time, individuals or departments may have completely controlled information technology and databases within an organization, thereby accruing considerable power. Now however, this technology and a greater amount of information can be made widely accessible in an organization, increasing the distribution of this source of power to more individuals (Morgan, 2006). Although there have been changes in organizational culture and technology that diffuse power more widely in an organization, particularly in such sectors as the high technology industry, there is still considerable hierarchy in many organizations, including health care organizations. As Pfeffer (2009) points out, hierarchies are still found everywhere in formal and informal groups and in social relationships, such as working relationships.

Power Relations in Organizations

As noted at the beginning of this chapter, many theories about organizations have ignored power and politics as a factor in how organizations actually operate. Pfeffer (2009) believes that many of us are ambivalent about power—we may be uncomfortable using the formal authority we have, are uneasy working in hierarchical relationships, are uncomfortable developing informal influence, or find politics to be stressful. Our culture may emphasize merit over political skill in achieving success or shape our views on justice and how we relate to others in a way that makes politics seem unacceptable. Kotter (1985) argues that there is a middle view between those who are naïve about power and influence in organizations (believing that they don't exist and all is harmonious) and those who are cynics (believing that organizations are rife with conflict and power struggles). He believes that, while some power processes and activities that are pathological to some extent may exist in all organizations, they do not operate in all organizations, and not in the best organizations.

Why do conflict and power struggles develop in the workplace at all? Kotter (1985) proposes that two factors—diversity and interdependence—set conditions that increase or decrease the likelihood of conflict and power struggles. In his view, it is the social environment that influences behaviour within the organizations, rather than the characteristics of individuals. First, there is diversity or differences among people around goals, values, and perspectives. Second, people are interdependent in that two or more actors are dependent on each other to some degree and therefore have power over each other. Groups or organizations that involve a lot of people who differ a great deal from each other (for example, in their profession, cultural background, age, and so on) are very diverse organizations. Most workplaces and organizations are very interdependent and therefore, participants are rarely able to act independently and many of their co-workers are able to stop or at least slow down decisions or actions that are unilateral. According to this scheme, when there are few people involved in a situation (low interdependence) and when differences between them are few (low diversity), it is easier to resolve conflicts efficiently and effectively. When there are many linked people with very different ideas, it is difficult to achieve agreement on decisions. Figure 3.2 illustrates these relationships.

Kotter predicts that when discussion fails to achieve agreement, people engage in other tactics to resolve conflict. This may include negotiation of a compromise, the formation of

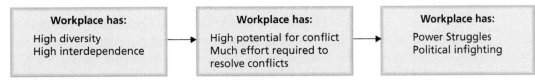

Figure 3.2 Factors in Organizational Conflict and Power Struggles

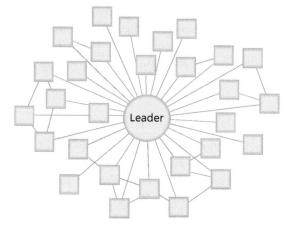

Figure 3.3 The Complex Relationships of a Leader

alliances, forcing a decision on others, manipulation of other parties, or other approaches, some of which can have negative consequences. A compromise may not be the best answer to a problem, a forced decision might lead to future resistance or retaliation, and manipulation will result in a loss of trust. Trends in the world of work increase the likelihood of working in an organization with the potential for conflict. Our society is more multicultural than in the past, meaning that there is greater cultural diversity in the workplace. Many health care teams now draw on a wide range of health care disciplines so that health care recipients benefit from the knowledge and skills of many experts who may have differing perspectives on how health care should be delivered or what the priorities of the organization should be. In addition, those participants are increasingly dependent on each other for achieving the results and benefits they seek. You may already have experienced the results of these differing perspectives. Note that it is the structure of the social milieu rather than the characteristics of the individual participants that set the conditions for greater conflict. At one time, leaders in the workplace related to a relatively small group of other people via the chain of command, illustrated in the rigid hierarchy depicted in Figure 3.1. In our more modern workplaces, in organizations of all sizes, the diversity of relationships and interdependencies is more like that in Figure 3.3. Kotter notes that strong leadership is needed in more diverse and interdependent organizations to resolve conflicts in a productive manner and he considers this ability to be a high-level skill required of leaders.

Systems of Influence in Organizations

Henry Mintzberg of McGill University wrote extensively about power in organizations. Rather than focusing on the power of individuals, Mintzberg (1983) described power in organizations in terms of groups and **systems of influence** that operated in the internal coalition that is, among and between key groups within the organization. The **internal coalition** consists of six groups of influencers, whose names may vary somewhat by the type and size of the organization. These groups are the top management (CEO and senior management team); operators (workers who produce goods or provide services, for example, nurses and doctors in a hospital); line managers (managers in a hierarchy with one or more levels between top management and operators); analysts (staff specialists, who design and operate systems, such as accountants, human resource specialists); and support staff (staff people who provide indirect support to operators and others, such as legal staff, mail room, cafeteria). Systems of influence are the ways in which power operates within the organization and different groups may have power through different systems of influence. Mintzberg identified four of these systems as follows:

- The System of Authority refers to the formal power that accrues to the holder of an official position, legitimate authority. The CEO and top management establish and design the hierarchy or chain of authority, with power flowing through the various levels of line management. This is one of the ways in which the work of the internal coalition members is co-ordinated to achieve goals.

- The System of Ideology refers to a system of beliefs about the organization that integrates personal and institutional goals, so that this ideology has an influence on the way that members think and act. This system involves a sense of mission and shared goals, traditions, identification, socialization, and loyalty. Identification may be the strongest way in which individual and organizational goals are integrated; however, when ideology is strong, the other systems may be weak.

- The System of Expertise arises in organizations that rely on professionals for the complex work required in the organization, such as a hospital. Since a system of authority that relies on bureaucratic controls and supervision is not appropriate or feasible with highly trained staff, a less bureaucratic form of organization with an informal system of expertise serves to coordinate the efforts and influence behaviour.

- The System of Politics arises in organizations because employees have delegated power that gives them the discretion to make decisions at some level. This discretion in their work makes the use of political power possible. This system of influence is discussed further in the next section.

Politics in Organizations

Among those who acknowledge the existence of politics in organizational decision making are those who view it as deviant and illegitimate because they define political behaviour in terms of self-interest that is not in line with organizational goals. Lee and Lawrence (1991) refer to this as the "political managerialist model" or perspective, in that it views pursuit of any goals other than the organizational goals to be political behaviour and dysfunctional. Those who hold this view of politics tend to see the processes and outcomes as negative for the organizations. When there is heightened politics in an organization, it may overtake the key purpose and work of an organization, divert the time and energy of organizational members, create turmoil and a poisonous climate of distrust, and damage an organization beyond repair. However, this outcome is not the typical result of the level of politics that is found in most organizations.

Mintzberg (1983) describes political power as a specific kind of power, and he says it arises inside of organizations as one of the systems of influence that he calls "the system of politics." He distinguishes it from the systems of authority, ideology, and expertise that operate as systems of legitimate influence to the extent that they meet the needs of the organization as a whole. His view of politics is negative and he makes the following points about what he means by politics:

1. Behaviour outside of the legitimate systems of influence (or at least outside their legitimate uses), and often in opposition to them, in other words behaviour that is technically illegitimate, and often clandestine

2. Behaviour designed to benefit the individual or group, ostensibly at the expense of the organization at large, (although…not always)

3. As a result of points 1 and 2, behaviour typically divisive or conflictive in nature, pitting individuals or groups against the organization at large, or against each other. (p. 172)

In contrast, some see the individuals and groups in an organization as having their own interests and who will try and get the decisions they want, without making a judgement that an individual or group is being deviant. In this view, which Lee and Lawrence refer to as the "radical political model," the actions and activities to achieve a person's interests is considered the way in which organizations normally function. They do not judge it as right or wrong, just the way that humans function in organizations. They recognize that even when there is agreement about high-level goals and overall values in an organization, there will be differing interests and views on how you should go about meeting goals. The strategies that are used to pursue goals constitute political behaviour, and this behaviour is the way in which key decisions are made, resources are allocated, conflicts about decisions are resolved, and directions for the organization are set. This view does *not* mean however, that any kind of behaviour, however unethical, is acceptable.

Those who view political behaviour as normal take the view that one ought to learn how politics operates in organizations and learn how to develop and use political power to influence others. They advocate the recognition and use of political strategies to achieve goals. Those who view politics as illegitimate in organizations, insofar as it subverts the legitimate goals of the organization in favour of particular interests, also advise that you ought to recognize the reality of political behaviour and the "political games" that they can encounter in organizations.

Political Strategies

Political strategies are the ways in which people develop and use power to their advantage to influence a decision and/or achieve goals. Lee and Lawrence (1991) describe political strategy as the development and mobilization of a person's power bases and the assessment of others' as two or more actors interact in a political situation. The actors in a political process consider their own sources of power and that of others, and develop their strategies based on that assessment in light of their goals and those of others. They describe the following kinds of strategies:

- Push strategies that threaten or force others to change behaviour through assertiveness, sanctions, or blocking through non-cooperation

- Pull strategies that use positive motivation to influence behaviour through recognition, benefits, or the satisfaction of needs and goals

- Persuasion strategies that appeal to logical reasoning or convincing others about behaviour in relation to goals

- Preventive strategies designed to prevent an issue from arising and may involve focusing attention elsewhere, avoiding a topic, or leaving it off an agenda

- Preparatory strategies aimed at preparing the ground or creating the conditions favourable to other strategies and range from the way in which someone dresses to create an impression to ordering the agenda in a favourable way to, simply, pouring on the charm

Push strategies are ones that can backfire and have negative results, so these must be used with caution. All of these strategies are used to gain influence with someone or some group and therefore in each situation you have to give consideration to your goals, the person/group that is to be influenced, and the most useful strategy to achieve influence at a particular time. An example of how nurse practitioners in Alberta utilized persuasion strategies with other health professionals in a variety of health care settings is presented in the Related Research.

Political Games

One way in which political behaviour is manifested in organizations is through the use of "**political games**." Political games are a pattern of behaviours engaged in by political actors who attempt to achieve their own ends, rather than the overall good of the whole organization. The metaphor of the game is used because the pattern reflects a set of rules that may or may not be explicit, but that involves positions and moves by the players who set out with similar bases of power as they seek to "win" through mobilizing strategies as the game develops. Mintzberg (1983) identifies a number of games that are played for five purposes: to resist authority, to counter the resistance to authority, to build power bases, to defeat rivals, and to obtain organizational change. These games may coexist with legitimate systems of authority, they may be antagonistic to them, or they may substitute for them. When the system of politics dominates in the organization, it weakens other, more legitimate systems of influence and can subject the organization to divisive conflict and damage. Most often however, these political games are used along with legitimate authority. One of the earliest games to be identified was "the budgeting game," because it is often more openly played and by more people in the organization (Mintzberg, 1983; Vigoda, 2003; Wildavsky, 1968). At the time the annual budget is developed, key actors, usually managers, present their budgets, make their cases, and bargain with others in an effort to get what they want to achieve their goals. Strategies, such as requesting more than is needed in anticipation of the request being cut, selecting evidence, and rational arguments are standard moves.

POWER AND POLITICS IN HEALTH CARE ORGANIZATIONS

There are several features of health care organizations that make them different from other ones, such as business firms. The largest health care organizations are hospitals, and therefore, we know more about them because they have been studied the most. Nevertheless,

Strategies of Persuasion: The Efforts of Nurse Practitioners in Institutionalizing a New Role (2008)

In 1995, new legislation in Alberta enabled the introduction of a wider scope of practice for nurses with additional training in medically underserviced areas. These nurses began to work on a trial basis in more areas, including hospitals, long-term care setting, and primary health care clinics. In 2003 legislation was introduced to protect the title of "nurse practitioner" for all of these nurses. Reay and Golden-Biddle noted that most studies of change in organizations focused on the role of the institution, but they were interested in how individuals influenced change at the front line and brought about institutionalization of a new practice or way of working. They engaged in a five-year study of how nurse practitioners persuaded other health professionals to accept the introduction of the new role and to change their behaviour in doing so. Over a four-year period they conducted 60 interviews with nurse practitioners, both men and women, in their workplaces; and toured the workplaces, collecting documents such as meeting minutes, archival material, and meeting observations. They analyzed the data to examine the processes NPs used to convince others to change their behaviours.

The researchers identified two strategies that were used by NPs to convince others to change their behaviour in a way that allowed NPs to work effectively. On a one-on-one basis, the NPs (1) explained their role and the advantage of their role to others and (2) improved work for others by ensuring few disadvantages and many advantages through acceptance of the NP on the team. They continued to use these strategies throughout the study period in a persistent manner, even in sites where the acceptance was slow and personally frustrating. The strategies involved repeatedly explaining their role and they

did not expect others to understand without detailed descriptions and repeated explanations. The researchers found that the role became more institutionalized over time and NPs became a normal part of the health care team in many of the settings. The NPs believed that they had to prove their value to others, particularly physicians, and therefore their second strategy was used to demonstrate how they could make things work better for them, for example, by reducing their hours of work and easing the burden of others. They did this carefully, in a low-key way, without "showing off" and initially it was generally easier to convince medical colleagues other than nursing ones to accept NPs, until they began to use this second strategy with nurses as well. In some cases, this resulted in undesired results in that prolonged persuasion efforts were needed and making things easier for others led to the view of NPs as helper or handmaiden rather than an independent professional.

The researchers concluded that the political efforts of individuals at the front line can be important in bringing about institutional change, as these individuals are very knowledgeable about the context and as change agents can guide the course of change in a low-key way. They noted that in some instances, particularly where acceptance is slow or limited, institutional change may require more strategies at the organizational level to move the new practice from legitimacy to fully institutionalized.

Source: Original article: Reay, T. & Golden-Biddle, K. (2008). Strategies of persuasion: The efforts of nurse practitioners in institutionalizing a new role. In L. McKee, E. Ferlie & P. Hyde (Eds). *Organizing and reorganizing. Power and change in health care organizations.* New York: Palgrave Macmillan.

some of what has been learned about power and politics in hospitals is applicable to other, smaller organizations.

Traditionally, three groups have been described as being powerful or influential in hospital decision-making (Brooks, 1994; Lemieux-Charles & Leatt, 1992). This triad consists of the board of trustees or directors, the senior administration of the hospital (CEO and senior management team), and senior physicians (heads of departments and officials). Mintzberg (1983) categorizes hospitals as "meritocracies," a kind of organization that features reliance on expertise, complex technology, and autonomous professionals who gain power because of their skill and knowledge. In his view, power in these organizations in distributed unevenly, because members have varying levels of the knowledge and skill that are critical to the organization. In meritocracies, the CEO cannot depend on positional power alone, as the authority system is a weak one; instead, the CEO's power depends on political skill and the ability to negotiate with groups that have conflicting goals. Thus power relationships are "fluid" and influence in decision-making in hospitals may shift over time.

In the normal course of your work in an organization, you may be relatively unaware of the use of power and politics. However, there are certain conditions and events that are more apt to give rise to political behaviour and it is likely that you will engage in the exercise of power and politics at some point in your career as a member of a health care organization. According to Alexander and Morlock (2000), power and politics arise "when goals are in conflict, where power is decentralized or diffused throughout the organization, where information is ambiguous, and where cause and effect relationships between actions and outcomes are uncertain or unknown" (p. 248). Some of the situations in which you may become more aware of political activity in your own work group or organization are:

- strategic planning processes
- budgeting processes (both capital and equipment. See Chapter 13)
- capital planning processes (especially large capital projects, like new buildings)
- periods of constrained resources in health care, "downsizing"
- leadership change
- implementation of a change in work, reorganization, re-engineering
- any process involving allocation of resources, such as space and equipment

As mentioned earlier in this chapter, when there is great diversity and great interdependence in the workplace, you can anticipate more conflicting views on what should be done and how it should be done. Therefore, the exercise of power and politics, which might have been under the radar, will become more overt and public.

Nursing and Power in Health Care Organizations

No matter what kind of health care setting you work in, nursing is likely to play a substantial role in the provision of care. Nurses are central to the provision of health care services in the full range of levels mentioned in Chapter 2—primary, secondary, tertiary, and quaternary health care. In large and small organizations, nurses provide core services that are central to the mission of the institutions in which they work. Since power and politics do play a role in the decision making that affects nurses, it is not surprising that nurses are interested in the topic. That interest has focused on three levels of analysis—the micro, meso, and macro level.

Authors, both nurses and others interested in nursing, address power and politics from the perspective of the individual nurse, nursing as a group within organizations (usually hospitals), and nursing within society. Table 3.2 illustrates the levels at which one can analyze nursing politics.

Thus far in this chapter, we have discussed the personal aspects of power and power in terms of the interaction between individuals. We have also discussed positional power in relation to organization hierarchy and the way in which power flows in organizations. In this section, we continue to focus on these levels, both micro and meso, as we discuss nursing within health care organizations. Although we do not directly address the macro level, that of the power and politics of the nursing profession within society generally, it should be noted that there are no rigid boundaries between these levels and that what happens at one level affects another.

Nursing Power and Powerlessness

The issue of the power of nursing in health care has been a recurring theme in the nursing literature. Most often, especially in early studies, the focus was nursing in hospitals and the conclusion was that nurses and nursing were lacking in power in those institutions. For example, Prescott and Dennis (1985) analyzed staff nurses' perceptions of their role in policy formation in a U.S. study using data from 250 nurses in 90 hospital units in 6 cities. They found that staff nurses as a group had limited involvement, with their role somewhat

Table 3.2   A Multi-Level Framework Reflecting Nursing Politics

Level	Activity/Form
Interpersonal	Relationships with patients
	Relationships with colleagues
	Negotiation
	Power in interaction
Organizational	Dominant groups and coalitions in organizations
	Institutional policies
	Power of the institution
	Organizational hierarchy
External	National/governmental policies
	Political action to influence policy

Source: Hewison, A. The politics of nursing: A framework for analysis, in *The Journal of Advanced Nursing, 20,* 1170-1175. Reprinted by permission of John Wiley and Sons.

limited to providing suggestions to nurse administrators who developed the policies. Based on comments from the nurses, the authors concluded that there was a sense of powerlessness that stemmed from structural and attitudinal factors. In part, there was a lack of awareness of the power the nurses did have and a lack of understanding how it could be used. When asked about the power of the nursing department, about one third of staff nurses thought it had a lot of power, but another third reported that they "didn't know." The higher up the hierarchy however, the more nurses thought that the nursing department had power. Based on their study results, the authors thought that the power of individual nurses and nursing departments was undeveloped.

Some studies have identified a great deal of power among nurses and nursing groups within organizations. Salhani and Coulter (2009) conducted an ethnographic study in a Canadian psychiatric hospital and explored the politics of an multidisciplinary mental health team on a new unit. Their sources of data included intense observations of interactions and functioning, formal interviews involving 48 people from a range of professions and positions, notes from informal gatherings, and documents from the organization. Their analysis revealed conflicting views and ideological and organizational struggles initially between nursing and physician groups, but also involving administration, subgroups of nursing staff, and subgroups of professionals or team members from other disciplines. They describe how "work relations, including interprofessional collaboration, were constituted and reconstituted through the use of various forms of power" (p. 1227) and describe the political strategies and tactics used. They describe the nurses as using coercive power (with dissenting nurses), collaborative power (with allies), and other strategies to wage a "complex and at times subtle campaign with a clear foreknowledge that there would be political winners and losers" (p. 1227). The nurses in this study were able to establish psychosocial treatment on the unit, despite the preference of psychiatrists and administrators to treat the particular mental illnesses of those on the unit only through pharmacological approaches.

Despite the centrality of nurses in many health care organizations, nurses have often viewed themselves as powerless in organizations like hospitals (a major source of employment for nurses since the 1940s) due to historical patriarchal attitudes and behaviour and oppression by physicians and administrators (Sieloff, 2004). A high profile and devastating situation at the Winnipeg Health Sciences Centre in 1994 illustrated how nurses concerns are not taken seriously and their expertise and authority within hospitals can have tragic results. The case of deaths of children undergoing cardiac surgery and the concerns and attempts of nurses to draw attention to the situation and investigate resulted in a provincial inquiry into the deaths of 12 children that has been detailed in numerous reports and analyses (Ceci, 2004; Sinclair, 2000). Nurses are not alone in experiencing powerlessness and Kanter (1997) argues that where patterns of powerlessness emerge in organizations, there is a need to examine the positions and correct the problems. She identifies signs and symptoms of powerlessness in different organizational positions and these are presented in Table 3.3.

While significant improvements have occurred in the profession's power in and out of organizations, many nurses believe that **oppressed group behaviour** persists (Sieloff, 2004). Oppressed group behaviour stems from "the ability of dominant groups to identify

Table 3.3 Common Symptoms of Powerlessness for Three Key Organizational Positions

Position	Symptoms	Sources
First-line supervisors	Close, rules-minded supervision	Routine, rules-minded jobs with little control over lines of supply
	Tendency to do things oneself, blocking of subordinates' development and information	Limited lines of information
	Resistant, underproducing subordinates	Limited advancement or involvement prospects for oneself/subordinates
Staff professionals	Turf protection, information control	Routine tasks seen as peripheral to "real tasks" of line organization
	Retreat into professionalism	Blocked careers
	Conservative resistance to change	Easy replacement by outside experts
Top executives	Focus on internal cutting, short-term results, "punishing"	Uncontrollable lines of supply because of environmental changes
	Dictatorial top-down communications	Limited or blocked lines of information about lower levels of organization
	Retreat to comfort of like-minded lieutenants	Diminished lines of support because of challenges to legitimacy (e.g., from the public or special interest groups)

Source: Kanter, R.M. *Frontiers of Management.* Copyright ©1997, Harvard Business Publishing. Reprinted with permission.

their norms and values and the 'right ones' in ... society and from their initial power to enforce them" (Roberts, 1983, p. 22). Roberts believes that nurses often exhibit characteristic behaviours of an oppressed group in that they have internalized the values of physicians and seek to attain the professional status of that group, think of themselves as second-class citizens, and even exhibit self-hatred and dislike of their colleagues. Two behaviours that have frequently been described in nursing since the initial article by Roberts are those of "silencing the self" and "horizontal violence" (Roberts, Demarco, & Griffin, 2009). Horizontal violence is discussed further in Chapter 7 as it is a significant issue in health care organizations today.

Perron, Fluet, & Holmes (2005) challenge the notion that nurses are powerless in their analysis of the concept of bio-power as it applies to nursing practice. Using Foucault's perspective on power, bio-power, and bio-politics, they identify how nurses been considered agents of the state historically, and that places nurses in a position of authority with

Interview with Dr. Judith Shamian

Dr. Judith Shamian was elected President of the International Council of Nurses, a prestigious international leadership position, in May 2013. She is the President Emeritus and past President and CEO of the Victorian Order of Nurses, a professor at the Lawrence S. Bloomberg, Faculty of Nursing at the University of Toronto, and a co-investigator with the Nursing Health Services Research Unit. She is a past President of the Canadian Nurses Association and was the Executive Director of Health Canada's Office of Nursing Policy for five years. Prior to that position, she was Vice President of Nursing at Mount Sinai Hospital in Toronto. She is the recipient of three honorary degrees as well as numerous national and international awards for her contributions to nursing and health care.

Q: You have worked in different kinds of health care organizations. From your perspective, are there differences in the way power and politics operate in different kinds of organizations?

A. Yes, there are differences—I will comment on hospitals (both teaching and non-teaching ones) as they compare to community organizations (even large ones). There is a basic and profound difference between community organizations and hospitals. Although there is a medical aspect to home care and community care, physicians are not part of the power structure of community organizations in the way that they are in hospitals. That has an enormous impact on the power structure and the power play within these different kinds of organizations.

Q: Many nurses may be uncomfortable with the idea that power and politics influence health services decisions. What do you think a nurse needs to know about power and politics in their workplace?

A. The number one thing that they need to know is the way their work is structured, and what they can or cannot do is a direct outcome of power and politics. So, they had better get interested in power and politics in a hurry! If their scope of work is that they can do discharge planning, they can do IVs, they can do medication management, *or they cannot*, it's purely politics and power at play in the workplace. And when you look at different organizations having different practices, it's because of who plays politics and who has power. There is no question that nurses need to know how power and politics work. If in their clinical practice they say, "this is a good hospital" or "this is a good unit" and if you ask the question "why?," it goes back to the power play and or political play of either the system, or the specific manager, or an individual.

Q: What advice would have for a new nurse in an organization who wants to influence a policy or raise an issue within their workplace?

A. My advice is fairly simple. Number one, watch your environment and understand it. So, if this is your unit and there are 20 nurses, 20 other professionals, and there's a manager, get a sense of how that little microsystem works. Who seems to have the influence, who gets listened to?—and it's not only the formal, but the informal power also. And once you understand that, be purposeful and be strategic. So if I looked at that unit and I decided that the physiotherapist and the social worker and the nurse instructor seemed to be able to work together and advance an issue, I would start informal conversations to see what they think about this issue that bothers me. The point I am making is: 1) understand the environment and, 2) changes do not happen overnight. The fact that you walk into the office of the manager and say "you must change this" and you walk out—that's not how it works. It takes time, and it takes setting priorities, getting involved. If there is a committee on your unit, get involved. But even if you don't want to get involved, be purposeful and strategic about getting an issue addressed.

Q: What are some of the ways in which nurse leaders use power and engage in political activity within health care organizations? Can you give some examples?

A. Again, be purposeful and be strategic. Nurse leaders at any level have a position responsibility and accountability to do more than just manage efficiently. It is essential for them to also say "how can we make this place better and how can we achieve the goals for patient care and practice?" How do you go about it—if you are looking at skill mix, or at models of care, or at evidence-based practice. First of all you determine, through engaging others, what some of the issues are. If they are system issues and let's say you are going to go into a new nursing model of care, then it's a role you play within the nursing leadership community of that organization. Simultaneously, you prepare the ground with others outside of nursing. It's insufficient for the nurse leader to prepare all the work and assume that it's going to happen on a dime. So some of the very same principles which are relevant to the staff nurse are relevant in the senior levels and that notion of saying OK who else should be involved? Then of course, evidence becomes very important. As mostly women and as nurses we have still not been as effective and influential as we should be, so evidence is a very powerful tool to frame the desired change. And then the question is, who do you need in your camp? And it doesn't mean that you need to sell it to everybody else, because you might find that some of the other professions will not support it for self-serving reasons. If you think it needs to be sold to the CEO or to some others, then you need to be strategic about it. Each institution will be different—where does power lie and who are our allies?

I can give the example from Mount Sinai Hospital in Toronto. When I became the Vice President, there were two offices—a corner one away from the board room and a windowless office, but across from the board room. I chose the latter where I was more visible, connected, and had informal opportunities with board members that I wouldn't normally have because I wasn't the CEO. When it came to the issue of moving the organization to all-RN staffing, I knew that evidence and financial costs were key to the argument to push forward, so I put a lot of energy into the CEO and the Board. I missed the boat and I didn't put sufficient energy into other groups—the allied health group and so on and it backfired. I needed to back track and build some relationships, but by the time it backfired, I had established a power base for nursing and for me that the backfiring wasn't as damaging as if I had tried to do it from the get go – they wouldn't have supported it. Knowing the art and science of leadership and management in the context of the environment is absolutely a must.

citizens. Analysis using these concepts suggest that nursing is "profoundly" political to the extent that it uses power in shaping individual and collective behaviours, for example through health promotion interventions. O'Byrne and Holmes (2009) point out that nursing is "inherently political" (p. 161) and argue that nurses can and do improve health care by the thoughtful use of their power and political force.

SUMMARY

In this chapter we have provided an additional lens with which to consider your working life in an organization in your roles as both a leader and a follower. This lens is a political one, which you can use to explore how power and politics might operate in your workplace, your own use of power and politics to influence others, and how you think they can be used in an effective and responsible way to achieve your own goals and those of the organization in which you work. There are many systems of influence that flow in and around organizations that shape decisions about organizational goals and priorities, as well as about decisions that flow from these, such as the allocation of resources (equipment, facilities, people, budgets). Decisions about nursing practice, such as philosophies of care, the selection of nursing care systems, and guiding policies are also subject to influence within an organization, no matter how small or large. We believe that an understanding of power and politics can help you fully participate in your nursing role in the workplace, both as a leader and as a member of a team. We also believe that your use of power and politics in working groups and settings can be done in ways that promote the well-being of your patients/clients, your work colleagues, and yourself.

Leading Health Care Example

In 2006, the Ontario Ministry of Health and Long-Term Care (MOHLTC) awarded the first nurse practitioner-led clinic to two nurse practitioners (NPs), Marilyn Butcher and Roberta Heale from Sudbury, Ontario. This model of primary health care delivery was a new one in the province. It differed in that the community board of directors has strong NP representation, but is similar to some other models in that NPs delivered primary health care to registered clients, and physicians are contracted for consultation and services outside of the NP scope of practice. The clinic opened in 2007, a satellite site opened in 2010 and the staff of NPs, RN, two contracted physicians, and a part-time pharmacist was set to expand to include a social worker and dietician.

Heale and Butcher (2010) describe the development of this clinic as a health care innovation and in doing so, they highlight the many interacting factors that were key in their success. Among these factors, power and politics played a role and this example illustrates some of the key points made in this chapter:

- Leadership. Advanced practice nurses (APNs) such as NPs are expected to demonstrate leadership and generate change that improves health care—these are considered core competencies. Both of the nurses who proposed and developed the clinic demonstrated *expert power*—they had considerable experience as NPs, as clinical and administrative leaders, and had worked on numerous community and governmental committees across the province.

- Networking and Teamwork. Heale and Butcher note that their extensive work in the province and on committees gave them *access to an extensive network* that provided them with support. While the two of them worked as a core team, they had support from regional NPs who contributed information to be used with local and provincial government and attended public events to promote the idea of a clinic.

- Political skills. The NPs identified key leaders in the health care field and *networked with those who had the power to influence* decision-makers. Early in the project, the NPs involved the Registered Nurses Association of Ontario (RNAO), the professional association for registered nurses in the province.

(Continued)

RNAO is a voluntary organization of RNs that engages in professional activities, including lobbying government about health, health care, and nursing issues. This organization has an established relationship with the Ministry of Health and is influential with respect to health care. The other strategy involved communication with the media. NPs had *access to information* that few others in the public, media, or government had—the numbers of unemployed or underemployed NPs available in the area.

■ Control of resources is often a major source of power and in this case, the NPs had *access to talent*. Unemployed NPs were available in the Sudbury area. Approximately 30,000 citizens in this area did not have an attachment to a primary health care provider. The proposal provided a solution to a problem in Ontario's health care system—lack of primary health care services, especially in rural and more remote areas of the province (Sudbury is considered a northern location).

Heale and Butcher emphasize that their success did not occur overnight and that getting from idea to implementation took years of work. However, their success in part illustrates the importance of understanding the role of power and politics and using that knowledge to accomplish cherished goals.

Source: Heale, R. & Butcher, M. (2010). Canada's first nurse practitioner-led clinic: A case study in healthcare innovation. *Nursing Leadership* 23(3), 21-29.

Glossary of Terms

Chain of command refers to the formal system of authority in which one position links to increasingly higher positions within an organizational hierarchy. In traditional organizational structure, one must "follow the chain of command" in sending directives down the hierarchy or requests up the hierarchy and not break this orderly sequence of communication and authority.

Empowerment refers to workplace factors that give employees a sense of power and more influence in the organization, including the ability to act and to make decisions in their positions. This requires support (supplies, resources, education, and information) as well as delegation to the employee.

Formal authority system refers to rights and responsibilities of a formal position within an organizational hierarchy. These provide individuals or organizational units with a sphere of influence in which to operate.

Internal coalition refers to the groups of full-time employees of an organization, each group with its own particular interests and influence. These groups (top management, operators, line managers, analysts, and support staff) bargain and establish relatively stable systems of power in an organization.

Oppressed group behaviours refer to characteristics of groups that have been oppressed by dominant groups. Oppressed groups internalize the dominant norms and values and experience, identify with the oppressors and experience low self-worth and regard, which results in characteristic behaviours, including horizontal violence.

Political games refers to a pattern of behaviours engaged in by political actors who attempt to achieve their own ends, rather than the overall good of the whole. The game is defined in terms of a set of rules that may or may not be explicit, but that involve positions and moves by the players. For example, the "budgeting game" typically involves requesting more funds than really needed in anticipation that the request will be reduced somewhat.

Political strategies refers to the ways in which people develop and use power to their advantage in relation to those of others with whom they interact, to influence a decision and/or achieve goals. For example, one locates hard-to-obtain information and uses it at a critical time in a decision-making process to cast one's proposed solution as the most effective one.

Politics activity by participants attempting to influence decisions or actions.

Power the ability or capacity to influence others and to bring about outcomes.

Systems of influence the means or channels through which power is exercised; instruments used by influencers to produce outcomes.

CASE

You work as a Registered Nurse in a 100-bed privately operated nursing home, Bayside Manor, that is led by an Administrator, supported by a Director of Care, who is a nurse, and a Director of Finance, who has an accounting background. The home also has a Medical Director, who has a part-time position with the nursing home to advise on medical policy, although she also has a private medical practice. The staff at Bayside Manor consists of Registered Nurses, Licenced Practical Nurses, Health Care Aides, a Physiotherapist, an Occupational Therapist, a Dietician; as well as administrative, dietary, and maintenance and housekeeping staff. The Director of Care is retiring and you have been asked by the Administrator to join a committee involved in the recruitment and hiring of a new Director of Care. The Administrator, who is chair of the committee, has also asked the Medical Director and the Director of Finance to be on the committee. The mandate of the committee is to advise the Administrator on the requirements for the position and the advertisement for the position, to set a short-list of applicants to be interviewed, to interview candidates for the position, and to recommend which of the candidates should be hired. At the first meeting, discussion centres on the requirements for the position. The Medical Director believes that at least 10 years of nursing experience should be required, the Director of Finance states that a bachelor's degree in nursing and two years of experience in a hospital should be required, the Administrator would like both a bachelor's degree in nursing and 10 years of nursing experience, at least 2 years of which were in a leadership position. You would like to recommend that the new person have a master's degree with a specialization in gerontological nursing.

Questions

1. What would you identify as bases and sources of power for each of the committee participants, including yourself?
2. What factors about this committee might lead you to anticipate differences of opinion?

3. How might you influence committee members to consider and adopt your recommendation about the requirements for the position?

4. Can you anticipate other decisions that the committee will have to make as you proceed with your mandate? How might you prepare for each of them? What strategies and tactics might you use?

5. The committee did not decide to limit applications to those candidates with a master's degree. Your committee selects three candidates to interview, based on the applications received. The Medical Director seeks you out to discuss the candidates prior to the interviews and says that she favours the one who has a master's. She notes that your idea of this requirement was really a good one. How would you respond? Discuss this behaviour and your response in terms of power and politics.

Critical Thinking Questions and Activities

1. Identify a situation in which you exercised influence with a colleague or patient. Did you consider yourself to be using your nursing power? What approaches, strategies, or tactics did you use? Were you comfortable in the situation? If not, reflect on why you were uncomfortable.

2. Analyze a situation that you encountered in your workplace in which you thought power and politics were used by others. Who was involved? Identify the interests and goals of each actor in the situation.

3. Have you observed nurses who you consider to be powerful? If so, what behaviours did you observe that you consider indicative of power? What do you think are his or her sources of power?

4. Have you ever encountered a patient care situation involving health teaching in which you thought the person was resistant to the ideas you were presenting or recommending? Analyze the situation in terms of power and politics and think about how you would respond to the resistance.

Self-Quiz

1. Which of the following types of power is based on personal appeal?
   a. Referent
   b. Reward
   c. Legitimate
   d. Expert

2. Power struggles are apt to arise under which of the following conditions?
   a. Small organizations
   b. Diverse members
   c. Strong system of authority
   d. Strong system of ideology

3. Which of the following systems of influence is likely to operate in a health care organization due to the nature of these organizations?

   a. Ideology
   b. Politics
   c. Authority
   d. Expertise

4. As a member of a committee in a public health agency, you are preparing to vote at the next meeting on priorities for equipment for the next year's budget. The department responsible for immunization clinics circulates a memo to members of the committee that argues for equipment that they have requested, providing a summary of research studies that support the effectiveness of this equipment compared to what is currently used. The department's approach is an example of which kind of political strategy?

   a. Push
   b. Pull
   c. Persuasion
   d. Preventative

Useful Websites

Canadian Healthcare
Association
www.cha.ca/

Canadian Health Leadership
Network
www.chlnet.ca/front_page

Canadian Nurses Association
www.cna-aiic.ca

The Academy of Canadian
Executive Nurses
www.acen.ca

Canadian Health Services Research
Foundation
www.chsrf.ca/Home.aspx

Registered Nurses Association of Ontario
www.rnao.org/Storage/16/1067_BPG_Sustain_
Leadership.pdf

Canadian Association of Schools of
Nursing
www.casn.org

Harvard Business Review
www.hbr.org

References

Alexander, J.A. & Morlock, L.L. (2000). Power and politics in health services organizations. In S.M. Shortell & A.D. Kaluzny. *Health care management. Organization design and behavior*. 4th ed. (244–269). Albany, New York: Delmar.

Brooks, K.A. (1994). The hospital CEO: meeting the conflicting demands of the board and physicians. *Hospital & Health Services Administration, 39*, 471–485.

Buchanan, D., & Badham, R. (1999). *Power, politics, and organizational change. Winning the turf game*. London: Sage.

Butcher, D., & Clarke, M. (2002). Organizational politics: The cornerstone for organizational democracy. *Organizational Dynamics, 31*(1), 35–46.

Cartwright, D., & Zander, A. (1968). Power and influence in groups: Introduction. In D. Cartwright & A. Zander (eds.), *Group dynamics. Research and theory*. 3rd ed. (pp. 215–235). New York: Harper & Row.

Cavanagh, G. F., Moberg, D.J., & Velasquen, M. (1981). The ethics of organizational politics. *Academy of Management Review, 6*(3), 363–374.

Ceci, C. (2004). Nursing, knowledge and power: A case analysis. *Social Science & Medicine*, 59, 1879–1889.

Cho, J., Laschinger, H.K., & Wong, C. (2006). Workplace empowerment, work engagement and organizational commitment of new graduate nurses. *Nursing Leadership*, 19(3), 43–59.

Foucault, M. (1977). *Discipline and punish: The birth of the prison*. Harmondsworth: Penguin.

French, J.R.P., & Raven, B. (1968). The bases of social power. In D. Cartwright & A. Zander (Eds.), *Group dynamics. Research and theory*. 3rd ed. (pp. 259–269). New York: Harper& Row.

Heale, R. & Butcher, M. (2010). Canada's first nurse practitioner-led clinic: A case study in healthcare innovation. *Nursing Leadership* 23(3), 21–29.

Hewison, A. (1994). The politics of nursing: a framework for analysis. *Journal of Advanced Nursing*, 20, 1170–1175.

Kanter, R.M. (1997). *Frontiers of management*. Harvard Business Review Book.

Kanter, R.M. & Stein, B.A. (Eds.). (1979). *Life in organizations. Workplaces as people experience them*. New York: Basic Books.

Kotter, J.P. (1985). *Power and influence*. New York: The Free Press.

Lammers, J., & Galinsky, A.D. (2009). The conceptualiation of power and the nature of interdependency. The role of legitimacy and culture. In D. Tjosvold & B. Wisse (Eds.), *Power and interdependence in organizations* (pp. 67–82). Cambridge: Cambridge University Press.

Lee, R., & Lawrence, P. (1991). *Politics at work*. Cheltenham, England: Stanley Thornes.

Lemieux-Charles, L., & Leatt, P. (1992). Hospital-physician integration : case studies of community hospitals. *Health Services Management Research*, 5(2), 82–98.

Liu, Y., Liu, J. & We, L. (2010). Are you willing and able? Roles of motivation, power, and politics in career growth. *Journal of Management*, 36(6), 1423–1460.

Mintzberg, H. (1983). *Power in and around organizations*. Englewood Cliffs, N. J.: Prentice-Hall.

Molm, L.D. (2009). Power and social exchange. In D. Tjosvold & B. Wisse (Eds.), *Power and interdependence in organizations* (pp. 153–168). Cambridge: Cambridge University Press.

Morgan, G. (2006). *Images of organization*. London: Sage.

O'Byrne, P., & Holmes, D. (2009). The politics of nursing care. Correcting deviance in accordance with the social contract. *Policy, Politics, & Nursing Practice*, 10(2), 153–162.

Perron, A., Fluet, C., & Holmes, D. (2005). Agents of care and agents of the state: bio-power and nursing practice. *Journal of Advanced Nursing*, 50(5), 536–544.

Pfeffer, J. (1992). *Managing with power*. Boston: Harvard Business School Press.

Pfeffer, J. (2009). Understanding power in organizations. In D. Tjosvold & B. Wisse (Eds.), *Power and interdependence in organizations* (pp. 17–32). Cambridge: Cambridge University Press.

Polifroni, E. C. (2010). Power, right, and truth: Foucault's triangle as a model for clinical power. *Nursing Science Quarterly*, 23(1), 8–12.

Prescott, P.A., & Dennis, K.E. (1985). Power and powerlessness in hospital nursing departments. *Journal of Professional Nursing*, 1, 348–355.

Randolph, W.A., & Kemery, E.R. (2011). Managerial use of power bases in a model of managerial empowerment practices and employee psychological empowerment. *Journal of Leadership & Organizational Studies*, 18(1), 95–106.

Reay, T., & Golden-Biddle, K. (2008). Strategies of persuasion: The efforts of nurse practitioners in institutionalizing a new role. In L. McKee, E. Ferlie, & P. Hyde (Eds). *Organizing and reorganizing. Power and change in health care organizations*. (pp. 167–179). New York: Palgrave Macmillan.

Roberts, S. J. (1983). Oppressed group behavior: implications for nursing, *Advances in Nursing Science*, 5(4), 21–30.

Roberts, S.J., Demarco, R., & Griffin, M. (2009). The effect of oppressed group behaviours on the culture of the nursing workplace: a review of the evidence and interventions for change. *Journal of Nursing Management, 17,* 288–293.

Salhani, D., & Coulter, I. (2009). The politics of interprofessional working and the struggle for professional autonomy in nursing. *Social Science & Medicine, 68,* 1221–1228.

Sieloff, C.L. (2004). Leadership behaviours that foster nursing group power. Journal of *Nursing Management, 12,* 246–251.

Sinclair, M. (2000). *The report of the Manitoba pediatric cardiac surgery inquest: An inquiry into twelve deaths at the Winnipeg Health Sciences Centre in 1994.* Provincial Court of Manitoba, Winnipeg. Retrieved from www.pediatriccardiacinquest.mb.ca

Vigoda, E. (2003). *Developments in organizational politics. How political dynamics affect employee performance in modern work sites.* Northampton: Edward Elgar.

Wildavsky, A. (1968). Budgeting as a political process. In D. L. Sills (Ed.), *The International Encyclopedia of the Social Sciences, 2,* (pp. 192–199). New York: Crowell, Collier and Macmillan.

Chapter 4
Change and Culture

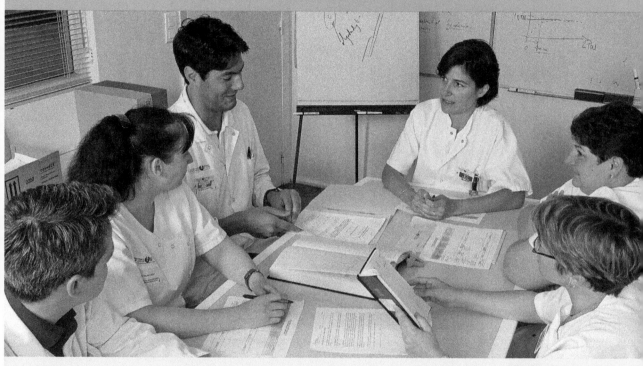

BSIP SA/Alamy

Learning Objectives

After reading, studying, and reflecting on this chapter's content, you will be able to:

1. Analyze how change theories could be used to help guide planned change in health care settings
2. Discuss how employees might respond to change and how resistance to change may be lessened
3. Define organizational culture and discuss aspects of the culture of an organization where you have worked
4. Define organizational climate and discuss aspects of the climate of an organization where you have worked
5. Discuss what is meant by the terms safety culture, culture of blame, culture of change, culture of continuous improvement, culture of empowerment, and culture of bullying
6. Identify the impact of organizational culture on employees and patients
7. Suggest strategies for changing an organization's culture

INTRODUCTION

A common expression is "the only thing that does not change is that things will always change." This expression seems particularly true for professionals working in today's health care settings. Recent changes in health care include the formation of large health care organizations from the merging of a number of smaller hospitals, long-term care centres, and/or community health centres; reduced length of stay for patients in acute care and rehabilitation hospitals; more acutely ill patients in all settings including the community; introduction of interprofessional teams and nurse practitioners; changes in the roles of registered or licensed nurses, licensed practical nurses, and nurse managers; and implementation of patient safety initiatives. In the past few decades, many innovations in how care is provided to patients were a result of budget reductions. For example, admitting patients on the same day of surgery rather than the day before, providing mental health services in the community and in emergency departments to reduce inpatient admissions, and educating persons about advanced patient directives are innovative practices driven by cost factors.

We need nurse leaders who are able to identify a vision for change and communicate this vision to nurses and other key stakeholders such as administrators and health care policy makers. However, in order for change to occur and endure, we need more than a vision and a sharing of this vision. We also need nurse leaders and nurse managers who have the skills required to implement these changes. Further, nurse leaders need to work with direct care nurses to help identify changes in the workplace that will improve work processes and patient care.

Many people resist change in the workplace. Nurse leaders need to help health care workers manage their feelings related to a change and adapt to new ways of working or providing care. While nurses in leadership positions have an important role in creating the vision for change, managing the implementation of change, and helping others to adapt to changes, all nurses have a role to play related to change in the workplace. Nurses need to be able to embrace changes that are part of the vision for improved ways of doing things, to engage in new work behaviours and to help their colleagues adapt and become committed to the change.

Organizational culture is a largely hidden aspect of an organization that influences the behaviour of its employees, including their responses to change. For a change to be successful, the organizational culture may need to be modified. Organizational climate is the perceptions employees have about aspects of their workplace, and these perceptions influence outcomes such as employees' affect, attitudes, and commitment.

In this chapter we will discuss a variety of theories and strategies for change. We will identify the role of leaders and followers in facilitating change. Then we will define the terms organizational culture and climate and discuss how organizational culture is a key factor to consider when implementing change.

THEORIES AND MODELS OF CHANGE
An Early, Landmark Theory of Change—Kurt Lewin's Theory

Many theories and models have been developed to explain how organizations change and to help managers implement change. An early theory of change that is still referred to today is Kurt Lewin's (1951) theory. Kurt Lewin (1890–1947) is often referred to as the father of social psychology. In his change theory, Lewin describes three stages of change: 1) unfreezing, 2) movement, and 3) freezing. For unfreezing to occur, individuals need to become dissatisfied with current practices and overcome their defensive response to change. The movement phase is a time of uncertainty and determining what the new way of doing things should be. Freezing occurs when the new way of doing things becomes habitual. While Lewin's theory is basic and not commonly used to guide major changes today, we have provided a brief overview of the theory because it is sometimes referred to and some later theories have built on this theory.

Now let us look at several theories or models of change that are currently in use and that we believe can help guide health professionals' efforts to effect change at the organizational or departmental level: Kotter's Eight-Stage Change Process, Diffusion of Innovations Theory, Action Research, Appreciative Inquiry, and Strategic Planning.

Kotter's Eight-Stage Change Process

Kotter's (1995; 1996) Eight-Stage Change Process is currently a leading model or guide for implementing changes in organizations. While Kotter developed his stages of change to explain how major transformations should progress in business organizations, his model is useful for planning departmental and organizational-wide changes in health care organizations.

Kotter identified eight stages of change (see Figure 4.1). He noted that, for a change to be implemented successfully, all of these stages need to be addressed, and in most cases the stages need to be worked through in the order they are listed. Kotter identified an error that is associated with each of the eight stages of change; making one of these errors can prevent a change from being implemented successfully (see Box 4.1).

The first stage of change in Kotter's change process is to establish a sense of urgency. The status quo can be very comfortable, so a leader may need to communicate that a crisis is at hand (Kotter, 1996). Kotter states that too much "happy talk" from senior managers makes employees believe they and the organization are successful, which serves

---

Box 4.1

Eight Mistakes Associated with Kotter's Eight-Stage Change Process

1. Allowing too much complacency
2. Failing to create a sufficiently powerful guiding coalition
3. Underestimating the power of vision
4. Undercommunicating the vision by a factor of 10 (or 100 or even 1,000)
5. Permitting obstacles to block the new vision
6. Failing to create short-term wins
7. Declaring victory too soon
8. Neglecting to anchor changes firmly in the corporate culture

Source: Kotter, J., Leading change: Why transformation efforts fail. *Harvard Business Review*, 61 (March-April): 57-67. Reprinted with permission of Harvard Business Publishing.

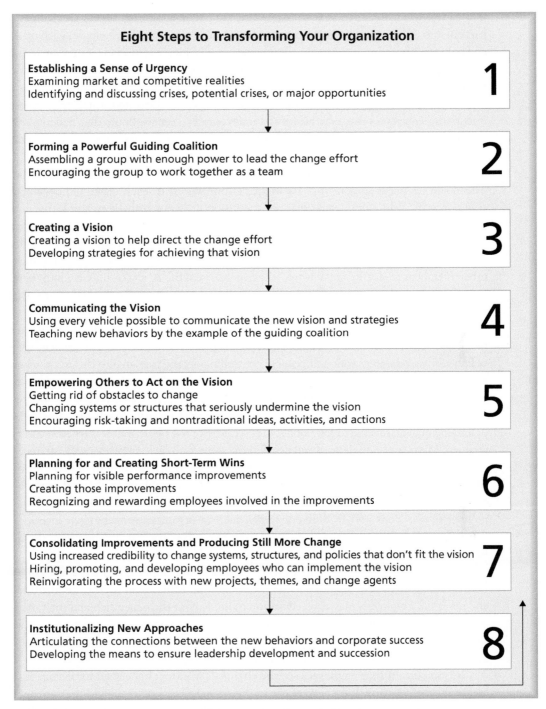

Eight Steps to Transforming Your Organization

Establishing a Sense of Urgency
Examining market and competitive realities
Identifying and discussing crises, potential crises, or major opportunities

1

Forming a Powerful Guiding Coalition
Assembling a group with enough power to lead the change effort
Encouraging the group to work together as a team

2

Creating a Vision
Creating a vision to help direct the change effort
Developing strategies for achieving that vision

3

Communicating the Vision
Using every vehicle possible to communicate the new vision and strategies
Teaching new behaviors by the example of the guiding coalition

4

Empowering Others to Act on the Vision
Getting rid of obstacles to change
Changing systems or structures that seriously undermine the vision
Encouraging risk-taking and nontraditional ideas, activities, and actions

5

Planning for and Creating Short-Term Wins
Planning for visible performance improvements
Creating those improvements
Recognizing and rewarding employees involved in the improvements

6

Consolidating Improvements and Producing Still More Change
Using increased credibility to change systems, structures, and policies that don't fit the vision
Hiring, promoting, and developing employees who can implement the vision
Reinvigorating the process with new projects, themes, and change agents

7

Institutionalizing New Approaches
Articulating the connections between the new behaviors and corporate success
Developing the means to ensure leadership development and succession

8

Figure 4.1 Eight Steps to Transforming Your Organization

Source: Kotter, J. (1995). Leading change: Why transformation efforts fail. *Harvard Business Review, 61*(March-April): 57–67. Reprinted with permission of Harvard Business Publishing.

as a barrier to change. We believe happy talk may be a significant barrier to change in particular to the nursing profession because the majority of nurses like to support each other and help the work team feel good about their accomplishments (especially if they are trying to avoid an oppressed group culture of horizontal violence and silence, as discussed later in this chapter in the section Types of Cultures and Climates in Health Care Settings). Nurses support their clients and expect their managers to support them and, therefore, a nurse leader who creates a crisis may be viewed unfavourably. Yet we know that patients and families are more apt to change when they experience a health crisis; so, similarly, we may be more apt to work differently if we experience a crisis.

The second stage of change in Kotter's change process is to create a guiding coalition. This coalition needs to consist of the right persons who trust each other and develop a common goal. While one leader may set the vision, it is not realistic to think that one person can be visible to everyone in a large organization as the change is implemented. Kotter says that the ideal coalition should avoid members who have huge egos or who are "snakes" (1996, pp. 59–60). A leader's ego cannot be so big that he or she cannot allow other members to act in areas where they have strength. A snake tells an individual something that another person has said or done that then turns the individual against this person. This type of communication creates distrust among team members.

Stage three of Kotter's change process is to developing a vision. The vision should not be spelled out in a way that it becomes **micromanagement**, which is the management style of frequently overseeing work and possibly controlling decisions related to this work, when this work is in the job description of a subordinate. Nor should the vision be presented as an authoritarian order. Rather, the vision should inform everyone exactly what the desired change is and motivate everyone in the organization to work towards this change. The leader or leadership team sets the vision but also sets **strategy** or the plan for how the vision can be attained. Managers and followers can develop the steps for how to implement the strategy.

After the vision is set, the fourth stage is to communicate the vision. The vision should be communicated in simple language, and using metaphors and giving examples can help people remember the vision (Kotter, 1996). The vision should be repeated on a number of occasions and in different forms, such as organization-wide town meetings, departmental meetings, emails, and daily interactions. Feedback about the vision should be solicited as employees may see potential issues and help refine the vision.

The fifth stage in Kotter's change process is to empower employees to act on the vision. Barriers that can prevent employees from working toward the vision need to be identified and removed. Employees may need education to implement the new vision and their managers may need to learn how to empower their followers to work towards the vision, rather than micromanaging them. When employees share a vision and are empowered to accomplish the vision, the odds of change being successfully implemented are increased.

It is important that employees see the change is working; hence the sixth stage is to create short-term wins. If employees are to continue to believe in the vision, they must be able to detect that it is working. Change is difficult, makes people feel uncomfortable, and can be just plain hard work. It helps when employees see short-term wins that illustrate the value of their efforts. Persons who have been negative towards the change, resisted the change, or neutral about the change may become convinced of the value of the change and become engaged. If the change was initiated by middle managers, senior managers will become or remain supportive of the change. Similarly, if the change was initiated by senior managers, the board of directors will remain supportive.

The seventh change in Kotter's change process is to consolidate improvements and produce more change. After change occurs, a sense of urgency to maintain the change should remain. It is fine to celebrate short-term wins but not to the extent that this makes people feel the hard work is behind them. Major changes in large organizations can require years to become entrenched and ongoing efforts are required. During this period, many other changes may be needed. If employees have been successfully empowered to develop and implement plans related to this change, senior leaders can work on a vision for another change, because in today's complex environment, organizations may need to engage in numerous changes simultaneously.

The eighth and final change in Kotter's change process is to institutionalize the changes, or to anchor them in the culture. **Organizational culture** refers to the shared assumptions, values, meanings, and beliefs that guide employees' interpretation of events and their behaviour within the organization. When changes become part of the organization's culture, the shared values and **norms** (norms are the acceptable attitudes or behaviours that are shared by a group) of members of the organization related to the change become permanent. If changes do not become part of the organization's culture, when efforts to promote the change end, the shared values and norms promote the way the organization operated before the change. When a change becomes anchored in the culture, the organizational values and norms will support this change.

Kotter notes that a common mistake made when implementing a change is to only do steps 5, 6, and 7. However changes that are made using only these three steps generally fail. Steps 1 to 4 are essential in preparing everyone for the change and step 8 is essential for making the change permanent (Kotter, 1996).

Kotter says that leadership is essential for change, and differentiates between leadership and management as follows:

> Management is a set of processes that can keep a complicated system of people and technology running smoothly. The most important aspects of management include planning, budgeting, organizing, staffing, controlling, and problem solving. Leadership is a set of processes that creates organizations in the first place or adapts them to significantly changing circumstances. Leadership defines what the future should look like, aligns people with that vision, and inspires them to make it happen despite the obstacles. (Kotter, 1996, p. 25)

Chapter 1, Leadership in Health Care, contains a discussion about the distinction between leadership and management.

For decades, our focus has been on educating managers to help make work processes in bureaucratic organizations run smoothly. It is easier to teach management skills than to prepare someone to be a leader; however, we need to prepare leaders who are capable of moving the direction of an organization (Kotter, 1996). Kotter notes that the work involved in the eight stages or changes is "70 to 90 percent leadership and only 10 to 30 percent management" (Kotter, 1996, p. 26). This is not to say that managers are not important; they are needed to manage the change. However, leaders are essential for motivating others and to lead the change.

Diffusion of Innovations Theory

Diffusion of innovations theory (Rogers 1962; 2003) is a marketing theory that was developed to explain how an innovation was adopted throughout a population. The innovation can be a new product, idea, or practice. Some people adopt the innovation early while others adopt it later. The first persons to adopt the innovation are referred to as *innovators*, then *early adopters* adopt the innovation, followed by the *early majority*, *late majority*, and *laggards* (see Box 4.2 on Categories of Adopters). Relatively few persons are innovators and they tend to be keen about trying anything new. Rogers states that early adopters tend to be **opinion leaders** or persons who are apt to change the opinions of others. Opinion leaders tend to be younger, and are persons whom others respect and observe to see if they find an innovation worthwhile. Persons in the early majority group tend to take more time to consider if they will try an innovation, while those in the late majority tend to adopt an innovation only after the majority of persons have done so. Laggards tend to be conservative and older and may never adopt an innovation.

While the adoption of an innovation starts with innovators and ends with laggards, the length of time for the majority to adopt the innovation depends on five features of the innovation (Rogers, 2003):

1. relative advantage
2. compatibility
3. complexity
4. trialability
5. observability

Relative advantage is the degree to which the innovation is seen as superior to the current product or practice. Compatibility measures whether the innovation is compatible with the other practices, beliefs, or values. Complexity is the degree to which people

---

Box 4.2

Categories of Adopters in Rogers' (1962; 2003) Diffusion of Innovations Theory

- Innovators—Innovators tend to be risk takers, young, and the first to adopt change.

- Early adopters—Early adopters adopt change after the innovators and also tend to be young. They tend to be respected by others, and therefore they motivate the early majority to adopt the change.

- Early majority—The early majority tend to be slower to adopt changes

and they are not considered opinion leaders.

- Late majority—The late majority tend to adopt a change only after the majority of other persons have adopted the change.

- Laggards—These persons tend to resist change, be older, and are conservative.

Source: Based on Rogers, E. (1962, 2003). *Diffusion of Innovations*. 5th ed. New York: Free Press.

---

can understand the innovation and are able to implement it. Trialability is the extent to which people can try the innovation. Observability is whether people can observe the innovation.

The diffusion of innovations theory has been used to explain how a change in health behaviour is adopted throughout a population following a health campaign or health promotion program (Haider & Kreps, 2004). In this case, the new health behaviour is considered the innovation. Similarly, the diffusion of innovations theory has been used to explain how change is accepted throughout an organization, and, in this case, the change is considered the innovation.

Whether the diffusions of innovations theory is used to promote the purchase of an innovative product by a population or to promote a change in a health care organization, early adopters are targeted because they are the opinion leaders who will help motivate the early majority. After the early majority have adopted the change, it becomes more pervasive and the late majority tend to follow. Ultimately in a health care setting, if senior management has endorsed a change and the majority have adopted the change, we believe a laggard could be considered a misfit for the organization. In some cases, it may be that an employee has been through a number of changes and no longer wishes to engage in another round. From our observations, it seems that when someone reaches this stage, he or she often realizes it is time to retire.

Kovach and colleagues (2008) describe how they used the five features that determine the speed of adoption of an innovation to promote an innovation in nine nursing homes in Wisconsin. The innovation that was introduced to nurses in the nursing homes was an assessment and treatment protocol for residents with advanced dementia. Strategies related to the features that have an impact on the speed of an innovation were used to promote the adoption of the new protocol, and these include but were not limited to the following examples. The relative advantage of the protocol was discussed in training about the protocol. Compatibility was enhanced by examining how the new protocol related to current policies and procedures. Complexity was managed by providing handouts and working through learning exercises. A test of the protocol with only five residents was done for trialability. A pilot implementation of the protocol allowed for observability of the intervention.

Using case study methodology, Randolph and colleagues (2012) describe the efforts of employees in a public health agency in North Carolina to create a culture supportive of continuous quality improvement (CQI). (See Chapter 11, Quality Improvement, for a more detailed discussion of continuous quality improvement.) CQI efforts had started in the agency ten years earlier. Telephone interviews were held with nine employees: two quality improvement leaders, three senior managers, and four frontline staff. Employees were asked to discuss their experiences at the agency over the past 13 years or so, or since they had started to work at the agency. Analysis of the interview data found support for a number of propositions in Rogers' diffusion of innovations theory (1962; 2003). For example, the importance of communicating the advantages of the new approach, ensuring the new approach was observable, communicating successes, making the change easy to implement, and demonstrating successful projects were all described as factors leading to the agency's successful adoption of CQI.

Action Research

Action research refers to research where members of a group study a problem that is a concern to them, with the goal of improving the quality of their lives (Calhoun, 1993; Stringer, 2007). Action research has been widely used with groups of educators in areas such as curriculum development and classroom processes (Stringer, 2007). Action research has also been used to help develop or change health and social services programs and with change and program development in organizations (Stringer, 2007).

Action research differs from other types of research in that the researcher does not control the process and participants are not just respondents. Instead, the members of the group identify an issue they would like to improve. The researcher works in an advisory capacity with the members of the group as they investigate the issue through data collection and analysis, with the goal of using what they learn to improve the issue (Stringer, 2007). While different theories or procedures have been developed for action research (for example, Argyris, Putnam & Smith, 1985; French & Bell, 1973; Kemmis & McTaggart, 1988), we will focus our description of action research on Stringer's (2007) process that he calls the "look, think, act" routine for community-based action research.

In the "look" phase of Stringer's routine for action research data or information is gathered to describe the issue community members would like to improve. Next, in the "think" phase the data or information is analyzed and interpreted to explain why the issue is the way it currently is. Following this, in the "act" phase community members develop a report and evaluate it. The process is cyclical and does not end with the "act" phase because the evaluation done during the "act" phase becomes the "look" phase of the next cycle.

Action research can be used in health care settings to develop or change practices at a departmental or organizational level. For example, a team of health professionals who feel the needs of certain patients were not being met could use the action research process to develop a plan to improve care. In another example, if the morale of employees within a health care organization was low, members of this organization could investigate sources of the low morale and work to improve it.

Appreciative Inquiry

Appreciative inquiry is an approach to organizational development or change that identifies what is working well (Cooperrider & Srivastva, 1987; Cooperrider & Whitney, 2008; Cooperrider, Whitney, & Stavros, 2003). Rather than looking at what is wrong in an organization, the developers of the appreciative inquiry model suggest that change starts with focusing on what the organization is doing right and what there is the potential to do even better. An assumption of this model is that every organization and every person within the organization has strengths and does certain things well. Change occurs by building on these strengths rather than trying to fix what is wrong. Employees are encouraged to discuss stories that describe their personal successes or the successes of others within the organization in order that everyone can try and build on these.

The appreciate inquiry model is known as the **4-D Cycle** since all of the stages start with the letter D: discover, dream, design, and destiny (see Figure 4.2). The AI process starts in the centre of the model shown in Figure 4.2 with the **affirmative topic choice**,

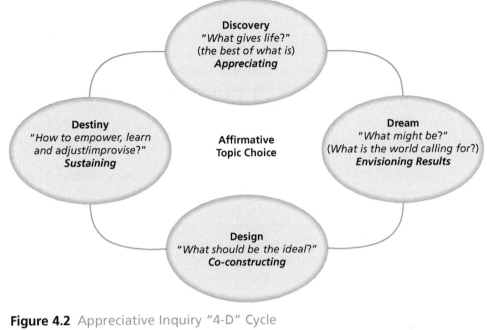

Figure 4.2 Appreciative Inquiry "4-D" Cycle
Source: Reprinted by permission of Dr. David Cooperrider.

or the topic from which a question is developed for everyone in the organization to think about and about which employees are interviewed. When major change is desired, generally three to five topics are identified to work on. In the discover stage, examples of successes related to the affirmative topic choice are shared. In the dream stage, a vision is developed for what the employees would like the organization to be like. After the dream is articulated, the design stage can begin and strategies to reach the dream are developed. While many change processes include a stage when strategy to obtain an objective is formed, the design stage in appreciative inquiry differs because the positive examples that have already occurred in the organization are used to help guide the design. Ultimately everyone's full potential is maximized in the destiny stage.

The most important decision for the success of appreciative inquiry is to determine the question for the affirmative topic choice. It is this question that everyone in the organization is asked to think about in the first or discover stage of appreciative inquiry. In this phase, employees ask this question when they interview other employees to discover positive examples or stories related to the affirmative topic choice. It is very important to frame the question that you want everyone to think about in a positive light because "... human systems grow in the direction of what they persistently ask questions about...." (Cooperrider & Whitney, 2008, p. 3). Unfortunately, health care professionals are trained to look for problems and when they do this at their workplace, they focus on deficiencies which results in an escalating negativity.

The following example discussed by Cooperrider and Whitney (2008) illustrates the importance of framing the question to be investigated in a positive light. The example concerns how appreciative inquiry can help an organization that has had numerous complaints about sexual harassment. If the question asked was how sexual harassment can be decreased (and this type of problem-solving approach is what managers have typically learned), then everyone focuses on the negative instances of sexual harassment. In contrast, with an appreciative inquiry approach, the goal of the organization was framed as the organization becoming "...a model of high quality cross-gender relationships in the workplace..." (p. 5). In the discover stage, many examples of these high quality cross-gender relationships were uncovered and shared throughout the organization. In the dream stage, employees identified ways that they could become even better. For example, they envisioned ways to improve gender equality in all aspects of organizational life, such as compensation, promotion, and representation at internal and external meetings.

When everyone in the organization commits to appreciative inquiry, the result can be a positive way for the organization's goals to be attained and for employee life to be enjoyable. It is a major paradigm shift from a focus on problems and deficits that breeds negativity and from the adversarial relationships that can develop when union members and managers bring opposing views to the table. We note that, in order to provide good nursing care, nurses develop critical thinking skills and seek out things that go wrong with patients and families. It is no wonder that they bring these skills to looking at issues in their workplace and with their colleagues, and perhaps this is one reason why there is so much negativity in many nursing work environments. Therefore, we think appreciative inquiry may be particularly beneficial in nursing environments, not only to bring about desired change but also to break a cycle of negativity. As such, it may not be embraced by persons who enjoy being negative, but then again, someone who enjoys a culture of negativity may not embrace any change.

We also note that the appreciative inquiry approach to building on strengths is similar to the approach suggested by some nursing theorists about how nurses should work with clients and families. For example, the McGill Model of Nursing developed by Moyra Allen guides nurses to work with families to identify and build on their strengths (Gottlieb & Ezer, 1997). If nurse managers and leaders hope that direct care nurses provide nursing care in a certain way, leaders need to interact with these nurses in a similar way. Therefore, we suggest that appreciative inquiry is a particularly beneficial change model to use in health care settings that promote a model of care where nurses build on clients' strengths.

Appreciative inquiry was used in two interdisciplinary outpatient cancer teams in a multi-site university health centre in Quebec (Richer, Ritchie, & Marchionni, 2009). In this initiative, the researchers conducted the appreciative inquiry process and held 11 one-hour sessions with the two teams. Health professionals were engaged in the change process and innovative ideas were generated. Both the engagement of professionals and the identification of innovative ideas are important outcomes in today's health care context.

Strategic Planning

Strategic planning is the process of planning an organization's strategy or the directions an organization will take. Typically, in large organizations such as hospitals, strategic planning is done by members of the management team, although non-management employees may be consulted and the plan shared with them. In smaller organizations, such as community health centres, all employees may participate in strategic planning. Strategic planning usually starts with participants developing a vision statement and then a strategy, which may include long-term planning for the next five years or even longer. Generally, a long-term strategic plan is reviewed each year to make refinements as aspects of the organization's internal and external context change.

Strategic planning is often reviewed annually when the organization's operating budget is prepared. The strategic plan helps guide decisions about how to allot financial resources.

For a strategic planning process to be implemented, specific actions for each aspect of the plan should be developed along with target dates and the name of the person(s) responsible for implementing the strategy. Including everyone in the organization in the development of the strategic plan and in the accountabilities can also help implement the plan. Leaders have traditionally been educated in how to develop strategic plans, with less emphasis on how to implement them (Shirey, 2011), but leaders need to become adept at implementing the plan or motivate managers and other employees to engage in the plan, if change is to occur.

Strategic planning does not necessarily mean that the developed plan outlines a plan for change or innovative work products or processes; the plan may be about engaging more (or less) in certain activities. However, we mention strategic planning as an approach to change because, while other processes may need to be used to ensure change occurs, outlining the desired change is a good first step. Strategic planning is also discussed in Chapter 5, Decision Making and Management of Workflow.

Helping Individuals Adjust to Change in the Workplace

The theories and models of change that we have introduced focus on how to structure the change process. Regardless of which model(s) you select to help guide a change process, you will also need to consider how individuals respond to change. It is rare that all employees will embrace change. Rather, many employees will resist change in varying degrees from lack of enthusiasm to attempts to sabotage the new way of doing things. Whether the change is relatively small, such as a change in the unit nurse manager, or relatively large, such as changing the mandate of a health care organization and the job responsibilities of employees, people have an emotional response to change and need time to adjust.

It is important to determine the reasons for this resistance, which may differ among employees. Determining the reasons can help you to work with employees to help them adjust to the change. Individuals may fear that they will not be able to perform as well when things change, experience a sense of loss of the old way of doing things, feel a new way of doing things means their current ways are not good and this is a reflection on them, and/or not understand why a change is needed. In their review of the literature on organizational change, Austin and Claassen (2008) identify three ways employees may respond to change. They state:

> Staff within organizations can experience change in one or more of the following three ways: (1) personal loss and feelings of inadequacy (Diamond, 1996), (2) lack of competence and self-confidence (Pearlmutter, 1998; Kayser, Walker, & Demaio, 2000), and (3) frustration related to a lack of understanding and knowledge (Tozer & ray, 1999; Zell, 2003). (p. 332)

Some potential reasons for resistance to change in the workplace are:

- Fear that they may be unable to perform as well
- Belief that they may not be able to do things now required
- Sense of loss experienced about the former way of doing things
- Perception that this means previous practices were not good
- Not understanding or knowing how to do things differently
- Not understanding the need for change

Employees may need to work through their feelings about the loss of the old way of doing things and determine how to adjust to the change or new way of doing things. This is similar to how clients work through their feelings when they adjust to new health behaviours, therapeutic regimes, or changes in their family. At a conference, a nurse leader whose name is, unfortunately, now forgotten, spoke about nurse managers who were unable to adjust to a structural change that had resulted in role changes for them. The manager told them to meet her in the front lobby the next morning. When they arrived the next day, she had a bus waiting for them and they drove off without knowing where they were headed. Their destination was a funeral parlour. She then asked everyone to write down several things they liked about the old way of doing things and then each manager was asked to stand up and say what they would miss and put their list in a box. When they were done, the box was put to rest, the idea being that it was time to stop talking about the old ways of doing things and implement the change.

The nurse leader who described this example said it greatly facilitated the change process, and we share it with you because it may be a strategy you find useful for helping people to work through their feelings about a change. Another strategy is to link some of the desirable, old ways of doing things with the new change. Austin and Claassen (2008) note, "If the change is presented as a *continuation of previous practice*, the resistance can be decreased" (p. 331). This can prevent employees from feeling bad about their former practices and also increase their confidence that they can do things differently because the new ways have something in common with the old ways.

Summary

There are many theories and models in general management and nursing management literature that suggest how we can effect change in an entire work organization or within a department of that organization. We have introduced only a few of those theories and models, specifically Kurt Lewin's three stages of change; Kotter's Eight-Stage Change Process; Diffusion of Innovations Theory; Action Research; Appreciative Inquiry; and Strategic Planning. Similarly, there are many theories and models in the nursing literature that suggest how we can promote change in individuals, families, and communities.

Whether you wish to guide a change in a health care setting or in your work with clients, there are some commonalities that we suggest you consider. First, rather than just hoping a change happens, select a theory or model of change, learn about this theory or model in detail, and use it to guide change strategies and processes. Engage everyone in the change from the beginning as they will need to buy into the change. Share a vision for the change with everyone and make the vision exciting so that employees and all stakeholders are motivated to attain it. Transformational leaders provide a type of leadership that is useful when change is needed as they share a vision and motivate others to share this vision (transformational leadership is discussed in Chapter 1). Help people see the need for change and show them data that suggests things need to change or provide them with **benchmarks** (benchmarks and benchmarking is discussed in Chapter 11). Identify key supporters of the change and provide them with what they need to help promote the change. Expect resistance to change and identify strategies to deal with resistance, but ultimately someone who tries to sabotage a change despite widespread support for this change, may not be a good fit for the organization. Communicate frequently during the change process to reduce the spread of rumours and negativity. Realize that it is important to have leaders who identify the vision for change, but managers who can help implement the change are equally needed.

Ultimately, whether the change is within an individual's health behaviour such as an increase in physical activity or within the way an organization operates, the hardest part of change is sustainability over time. Sustainability of a change requires ongoing efforts until the change becomes a normal part of an individual's behaviour or an organization's way of operating. When a change is adopted in an organization, it becomes part of the organization's culture.

In the next section, we describe organizational culture, how culture can support or hinder a change, and why culture may need to be changed for an organization to move forward with new initiatives.

ORGANIZATIONAL CULTURE AND CLIMATE
Organizational Culture

There are numerous definitions of organizational culture. For example, Cameron and Quinn (2011) say organizational culture:

> . . . encompasses the taken-for granted values, underlying assumptions, expectations, collective memories, and definitions present in an organization. It represents "how things are around here." It reflects the prevailing ideology that people carry inside their heads. It conveys a sense of identity to employees, provides unwritten and often unspoken guidelines for how to get along in the organization, and it helps stabilize the social system that they experience. (p. 19)

Schein (1987), a well known theorist in the area of organizational culture, defines culture as:

> . . . the pattern of basic assumptions which a given group has invented, discovered or developed in learning to cope with its problems of external adaptation and internal integration . . . it is the assumptions which lie behind values and which determine the behavior patterns and the visible artifacts such as architecture, office layout, dress codes, and so on. (p. 383)

Bellot (2011) suggests that there are several definitions of organizational culture because organizational culture is something that is not seen and because organizational culture has been defined by a variety of disciplines including anthropology, social psychology, sociology, and business. As well, organizational culture is an emerging area of research. However, she notes that there are four themes in the literature that describe organizational culture. First, while organizational culture is largely invisible, it does exist and as such, it does have an impact on outcomes that we will discuss later in this chapter. Second, because culture is largely invisible, it is intangible and ambiguous, leading to confusion about what it is and difficulties in measuring it. Third, organizational culture is based on the shared experiences of its members or is "socially constructed." It is a group phenomenon that helps members of the group make sense both of their workplace and their work experiences (Siehl & Martin, 1983, cited in Bellot, 2011). Fourth, each organization has a unique culture that evolves over time.

Organizational culture is something that we cannot see, and we may only become aware of the culture in our workplace when someone from another organization starts to work with us and we are surprised by aspects of this newcomer's behaviour. For example, we may be surprised by how the newcomer dresses for work or the informality or formality that he or she uses when talking with managers, colleagues, or customers. Similarly, if we accept a job in a new organization, we may be surprised when others give feedback about behaviours that were normal in our former workplace. We end up learning the culture of our new workplace during orientation but also through **socialization**, the process of learning values, norms, traditions and behaviours required to function within the culture.

Aspects of culture such as assumptions and norms are hidden and therefore employees may not be aware of these aspects of a culture. Other aspects of a culture such as artifacts are more visible. Examples of artifacts are the organization's logo, type of furniture, pictures or awards on the wall, and so on. Visible aspects of culture include how employees behave toward each other, behaviour at meetings, interactions between managers and employees, and so on. Figure 4.3 illustrates the observable and unobservable

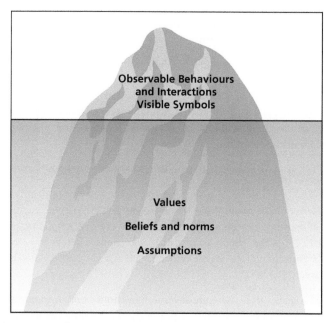

Figure 4.3 Elements of Organizational Culture

Source: Cameron and Quinn, "Nine Steps for Changing an Organization's Culture," in *Diagnosing and Changing Organizational Culture*, 3e, © 2011 by Jossey-Bass, Inc., a division of John Wiley & Sons. Reprinted by permission.

parts of an organization's culture. Organizational culture is often referred to as similar to an iceberg, with only the tip being observable (Schein, 1992).

Organizational Climate

Organizational climate refers to how employees feel in their workplace and their perceptions of different aspects of the workplace; for example, their perceptions about leadership, reward systems, conflict, or safety practices. There are a variety of definitions of organizational climate and about whether organizational climate is really different from organizational culture. Schneider defines organizational climate as different from organizational culture and says organizational climate refers to more temporary employee perceptions about organizational routines and rewards as these relate to a particular function of the organization, such as safety (Schneider, 1990). Rousseau defines organizational climate as employees' perceptions of practices within the organization (1988; 1990). She says organizational climate and culture overlap because climate emphasizes employees' perceptions of behaviours in the workplace and organizational culture includes the norms and patterns of behaviours in the workplace (1988). She notes that organizational climate or employees' perceptions of their workplace are often described as positive and negative; however different persons viewing the same aspect of the workplace, for example a particular leadership style, may see this differently (1988).

The Competing Values Framework

While a number of dimensions of and frameworks for organizational culture have been developed (for example, Deal & Kennedy, 1983; Denison, 1990; Earnst, 1985; Hofstede, 1980; Martin, 1992), we will focus our discussion on the framework that is most commonly used today for assessing organizational culture, the competing values framework (Cameron & Quinn, 2011). This framework comprises two dimensions. The first dimension is based on a continuum from "flexibility, discretion, and dynamism" to "stability, order, and control" (Cameron & Quinn, p. 38). The second dimension is based on a continuum from "an internal orientation, integration, and unity" to an "external orientation, differentiation, and rivalry" (p. 38–39). The framework reflects four types of organizational culture, based on whether the culture is high or low on each of the two dimensions. The four types of culture are known as: 1) clan (collaborative), 2) adhocracy (create), 3) hierarchy (control), and 4) market (compete). Figure 4.4 illustrates the two dimensions and the four types of culture in the competing values framework.

The hierarchy (control) culture is one with stability and control and an internal focus and integration. These organizations are bureaucratic, with a hierarchy, rules, and specialization of roles or functions (Cameron & Quinn, 2011). Much of the work in organizations with this type of culture is dictated by policies and routines, with the work of managers being to ensure policies are followed and work is accomplished smoothly because control and efficiency are important in these organizations.

Most large hospitals and health care organizations function in a hierarchy (control) culture. Further, nursing culture within the larger culture of health organizations has traditionally

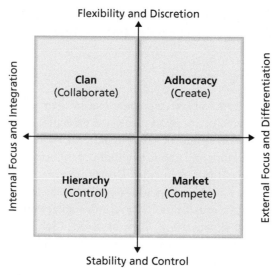

Figure 4.4 Competing Values Framework

Source: Cameron and Quinn, "Competing Values Framework," in Diagnosing and Changing Organizational Culture, 3e, © 2011 by Jossey-Bass, Inc., a division of John Wiley & Sons. Reprinted by permission.

been this type of culture, with an emphasis on nursing policies and procedures, and a hierarchy of roles (for example, staff nurse, assistant head nurse, head nurse, nursing supervisor or coordinator, director of nursing). Today, the job titles (although probably not the culture) within the hierarchy of roles have changed (for example, direct care nurse, patient care coordinator, nurse manager, director of nursing, vice-president of patient care services).

The market (compete) culture is one with stability and control and an external focus and differentiation. Like hierarchy (control) cultures, the market (compete) culture is associated with centralized control. However, the market (compete) culture is typical of organizations in which employees interact more with persons outside of the organization that with coworkers. This type of organization is focused on securing customers, on performing better than competing organizations, and on results and profitability (Cameron & Quinn, 2011).

In the Canadian health care context, we think that the type of organization associated with a market (compete) culture is uncommon. Some examples might be private clinics where elective surgery such as plastic surgery is performed, or private nursing home care services. However, now that provincial governments are comparing hospitals' outcomes, such as infection rates, wait times, and costs for procedures; then requesting hospitals attain the best outcomes or lowest costs may increase market (compete) cultures in health care.

The clan (collaborate) culture is one with flexibility and discretion and an internal focus and integration. These organizations operate as families, emphasizing relationships with other employees and customers, and teamwork, commitment, and loyalty. The participation and development of employees are important (Cameron & Quinn, 2011).

We would place organizations such as private nursing homes or small or medium health centres where many employees know each other and remain with the same organization for years as organizations that may have a clan (collaborate) culture. Further, this type of culture can exist with many health care teams within a larger organization. For example, oncology, mental health teams, and maternal-child teams often form close units within a large organization. Employees in these settings may have highly specialized skills and function largely within their specialized units.

The adhocracy (create) culture is one with flexibility and discretion and an external focus and differentiation. This type of culture is typical of organizations where innovation and adaptation are required for success. This type of organization needs to be responsive in providing innovative services to customers. Power is not centralized; instead work teams develop to meet the needs of the project employees are currently working on (Cameron & Quinn, 2011).

We think that it would be beneficial for a nursing research unit to have an adhocracy (create) culture. Nurse researchers have to be innovative in developing projects, but they also have to base their research on areas that will help practising nurses. Further, we think that services such as community health services and health promotion activities would function well within an adhocracy (create) culture. Community-based health centres that respond to the needs of the community need to be flexible in providing the services their community requires, and in changing the programs that they offer as the community's needs change.

Types of Cultures and Climates in Health Care Settings

In recent years, different types of cultures have been referred to in the health care literature, for example a safety culture (Ruchlin, Dubbs, & Callahan, 2004), a culture of blame (Scott-Cawiezell et al., 2006), a just culture (Marx, 2001), a culture of accountability (O'Hagan & Persaud, 2009), and a culture of bullying (Hughes & Clancy, 2009). O'Hagan and Persaud describe a culture of accountability as one that has:

> . . . a set of common elements wherein the common belief is continuous learning and improvement at the individual, unit or department, and organizational levels; wherein decisions regarding care and direction are guided by evidence-based protocols and clinical practice guidelines (CPGs) but not by individual preference; wherein performance measurement is an essential element in assessing outcomes and guiding improvement initiatives; wherein reporting errors is encouraged and not punished; and wherein there is collaboration and coordination among and between all levels of the organization and across all specialties. (p. 125)

These cultures are described as promoting outcomes that are either beneficial or harmful for organizations and employees.

A culture of bullying is one where horizontal and/or vertical violence is endemic. Chapter 10, Team Building and Managing Conflict, has a more detailed discussion of horizontal and vertical violence. Roberts, Demarco, and Griffin (2009) reviewed the nursing literature on oppressed group behaviour and discuss two concepts associated with it: horizontal violence and silencing. As a group, nurses do not feel particularly empowered in hospital settings because physicians control decision making (Roberts, 1983; 2000 cited in Roberts et al., 2009). Like other oppressed groups, the anger they experience because of the control held by a powerful group is turned inward, toward other members of their group resulting in horizontal violence (Fanon, 1963, cited in Roberts et al., 2009). Nurses who feel powerless may be silent when they disagree with persons who hold power. Nurses' silence about their accomplishments decreases their visibility, thereby preventing their group from gaining power (Buresh & Gordon, 2006). Given the importance of speaking out about potential risks and patient safety issues, nurses, health care administrators, and the public alike should be concerned about this feature of a nursing culture. Learning about oppressed group behaviours and how this can lead to a culture of horizontal violence and silence may be a first step in nurse leaders and nurse followers taking responsibility for changing this culture. We need to support each other rather than look for deficiencies in our colleagues and this support for our colleagues means we should not try and silence them when they speak out, even when we don't agree with what they say.

Different types of cultures have an associated climate. For example, a safety climate refers to employees' feelings and perceptions about how safety issues are managed in their workplace.

Subcultures

A **subculture** is the shared assumptions, values, meanings, and beliefs that guide the interpretation of events and behaviour of a smaller group of employees within the organization. Members of a subculture identify with other members and behave according to their shared beliefs (Hatch & Cunliffe, 2006). Examples of subcultures within a health care organization may be the subculture of an intensive care unit or the subculture of members of the nursing profession.

Members of this smaller group also share the assumptions, values, meanings, and beliefs held within the entire organization, the exception being a **counterculture**. When counterculture is used to describe a subculture within an organization, it describes a group in which members share values, meanings, and beliefs that are opposite of those of the larger culture (Hatch & Cunliffe, 2006; Siehl & Martin, 1983). An example of a counterculture in health care might occur when a particular professional group holds values that they believe are contrary to those of the organization, for example, if physicians believe they should be in charge of all decision making including length of patient stay. Another example is union groups, particularly in organizations where unions and managers have not decided to work together and so the union acts as the official opposition to the ruling party (managers).

While subcultures may flourish in a democratic society, employees working in organizations have contracts that stipulate required work and behaviour. Canadians value democratic principles, and many Canadian health care settings encourage employee participation in decision making. Nevertheless, regional health authorities and boards of directors for health care settings hold senior executives accountable for decision making. Therefore health settings do not operate as democracies, and senior executives may sometimes make decisions that the majority of employees disagree with. Further, organizations that have a strong culture may have minimal acceptance of a counterculture that goes against strongly held aspects of the organization's culture.

Importance of Organizational Culture

Organizational culture is important to us because researchers have found it has an impact on employee productivity, commitment, and morale (Kozlowski, Chao, Smith, & Hedlund, 1993). Organizational cultures where employees are treated fairly and respectfully have been associated with higher employee productivity and helpful behaviours, and lower rates of absence from work (Colquitt, Noe, & Jackson, 2002; Naumann & Bennett, 2000).

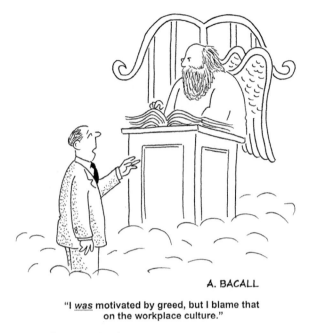

A. BACALL

"I _was_ motivated by greed, but I blame that
on the workplace culture."

A. Bacall/CartoonStock.com

Alvesson (2002) discusses four views about how an organization's culture may have an impact on the performance of an organization. First, a strong culture, or one where members of the organization identify strongly with the shared assumptions, values, and beliefs, may increase employee commitment to the organization and their motivation to perform well. Second, it may be that instead of a strong culture leading to higher performance, the observed rewards of seeing high performance lead to a strong culture, where members see the organization as successful. Third, different types of cultures may be more or less successful at different times or in different contexts. For example, an innovative culture may be beneficial when innovation is needed for success, but a bureaucratic culture may be needed at other times for high performance. Fourth, adaptive cultures or cultures that can respond rapidly to changing conditions are more apt to be associated with high performance.

There is some support in the nursing literature for organizational culture to have an effect on the quality of nurses' work life and their nursing care. In a cross-sectional study of Korean hospital nurses, organizational culture was significantly correlated with the quality of nurses' work life and organizational effectiveness, with organizational effectiveness measured by five items, of which two measured job satisfaction, and the other three measured organizational involvement (An, Yom, & Ruggiero, 2011). A study in four private and four public hospitals in Istanbul included 1,289 physicians and 1,778 nurses who completed questionnaire measures of organizational culture and attitude toward change. Findings included the conclusion that the private hospitals were associated with a cooperation culture or a culture where teamwork and team management are valued, and the public hospitals with a power culture, or a culture where power and authority are centralized. Moreover, employees who worked in the hospitals with a power culture had lower scores on the attitudes toward change measure than those who worked in a cooperative culture, suggesting that culture can impact employees' willingness to participate in change (Seren & Baykal, 2007). A cross-sectional study of 200 hospital nurses in Taiwan found that organizational culture correlated with leadership behaviour and job satisfaction (Tsai, 2011).

Shirey (2009) examined how organizational culture was related to authentic leadership and healthy work environments in a qualitative, descriptive study. Authentic leaders have a number of characteristics including being genuine and trustworthy. (In Chapter 1, Leadership in Health Care, you can find a description definition of authentic leaders.) Shirey interviewed 21 nurse managers employed by three hospitals in the United States. The nurse managers were asked to talk about stressful situations they experienced at work, how they coped with these situations, their health outcomes, and the decision processes they used in these stressful situations. One of the probes used was, "Tell me about the organizational culture at your facility" (p. 191). From the responses to this probe, Shirey decided if the nurse manager worked in a positive (n = 12) or negative (n = 9) culture based on whether the manager's responses suggested the hospital met specific standards of healthy work environments. She found managers who worked in negative cultures said they were less free to talk about their ideas, felt less support from their leaders, and found the punitive environment of their workplace drained their energy. Managers who worked in positive cultures were more apt to use an authentic leadership style. The findings of this study suggest the hospital's culture has important outcomes for how nurse managers feel and act, which ultimately has an impact on the experience of the employees they manage.

CHANGING THE ORGANIZATION'S CULTURE

Making any change in an organization can be difficult, but changing the organization's culture is particularly challenging. Culture is pervasive and largely hidden from employees and managers, and it is hard for anyone to change something they are unaware of. Further, one aspect of culture is values. Individuals keep their values over time and do not change them readily. Although it is difficult to change an organization's culture, when this culture no longer helps the organization to be effective, the leader or leadership team needs to focus on what the desired culture should be and how to move toward this culture.

Several approaches to culture change are suggested in the literature (for example, Khademian, 2002) but Cameron and Quinn (2011) described a nine-step process that is based on their Competing Values Framework. In the first step, a group of key employees in the organization, including those responsible for implementing the change, is formed. In subsequent steps the group collect input and reach agreement of the current organizational culture, come to an agreement on a preferred future for the organizational culture, identify discrepancies between the actual and the ideal culture, and figure out what they would like to keep and what they would like to change to shift the culture. The group develops a strategic action plan and helps employees in the whole organization ready themselves for change. Beginning with aspects of cultural change are easy, small changes are celebrated. Leaders develop their skills in leading change. The group measures its progress in achieving cultural change by identifying measures and milestones of change. Ways to communicate change are identified and such items as new logos, slogans, and stories are used to help employees become aware of how things have changed. An example of Cameron and Quinn's nine steps for changing an organization's culture is given in Box 4.3.

Box 4.3

Application of Cameron and Quinn's Nine Steps for Changing an Organization's Culture to Create a Culture of Safety in a Health Care Organization

The Chief Executive Officer of a non-teaching hospital located five hundred kilometres from a major Canadian city wanted to improve patient safety. She put together a team of 10 persons consisting of the Vice President for Patient Care Services, three managers, two union representatives, and four health care professionals and told them she would like the organization to have a strong culture of safety. She gave this group the mandate to identify what aspect(s) of the organization's culture needed to change to create a culture of safety. She also recommended that the group work through Cameron and Quinn's nine steps for changing an organization's culture.

The group reviewed Cameron and Quinn's nine steps, and decided to start by completing the OCAI questionnaire. By summarizing everyone's questionnaire responses, they were able to discuss aspects of their organization's actual culture (Step 1). They then went on and discuss what their ideal culture of safety would look like (Step 2). They plotted the questionnaire responses on Cameron and Quinn's Competing Values Framework (see Figure 4.4). While they noted a number of aspects of their culture that could shift to facilitate a culture of safety, we will limit our discussion to the finding that their organization's culture was one of order and control. They discussed how care was often routinized rather than considering individual patients' and families' needs. They also discussed how health professionals sometimes acted as if other professionals were the customers more than the patients. For example, nurses and physicians took care to exchange information with other nurses and physicians but did not always exchange information with patients and family members. They knew that for patient safety, it was important to communicate well with patients and designated family members who should be key team members.

Group members decided that including the patient/family as team members was an important part of a culture of safety (Step 3). This represented a major change in how they practised, so they decided to pilot the change on the cardiology unit. The cardiology staff shared examples of how including the patient as a team member led to preventing a particular error (Step 4).

The group discussed their suggestions for the need to have a more flexible culture with the CEO, and the CEO incorporated this message into speeches she made to employees, and shared stories of improved patient safety in the cardiology department (Step 4). The group met with the strategic planning committee, which began to revise the organization's mission statement, values, and strategic plan to include both the organization's commitment to patient safety and to having the patient/family as team members (Step 5).

The cardiology unit regularly surveyed patients after discharge about their satisfaction with care, and found a major improvement after the initiative to make the patient/family key members of the team. They also looked at their medication error rate, and found it had decreased.

(Continued)

Box 4.3 *(Cont.)*

The group shared the improvements in the cardiology unit with all employees (Step 6). The CEO and group members met with the cardiology staff and listened to them discuss some difficulties they had with this change, and the CEO asked how she could support them (Step 7).

The group then identified what other aspects of the culture should be shifted to facilitate a culture of safety, and assigned person(s) to be accountable for implementing different activities, including initiating the change of having the patient/family as a team member on other units (Step 8). They also developed a communication strategy that included sharing success stories related to the strengthening of the culture of safety (Step 9).

Source: Cameron and Quinn, "Nine Steps for Changing an Organization's Culture," in *Diagnosing and Changing Organizational Culture*, 3e, © 2011 by Jossey-Bass, Inc., a division of John Wiley & Sons. Reprinted by permission.

RELATED RESEARCH

Summary of a Study of the Culture of Four Home Care Organizations and Its Impact on the Adaptation of Continuous Quality Improvement

Firbank (2010) explored the culture of four home care organizations in Quebec, Canada, to investigate if their cultures influenced how readily each setting was able to adopt continuous quality improvement (CQI). (See Chapter 11, Quality Improvement, for a more detailed discussion of continuous quality improvement.) The four home-care organizations were 1) a local community services centre that was publically funded to provide primary health care and social support services, known in Quebec as a CLSC; 2) a non-profit social economy enterprise that provided home cleaning and meals, known in Quebec as an EESAD; 3) a private agency that was a for-profit, family business that provided mainly personal care and respite services but also some nursing and rehabilitation services; and 4) a non-profit community organization staffed primarily by volunteers, that provided home support programs such as meals-on-wheels, special transportation, and telephone security check calls but also had a small residential care unit.

In this study, a qualitative, multiple case-study approach was used to describe the culture of the four home care settings and to describe how readily CQI was adopted in each setting. Data were collected from a number of sources:

1. Written documentation from each setting about their mandate, policies, previous involvement in quality improvement, and so on;

2. A member of the research team was a participant observer at all CQI meetings, approximately 300 hours at each site over 9 months on average;

3. Minutes from all CQI meetings;

4. Assessments completed by CQI team meetings at three times over 9 months; and

SUMMARY

Some cultures may make change within the organization more difficult or may be more or less beneficial for the success of the organization. Therefore, senior managers may sometimes wish to change the organization's culture. Culture is not easy to change as it is created over time. One way to change the culture is create new history and values, as a leader can do when he or she shares a story that is in line with the desired culture, or informs employees what his or her values are. Of course, if the leader does not behave in ways that match the desired culture or behaves in ways that are contrary to the values, this can lead to lower morale. For example, when a leader says innovation is required but then does not support another leader who attempts an innovation, or when a leader says he or she values transparency but then hires and promotes employees in a way that is not visible and is seen as unfair, these leaders are behaving in a way that does not support a culture of change or transparency.

5. Focus groups with CQI team members following the approximately 9-month implementation of CQI.

The CQI program was implemented at each setting by members of the research team. Firbank reviewed the literature and identified nine aspects of an organization's culture that may impact the implementation of CQI:

1. collegiality and teamwork,
2. organizational commitment of personnel,
3. organizational involvement of personnel,
4. degree of professionalization,
5. formalization of work,
6. centralization of decision making,
7. reward orientation,
8. organizational progressiveness, and
9. customer focus.

He compares how each of the four health settings rate from very low to very high on each of these nine aspects of the culture.

Firbank finds support that most of the nine aspects of the culture he identified impact how readily each home care setting adopts CQI. The cultural attributes of collegiality and teamwork, personnel organizational commitment, personnel organizational involvement, degree of professionalism, and organizational progressiveness, as well as *decentralization* of decision making contributed to the CLSC and EESAD adopting CQI more readily and CQI being more firmly established there at the end of 9 months.

Based on Firbank, O. (2010). Exploring the fit between organizational culture and quality improvement in a home-care environment. *Health Care Management Review, 35*, 147–160.

All nurses have a role to play in identifying and implementing changes that will improve client care and improve nurses' work life. All nurses have a role to play in helping to create the type of culture that they want to work in. In this chapter we have introduced theories of change and discussed how culture may impact behaviour and how dysfunctional aspects of the culture may be changed over time. As nurses become more educated in theories of change and culture, they will be able to take an active role in managing health care systems and environments.

Glossary of Terms

Action research is a type of research where members of a group study a problem that is a concern to them, with the goal of improving the quality of their lives.

Affirmative topic choice In appreciative inquiry, the affirmative topic choice is the topic from which a question is developed for everyone in the organization to think about and about which employees are interviewed.

Appreciative inquiry Appreciative inquiry, also referred to as AI, is an approach to organizational development or change that identifies what is working well in the organization. The affirmative topic choice is at the core of the four stages of the appreciate inquiry model or 4-D Cycle: discover, dream, design, and destiny.

Benchmarking The process of comparing an organization's performance with other organizations. Generally, the comparison is made with an organization that is performing higher, with the goal of trying to establish what the organization is doing differently. The best performance becomes known as the benchmark.

Counterculture is a organizational subculture wherein members share values, meanings, and beliefs that are opposite of those of the larger culture.

Diffusion of innovations theory is a marketing theory that was developed by Rogers (1962; 2003) to explain how an innovation was adopted throughout a population, with *innovators* adopting the innovation first, followed by the *early adopters*, the *early majority*, the *late majority* and finally *laggards*.

4-D Cycle is the appreciate inquiry model and has four stages (discover, dream, design, and destiny). Affirmative topic choice at the core of the model.

Micromanagement refers to the management style of frequently overseeing work and possibly controlling decisions related to this work, when this work is in the job description of a subordinate.

Norms are the acceptable attitudes or behaviours that are shared by a group.

Opinion leaders In Rogers' diffusion of innovations theory (1962; 2003) opinion leaders are persons who are apt to change the opinions of others. They tend to be early adopters, younger in age, and are persons whom others respect and observe to see if they find an innovation worthwhile.

Organizational climate refers to how employees feel in the workplace and their perceptions of different aspects of the workplace.

Organizational culture is the shared assumptions, values, meanings, and beliefs that guide employees' interpretation of events and their behaviour within the organization.

Socialization is the process of learning values, norms, traditions, and behaviours required to function within the culture.

Strategic planning is the process of planning an organization's strategy or the directions an organization will take.

Strategy In an organization, the strategy is the plan for how the vision that is set by the leader or leadership team can be attained.

Subculture is the shared assumptions, values, meanings, and beliefs that guide the interpretation of events and behaviour of a smaller group of employees within an organization

CASE

The hospital recently replaced all the machines that monitored intravenous infusions. The nurses were getting increasingly frustrated by the new machines because they beeped all the time. As well, sometimes the intravenous infusion stopped running, but the machine did *not* beep. The nurses on one of the hospital's units discussed this situation with their manager, who said the machines were new and they could not be returned. The nurses on this unit decided to write a petition saying the machines were not safe, and they circulated this to nurses throughout the hospital, who all signed the petition. The local newspaper learned about this situation and published an article saying the hospital's nurses had protested unsafe equipment, and the newspaper asked the hospital's CEO to comment. The CEO said the equipment was safe and was used at other hospitals, but the nurses did not know how to use the equipment and so more in-service training would be organized. This response infuriated the nurses.

Questions

1. Do you agree with the nurses' decision to start a petition? Are there other ways they could have managed this situation?

2. How else could the nurse manager have dealt with the issue the nurses brought to her attention?

3. How else could the CEO have responded?

4. The CEO's role includes a) helping the community become involved in the health care organization's activities, b) ensuring safe care for the community, and c) creating a positive image about the health care organization among internal and external stakeholders. How may the CEO's response have been influenced by these three aspects of the role? How may the CEO's response have led to a positive and/or negative impact on these three areas?

5. What effect, if any, do you think the CEO's response had on the organization's culture? What effect, if any, do you think the nurses' actions had on the organization's culture?

6. The nurses were infuriated that the CEO suggested they did not know how to use the machine. However, more in-service training was offered and the nurses learned that these machines had different settings from their previous machines. As a result, the problems they experienced with the machines were alleviated. Does this change how you feel about how the nurses, the nurse manager, and the CEO responded in this situation?

Critical Thinking Questions and Activities

1. Think of a problematic issue that you would like to change, either in an area where you have done clinical work or where you are studying nursing. Instead of wording this as a problem, can you reframe it as an affirmative topic choice that would be used in appreciative inquiry? What question(s) would you use to interview others in the organization, to elicit positive examples of the affirmative topic choice?

2. Identify a change you would like to see in an area where you have done clinical work or where you are studying nursing. Which theory or model presented in this chapter would you find useful to help guide the change? Discuss.

3. Think of a change that was introduced in your workplace or school of nursing. How did you respond?

4. Describe the climate in an area where you have done clinical work or where you are studying nursing.

5. What aspects of the organizational culture can you identify in an area where you have done clinical work or where you are studying nursing?

6. Thinking of an area where you have done clinical work, complete one of the safety attitudes instruments and the safety climate instrument (Sexton et al., 2006) that are used to measure safety culture and climate, and are available at this web site:www.uth.tmc.edu/schools/med/imed/patient_safety/questionnaires/SAQBibliography.html. What have you learned about the safety culture and climate of the organization where you have done clinical work?

Self-Quiz

1. All of the following are true about appreciative inquiry *except*:
   a. Starts with an affirmative topic choice
   b. Focuses on a problem in the organization
   c. Focuses on strengths
   d. Includes a 4-D Cycle

2. Which of the following is true about organizational culture?
   a. It is largely invisible
   b. It refers to employee perceptions of aspects of the workplace
   c. It is consistent with the McGill Model of Nursing
   d. It is largely determined by the organization's context

3. All of the following are true about change in work settings *except*:
   a. Change is inevitable
   b. Change is met with resistance
   c. Leading change is a major role function of leaders
   d. Change is less important for health care organizations that have received accreditation

4. Which of the following is a good example of how to create a culture of quality?
   a. During orientation of new employees, the CEO discusses that the organization is planning to have zero tolerance for bullying in the workplace
   b. The organization's administration decides to commit an increase of funds for staff development

c. The organization's administration initiates discussion with administrators of similar organizations to discuss how they could share resources

d. The CEO is supportive of all countercultures within the organization

Useful Websites

ICN (International Council of Nurses) Leadership for Change Program www.icn.ch/pillarsprograms/leadership-for-change/

Safety attitudes instruments and safety climate instrument (Sexton et al., 2006)

are used to measure safety culture and climate, and are available at: www.uth.tmc.edu/schools/med/imed/patient_safety/questionnaires/SAQBibliography.html

References

Alvesson, M. (2002). *Understanding organizational culture*. Thousand Oaks, CA: Sage Publications.

An, J., Yom, Y., & Ruggiero, J. (2011). Organizational culture, quality of work life, and organizational effectiveness in Korean university hospitals. *Journal of Transcultural Nursing, 22*(1), 22–30.

Argyris, C., Putnam, R., Smith, D. (1985). *Action science: Concepts, methods and skills for research and intervention*. San Francisco, CA: Jossey-Bass.

Austin, M., & Claassen, J. (2008). Impact of organizational change on organizational culture. *Journal of Evidence-Based Social Work, 5*, 321–359.

Bellot, J. (2011). Defining and assessing organizational culture. *Nursing Forum, 46*, 29–37.

Buresh, B., & Gordon, S. (2006). *From silence to voice*, 2nd ed. Canadian Nurses Association, Cornell University Press, Ithaca, NY.

Calhoun, E. (1993). *Action research: Three approaches*. Educational leadership, 51(2), 62–65.

Cameron, K., & Quinn, R. (2011). *Diagnosing and changing organizational culture*, 3rd ed. San Francisco, CA: Jossey-Bass.

Colquitt, J., Noe, R., & Jackson, C. (2002). Justice in teams: antecedents and consequences of procedural justice climate. *Personnel Psychology, 55*, 83–109.

Cooperrider, D. & Srivastva, S. (1987). Appreciative inquiry in organizational life. In W. Pasmore & R. Woodman (eds.), *Research in Organization Change and Development, 1*, 129–169. Greenwich, CT: JAI Press.

Cooperrider, D. & Whitney, D. (2008). A positive revolution in change: Appreciative inquiry. Retrieved from http://appreciativeinquiry.case.edu/uploads/whatisai.pdf

Cooperrider, D., Whitney, D., & Stavros, J. (2003). *Appreciative inquiry handbook*. Bedford Heights, OH: Lakeshore Publishers.

Deal, T., & Kennedy, A. (1983). Culture: A new look through old lenses. *Journal of Applied Behavioural Sciences, 19*, 498–506

Denison, D. (1990). *Corporate culture and organizational effectiveness*. New York: John Wiley & Sons.

Diamond, M. (1995). Organizational change as human process, not technique. *National Institute of Drug Abuse Research Monograph, 155*, 119–131.

Ernst, R. (1985). Corporate cultures and effective planning: An introduction to the Organizational Culture Grid. *Personnel Administrator, 30*, 49–60.

Fanon, F. (1963). *The wretched of the earth*. Grove Press, New York, NY.

Firbank, O. (2010). Exploring the fit between organizational culture and quality improvement in a home-care environment. *Health Care Management Review, 35,* 147–160.

French, W. & Bell, C. (1973). *Organization development: behavioral science interventions for organization improvement.* Englewood Cliffs, N.J.: Prentice-Hall.

Gottlieb, L. & Ezer, H. (Editors). (1997). *A perspective on health, family, learning, and collaborative nursing: a collection of writings on the McGill model of nursing.* Montreal, Canada: McGill University, School of Nursing.

Haider, M., & Kreps, G. (2004). Forty years of diffusion of innovations: Utility and value in public health. *Journal of Health Communication, 9,* 3–11.

Hatch, M. & Cunliffe, A. (2006). *Organizational theory,* 2nd ed. New York: Oxford University Press.

Hofstede, G. (1980). *Culture's consequences.* Thousand Oaks, CA: Sage.

Hughes, R., & Clancy, C. (2009). Complexity, bullying, and stress. Analyzing and mitigating a challenging work environment for nurses. *Journal of Nursing Care Quality, 24,* 180–183.

Kayser, K., Walker, D., & Demaio, J. (2000). Understanding social workers' sense of competence within the context of organizational change. *Administration in Social Work, 24*(4), 1–20.

Kemmis, S. & McTaggart, R. (1988). *The action research planner.* Geelong, Victoria, Australia: Deakin University Press.

Khademian, A. (2002). *Working with culture: How the job gets done in public programs.* Washington, DC: CQ Press.

Kotter, J. (1995). Leading change: Why transformation efforts fail. *Harvard Business Review, 61*(March–April): 57–67.

Kotter, J. (1996). *Leading Change.* Boston, MA: Harvard Business Press.

Kovach, C., Morgan, S., Noonan, P., & Brondion, M. (2008). Using principles of diffusion of innovation to improve nursing home care. *Journal of Nursing Care Quality, 23,* 132–139.

Kozlowski, S., Chao, G., Smith, E., & Hedlund, J. (1993). Organizational downsizing: Strategies, interventions, and research implications. *International Review of Industrial and Organizational Psychology, 8,* 263–332.

Lewin, K. (1951). *Field theory in social sciences: Selected theoretical papers.* D. Cartwright (Ed.). New York: Harper & Row.

Marchionni, C., & Richer, M. (2007). Using appreciative inquiry to promote evidence-based practice in nursing: The glass is more than half full. *Nursing Leadership (CJNL), 20*(3), 86–107.

Martin, J. (1992). *Cultures in organizations.* New York: Oxford University Press.

Marx, D. (2001). *Patient safety and the "just culture": A primer for health care executives.* New York City: Columbia University.

Naumann, S., & Bennett, N. (2000). A case for procedural justice climate: development and test of a multilevel model. *Academy of Management Journal, 43,* 881–889.

O'Hagan, J., & Persaud, D. (2009). Creating a culture of accountability in health care. *The Health Care Manager, 28*(2), 124–133.

Pearlmutter, S. (1998). Self-efficacy and organizational change leadership. *Administration in Social Work, 22*(3), 23–38.

Randolph, G., Stanley, C., Rowe, B., Massie, S., Cornett, A., Harrison, L., & Lea, C. (2012). Lessons learned from building a culture and infrastructure for continuous quality improvement at Cabarrus Health Alliance. *Journal of Public Health Management Practice, 18,* 55–62.

Richer, M., Ritchie, J., & Marchionni, C. (2009). 'If we can't do more, let's do it differently!': using appreciative inquiry to promote innovative ideas for better health care work environments. *Journal of Nursing Management, 17,* 947–955.

Roberts, P., and Thomas, E. (2006). The safety attitudes questionnaire: Psychometric properties, benchmarking data, and emerging research. *BMC Health Services Research, 6,*44.

Roberts, S. (1983). Oppressed group behavior: implications for nursing. *Advances in Nursing Sciences, 5*(3), 21–30.

Roberts, S. (2000). Development of a positive professional identity: liberating oneself from the oppressor within. *Advances in Nursing Science, 22*(4), 71–82.

Roberts, S., Demarco, R., & Griffin, M. (2009). The effect of oppressed group behaviours on the culture of the nursing workplace: a review of the evidence and interventions for change. *Journal of Nursing Management, 17,* 288–293.

Rogers, E. (1962). *Diffusion of innovations.* Glencoe: Free Press.

Rogers, E. (2003). *Diffusion of innovations.* 5th ed. New York: Free Press.

Rousseau, D. (1990). Assessing organizational culture: The case for multiple methods. In B. Schneider (Ed.), *Organizational climate and culture* (pp. 153–192). San Francisco: Jossey-Bass.

Rousseau, D. (1988). The construction of climate in organizational research. In C. Cooper, & I. Robertson (Eds.), *International review of industrial and organizational psychology* (Vol. 3, pp. 139–158). New York: Wiley.

Ruchlin, H., Dubbs, N., & Callahan, M. (2004). The role of leadership in instilling a culture of safety: Lessons from the literature. *Journal of Healthcare Management, 49,* 47–58.

Schein, E. (1987). Defining organizational culture. In J.M. Shafritz & J.S. Ou (Eds.), *Classics of organizational theory.* 2nd ed. (pp. 381–396). Chicago, IL: The Dorsey Press.

Schein, E. (1992). *Organizational culture and leadership: A dynamic view.* 2nd ed. San Francisco, CA: Jossey-Bass.

Schneider, B. (1990). The climate for service: An application of the climate construct. In B. Schneider (Ed.). *Organizational climate and culture* (pp. 383–412). San Francisco: Jossey-Bass.

Scott-Cawiezell, J., Vogelsmeier, A., McKenney, C., Rantz, M., Hicks, L., & Zellmer, D. (2006). Moving from a culture of blame to a culture of safety in the nursing home setting. *Nursing Forum, 41*(3), 133–140.

Seren, S., & Baykal, U. (2007). Relationships between change and organizational culture in hospitals. *Journal of Nursing Scholarship, 39*(2), 191–197.

Shirey, M. (2011). Addressing strategy execution challenges to lead sustainable change. *Journal of Nursing Administration, 41,* 1–4.

Shirey, M. (2009). Authentic leadership, organizational culture, and healthy work environments. *Critical Care Nursing Quarterly, 32,* 189–198.

Sexton, J., Helmreich, R., Neilands, T., Rowan, K., Vella, K., Boyden, J., Siehl, C., & Martin, J. (1983). Organizational culture and counter culture: An uneasy symbiosis. *Organizational Dynamics, 12*(2), 52–64.

Stringer, E. (2007). *Action research,* 3nd ed. Thousand Oaks, CA: Sage.

Tozer, C., & Ray, S. (1999). 20 questions: The research needs of children and family social workers. *Research, Policy and Planning, 17*(1), 7–15. Retrieved from www.whatworksfor-children.org.uk/docs/GAP%20STUDY/top%20questions%20asked.pdf

Tsai, Y. Relationship between organizational culture, leadership behavior and job satisfaction. *BMC Health Services Research, 11*:98. Retrieved from www.biomedcentral.com/1472-6963/11/98

Zell, D. (2003). Organizational change as a process of death, dying, and rebirth. *Journal of Applied Behavioral Science, 39*(1), 73–96.

Chapter 5
Decision Making and Management of Workflow

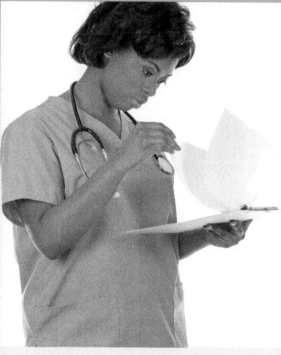

Zdenka Darula/Fotolia

Learning Objectives

After reading, studying, and reflecting on this chapter's content, you will be able to:

1. Identify different models and tools of decision making
2. Identify a variety of styles of management decision-making
3. Suggest how strategic planning could be used in a health care organization at both the departmental and organizational levels
4. Discuss how core values can be used to guide decision making in organizations
5. Discuss the roles of direct care nurses, their managers, and senior administrators in decision making, and everyone's accountability for their decisions
6. Be aware that rational decision-making models may have limited use in "wicked" contexts
7. Apply strategies for innovative decision-making
8. Compare different organizational and reporting structures, including shared governance, program management, and interprofessional teams
9. Discuss what and how nursing care can be delegated (or assigned) to other nurses and non-nurses

INTRODUCTION

Decision making and the management of workflow are important skills for direct care nurses and managers. Direct care nurses make many decisions each work day, for example, decisions about which nursing interventions will be effective for a client, what issues to bring forward in a staff meeting and how to present these, and what care to **delegate** or to assign to other employees and how to communicate with these employees. Managers and charge nurses' decisions include which patients to assign to which nurses, how to deal with client complaints, how to deal with requests from other employees, how to plan for future programs and services, what issues to bring forward to senior managers, what longterm plans to make for the department, and what feedback to give to staff members. Senior managers make decisions about the strategic plan for the organization and what responsibilities, including decision-making authority, to delegate to managers.

While different roles come with the authority to make different types of decisions, the quality of your decisions, the process you use to make decisions, and how you communicate your decisions are important for how effective you are in your role. Decisions made by your manager, the process your manager uses to make these decisions, and how he or she communicates decisions can make a huge difference in how well you are able to provide nursing care, as well as how you evaluate your workplace and your manager.

In this chapter we describe different models and tools of decision making, as well as the styles managers might use in decision making. We also discuss the importance of values in determining the numerous small decisions made daily in the workplace and the larger, strategic planning decisions. Different organizational structures such as centralized and decentralized structures, shared governance, program management, interprofessional teams, and **nursing care delivery models** are discussed because these structures relate to decisions about who does what work, or the flow of work in the organization. Finally, we outline what to consider when delegating work to others and how to communicate when delegating.

Some of the content in this chapter focuses on the types of decisions made by managers, and on the organizational structures that have an impact on workflow and are generally determined by managers or senior administrators. Direct care nurses need to learn about the work of nurses and senior administrators, in order that they can understand the organizational context or the "big picture" where they work. For those of you who may consider a management position in the future, learning about nurse management functions provides an introduction to the field of management.

DECISION-MAKING MODELS
Rational Decision-Making

Numerous models developed for making decisions in organizations assume organizational decision making is a rational, cognitive process. Rational decision-making models are developed on the assumption that a person determines the best course of action through logically thinking about all possible options. These models include steps, and, while the number of steps in different models may vary, in general these models include identifying

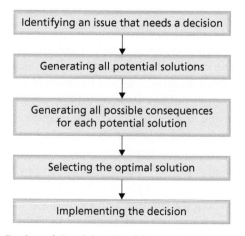

Figure 5.1 Steps in Rational Decision-Making Models
Source: Based on "Steps in Rational Decision-Making Models."

an issue about which a decision is needed, generating all potential solutions and their consequences, selecting the optimal solution, and then implementing the decision (see Figure 5.1).

Herbert Simon (1957) is well known for developing a different model of how decisions are made in organizations. He noted that it is not possible for us to identify all possible alternatives, nor to obtain all information about these alternatives and rationally determine the best solution. This is simply too much information for the human brain to process, and would also take too much time. Instead, we consider alternatives until we find one that will satisfy the problem. Simon referred to this as **satisficing**, or selecting an alternative that is satisfactory without spending additional time identifying the pros and cons of all possible solutions.

Decision Making Based on Patterns and Cues

In the mid-1980s Gary Klein looked at how fire fighters in the army made decisions and concluded they did not use the steps implied in rational decision-making models. Fire fighters make decisions under time pressure and with conditions changing quickly. He found that fire fighters identify a possible course of action, consider if it will work or not, and go with the first course of action that they believe will work. Klein established that, as employees in fast moving, complex, and changing environments gain experience at work, they recognize patterns and cues, and named his intuitive decision-making model the Recognition-Primed Decision Model. With experience, expertise is developed that is related to the ability to see patterns in situations. We may think we are acting on our intuition; however, this intuition may be our recognition of patterns and cues. In addition to studying fire fighters, Klein studied this type of decision making with members of other professional groups, including critical care nurses. Klein (2003) has gone on to suggest how we can use our intuition to our advantage.

Patricia Benner (1984) discusses the type of decision making that is based on the recognition of patterns in her well-known book *From Novice to Expert*. She found that novice nurses had to go through steps when recognizing patient care situations, while nurses with years of experience, who were experts in their field, recognized patterns and were able to make decisions quickly.

We suggest that nurses who are just starting out in leadership positions may benefit from working through steps of a rational decision-making model and using decision-making tools such as the ones discussed in this chapter (for example, decision trees, Pareto analysis, SWOT analysis, cost-benefit analysis). Further, if you take the time to work through the steps of a decision-making model or tool, you may select a better alternative even if you are an expert in an area. In complex situations, expert nurses may recognize patterns and select an effective alternative. However, you should realize that this effective decision is based on experience. As a new nurse, until you develop expertise, you have fewer "patterns" to draw on and may benefit from using decision-making tools and consulting experts.

Innovative Decision-Making

Innovative decision-making is often described as a decision-making process that requires "thinking outside the box." Thinking about a problem in different ways may lead to seeing the problem differently and to a new solution. In today's challenging and multifaceted health care environment, the current way we do something may no longer be effective.

There are a number of techniques that help both individuals and groups with innovative decisions. A commonly used technique is **brainstorming**, a process where everyone is encouraged to give ideas about the issue. To encourage everyone to give ideas, the others in the group are asked to not evaluate the ideas as they are presented. The idea is to generate a number of ideas that in turn may stimulate others to build on these ideas.

Brainstorming is a well-known and frequently used strategy. Yet surprisingly, research evidence has not supported claims that it results in more ideas than when a person works alone (Diehl & Stroebe, 1991). Perhaps this is in part because people wish to be credited individually for their own good ideas, rather than the group, or they may be reluctant to speak up in a group and have their ideas judged (Diehl & Stroebe, 1991). To help individuals share ideas with their work group, we need to consider giving rewards for group rather than individual performance. This requires a shift in the way we think, because our Western culture emphasizes the individual rather than the collective, and we typically reward individuals (for more discussion about rewarding the performance of groups versus individuals, see Chapter 7, Motivation and Performance). To help reduce the potential reluctance of group members to share their ideas, the group leader might ask each member to write one idea and collect these and read them to the group, and then continue by having members write another idea.

The most important advice we can offer to encourage innovative solutions is to respond with interest and curiosity when you are asked about the current way things are done, or when suggestions are offered. Even if your initial reaction is that the idea is silly or it has been tried before, by allowing discussion of the idea, you foster a culture of curiosity. At the same time, by demonstrating respectful verbal and nonverbal communication, you prevent the development of a culture of bullying or incivility. (Please see Chapter 4, Change and Culture, for more discussion about culture.)

Winona was in charge of client services at a large, urban community services organization. Although Winona was a nurse, she was in charge of not only registered nurses, licensed practical nurses, unregulated healthcare providers, and clerical workers, but also social workers and a dietitian. The community services organization had a mandate for public health, health education, and home care. As well, it provided clinical placements for nursing and social work students.

The home care division was having increasing difficulty in providing timely services to new clients. They were required to provide an assessment of referred hospital patients the day following discharge, but on several recent occasions they had not met this requirement. For several months at staff meetings, the home care nurses said they had too many clients and felt they were rushing away from visits without giving the clients and their family members enough time to discuss their concerns.

The social workers were concerned with what they believed was an increasing number of child protection cases, and, along with the nurses in the public health and health education divisions, they wanted to develop programs to prevent bullying and recognizing teens who were at risk to attempt suicide.

The CEO of the community services organization informed Winona that she must find a way to always meet the standard of assessing referred hospital patients the day after discharge within her current budget.

Discussion Questions

1. Using a rational decision-making approach, work through the steps that Winona could use to decide how to shift resources to the home care program.

2. Working in a small group of four to five students, brainstorm to identify possible ways to meet the required standard for home care assessments without having an impact on other programs. Did this method help you identify an innovative solution?

Values and Decision Making

Most organizations have developed statements about their values, and these are often posted on their websites along with their mission and vision statements. Decisions made in the organization should be consistent with these values. Employees and other onlookers consider decisions made by an organization's administrators or board of directors to be a reflection of the organization's actual values. Employees will feel cynical if they are told the organization has certain values but see opposing values in the organization's decisions. For example, an organization may list *respect* as one of its values, but if a manager speaks to an employee in an uncivil manner, this employee and any onlookers will doubt the organization is serious about respect. If a health care organization lists *teamwork* as one of its values, yet senior administrators are aware that some team members do not demonstrate respect for other members or will not work with them and that many departments do not even include the patient or client or resident on the team, employees will lose faith that this is really one of the organization's values.

Although there are many values that health care organizations can choose for their key values, some examples are respect, equity, accountability, collaboration, teamwork, transparency, caring, and participation. We will limit our discussion to two values that are held by many Canadians, *equity* and *transparency*. We do this to help you identify some of the difficulties organizations may have in implementing values, and how the views of nurses and other health care employees about what a particular value means may differ from how others interpret this value.

Equity

To some people, equity means everyone should have the same amount, while others believe that those who contribute more should receive more, or those with the biggest need should receive the most, or that fairness is not in the *outcome* but in the *process*. As an example, if a nurse manager has funding for only one nurse to travel to another province and attend a conference that many nurses in the department would like to attend, how should she make a fair decision? Should the nurse manager select the nurse with the most seniority, the nurse who has contributed the most to extra activities in the department, the nurse who has the most monetary need, the nurse who has identified the conference content in his or her performance appraisal as something he or she needs to learn, or should a name be drawn at random from a hat? Herein lies the difficulty in order for that nurse manager to be viewed as equitable; different people have different views about what is equitable in any situation.

Given that people hold different views about what is equitable or fair in a given situation, one thing that helps a nurse manager to be seen as fair is to communicate how a decision was made. When possible, communicating how a decision will be made *before* it is made will also help others believe the decision was equitable, especially if they can observe the procedure. It is important for nurse leaders to be fair, but that is not enough. It is also important for nurse managers to be viewed by others as fair. A nurse manager may be fair, but staff members

---

Box 5.1

Reflections of a Nurse Manager

I recall when I was a fairly new nurse manager, one of the staff nurses told me that she and a number of other nurses had been talking about what a good nurse manager I was, and went on to say that they felt I was a good manager because I was always fair. I was surprised with the reason that they gave, because I had expected the reason to be that I had a lot of clinical knowledge or they had learned a lot from me because I spent a lot of time mentoring the nurses. Being fair seemed like nothing to me. Why wouldn't I be fair? They all reported to me, and I wanted the best for all of them. The comment about being fair stuck with me, and I came to realize the importance of fairness for nurses' job satisfaction and

for their perception of a leader. I was struck with how often I heard the word fair being used when people were discussing whether someone was a good leader.

Questions

1. What are your own values as these relate to your interactions with others in the workplace? How do your values influence your interactions with others? How would they influence decisions you made if you were a nurse manager?

2. Look at the web site of the health care organization where you are doing clinical work to see the values of the organization. Do you see evidence of how these values influence decisions in that organization?

When Should Information Be Provided?

The CEO of a home care services centre had informed all employees when she became CEO that transparency was one of her key values. Several months later, she realized the organization was in financial difficulty. One way to balance the budget was to only approve overtime for nursing staff in very exceptional cases, and in those cases to approve time rather than salary. This was something she really did not want to do because she believed the nurses requested overtime because they wanted to provide quality care, and they require time to provide information and support, and to discuss issues with clients and family members. As well, the CEO knew the employees were already feeling dissatisfied because of other changes. She also felt confident she would be able to obtain additional funding, and would not have to restrict paid overtime. Her management team was aware that overtime might not be paid in the future but were asked not to share this with their staff. Several of the CEO's managers advised her to inform staff, because they had a right to know their working conditions might change in the future.

After several months, the CEO realized she could not obtain additional funding and announced that paid overtime would be discontinued. Employees were understandably upset, and one person asked when the CEO had first learned this might happen. The CEO replied she had known for several months, but had thought she could avoid the situation. Her thinking was that if the situation had been avoided, staff would have had several months being distressed about something that would never happen.

Discussion Questions

1. Which decision-making model did the CEO use in this case?

2. Given the CEO had said transparency was one of her values, do you feel she handled this situation appropriately? Why or why not?

3. Do you think that the CEO's decision to inform employees that transparency was one of her values would lead employees to feel more negatively toward how she handled this situation? Why or why not?

may not believe this, and so the manager has the reputation of not being fair. This has an impact on staff members' job satisfaction as well as how the nurse manager is seen as a leader.

Transparency

Transparency means being open about what is occurring and what decisions are made. This openness is associated with our need to see that others are accountable for their actions. We particularly believe that publicly funded organizations, such as Canadian hospitals and many long-term-care and community health centres, should operate with openness. In the past, employees in Canadian health care organizations did not necessarily believe they had the right to know why the administration made certain decisions, but this is no longer the case. Today, Canadian health care workers believe senior administrators should be transparent because they believe they are part of the organization and they should have input into how the organization functions. They also believe senior administrators should be transparent with employees because employees are also taxpayers with the right to see the organization is accountable for public funds.

It can be difficult for managers to be transparent in situations that require privacy, such as issues related to employees and patients. Managers may also delay providing information because the information isn't finalized, and informing employees about a situation may cause unnecessary distress (see Box 5.2). We suggest that whether or not transparency is a stated value of a manager or an organizational value, it is useful to communicate the boundaries of transparency. For example, certain information may not be able to be shared for privacy reasons, while other information may be withheld at the request of an external.

STYLES OF MANAGEMENT DECISION-MAKING

Autocratic Decision-Making

In autocratic decision-making, the manager makes a decision without input from others in the organization and then implements the decision. There are times when this type of decision making is beneficial, such as during an emergency when a decision(s) needs to be made quickly, or an opportunity will be lost if an offer is not immediately accepted.

Consultative Decision-Making

In consultative decision-making, the manager consults with employees, but after the consultation process, the manager makes the decision. This type of decision making should result in better decisions than autocratic decision-making because employees give the manager information that may help identify which alternative is needed or will work. This type of decision-making also helps employees feel involved and should increase acceptance of the decision, although not to the degree of collaborative decision-making.

Participatory Decision-Making

Participatory decision-making, sometimes referred to as participatory management, refers to decision making where the manger allows employees to share in the decision. Of course, the degree to which employees are allowed to participate may vary greatly, from providing information requested by the manager to a group of employees being allowed to make the decision themselves. There is much research support for the beneficial effects on staff of participating in decisions, for example, the reduction of absenteeism (Probst, 2005).

Collaborative Decision-Making

Collaborative decision-making is also known as group decision-making, and refers to when a decision is made by a group rather than an individual. An important advantage of collaborative decision-making is that group members have been involved in the process and should be more supportive of the decision. When a group makes a decision, there often is not 100 percent agreement. Frequently, the decision is decided by a vote as is commonly used in democratic societies.

One would think that decisions made by a group would be of higher quality than those made by individuals, the idea that "two heads are better than one." There is the potential for more creative decisions, particularly if the group strategizes to promote innovation. However, research has found that groups sometimes make worse decisions than individuals. For example, **groupthink** (Janis, 1982) refers to the tendency for group members not to speak out against the ideas of an influential group member(s) and go along with a poor decision. (For more discussion on groupthink, see Chapter 10, Team Building and Managing Conflict.)

Polarization refers to the finding that groups sometimes make more extreme decisions than an individual would make. Polarization can occur when, for example, a group interviews a nurse for a position. The group's decision may be a very strong "do not hire" or "hire," while an individual interviewing the same nurse may make the same recommendation, but not as strongly.

Consensus Decision-Making

Consensus decision-making is a type of collaborative or group decision making. What does it actually mean when we say we will make a decision by consensus? If you were to say this to a group of nurses, chances are the response would be that everyone would have to agree with the decision. In reality, there are many situations where it would be extremely difficult if not impossible for everyone to agree. Consensus decision-making refers to the decision-making process in which the group makes the decision and there is general agreement about the decision. Further, efforts are made to work through opposing positions and to try and lesson the amount or intensity of opposition by those who remain in disagreement with the decision. Consensus decision-making is particularly useful when the group's support of a decision is required for it to be effective (Dressler, 2006).

Consensus decision-making has definite benefits compared with autocratic decision making or decisions by majority vote. When a decision is made by majority vote, the decision can be made with 50 percent plus one vote. This can lead a large number of persons feeling dissatisfied with the outcome and potentially acting to sabotage what was voted on. Consequently, a valuable skill for a manager to have is consensus building, in which there is a clear majority who agree on the decision that is made.

If you inform a work group that they will be able to make the decision by consensus, we advise you to say that not everyone may agree with the final decision, but that dissenting views will be heard and the rationale for the final decision will be transparent. If group members believe a decision made by consensus means all are in agreement with the decision, then those who are not in agreement may feel betrayed.

Decision-making Tools

Numerous decision-making tools have been developed to help people make decisions, or to help them with rational decision-making. These tools are not meant to make the decision, but to provide a rational analysis of information for decision makers to consider. There are numerous decision-making tools, but here we describe four examples of these

Winona needed to decide how the standard to assess hospital patients the day following discharge could be met. She wanted to make this decision in a way that was consistent with the values she had informed her staff that she held as a manager—transparency, equity, and respect. She also wanted to make this decision in a way that was consistent with the stated values of the organization—which were respect, caring, quality, and accountability.

To begin her decision-making process, Winona decided to write guiding principles that were congruent with her values as a manager and the organization's values. Consistent with her value of transparency and respect, she shared the need to meet the standard and the guiding principles with her staff. One of the guiding principles she developed was that the all programs needed to provide quality services. Another guiding principle was financial accountability to the provincial government for how funds were spent.

Winona decided to reduce worked nursing hours in health education and increase nursing hours in home care.

She called a staff meeting, informed them of the problem and identified the guiding principles she had used. She said that persons working in health education might not find this equitable; however, she believed quality care could be maintained by providing health education to larger sized groups. She said she was sharing how she made the decision with staff, to help them understand the process.

Discussion Questions

1. What other guiding principles can you develop that are consistent with Winona's managerial values? With the organization's values?

2. Do you believe that Winona's decision was equitable in terms of outcomes for clients? Outcomes for staff members?

3. Winona shared her decision-making process with her staff members. Do you feel this contributed to process equity? How or how not?

4. What style of management decision-making did Winona use? Do you agree with how she made the decision?

tools, specifically decision trees, Pareto analysis, SWOT analysis, and cost-benefit analysis. These tools can help people make decisions in a number of different contexts, including nursing management and clinical decisions.

Decision Trees

A **decision tree** shows a tree-like path with branches showing the implications of taking a certain decision. Essentially, a decision tree shows an algorithm, with the branches indicating that a specific outcome will probably occur if that branch is followed (see Figure 5.2). Decision trees can be used in many different contexts. For example, a clinician could use one with a client to walk through the probable outcomes of deciding in order to select different treatments and/or health behaviours. A manager can develop a decision tree to help him or her work through the probable outcomes of different budget allocations, or the probable outcomes of bringing an issue to his or her manager.

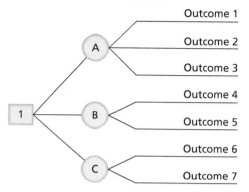

Figure 5.2 Decision Tree

1 is the point where the person needs to make a decision; A, B, C are the possible alternatives for the solution.

Source: Based on "Decision Tree."

Pareto Analysis

The **Pareto Principle** is also known as the 80–20 rule, and refers to the idea that 80% of the results come from 20% of the efforts. This principle is used to suggest a variety of things, when used in different contexts. For example, the principle is used to suggest where employees should decide to spend their time when it is said that 20% of their work will provide 80% of the results. Obviously, the amounts of 80 and 20% are not exact amounts and essentially mean that most of the results come from expending efforts in a few areas. When this principle is applied to employee relations, it refers to the idea that most of the employee-related problems in an organization come from a few of the employees. Therefore, this principle suggests that the manager should decide to correct issues with these few employees, for a major reduction of problems related to employees. This type of analysis, based on the Pareto principal, is known as Pareto analysis.

The Pareto principle is useful in considering problems related to quality. When this principle is used in quality improvement, it is said that 80% of the problems come from 20% of the causes. Pareto analysis involves identifying the 20% that will obtain the 80%; for quality improvement this means uncovering the causes and then pinpointing those that lead to the majority of problems. A manager or a quality improvement team can list the causes of quality-related problems. Next, the causes can be placed in order, from those that are the largest to the smallest cause of problems and a **Pareto chart** can be drawn. A Pareto chart is a bar diagram with each cause shown as a bar that indicates the approximate percentage of the problems associated with it, as well as a line to show the cumulative total of the causes (see Figure 5.3). This chart helps the manager or quality improvement team decide which cause to work on first.

SWOT Analysis

SWOT stands for strengths, weaknesses, opportunities, and threats. When doing a **SWOT analysis** for an organization, group members assess *internal* factors—the strengths and weaknesses of their organization—and they assess *external* factors—the opportunities for

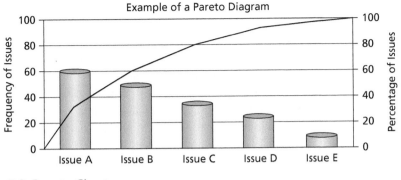

Figure 5.3 Pareto Chart

and threats to their organization. Two strengths might be that the health centre has a high retention of nurses, or that the health centre is known in the community for its excellent palliative care program. Weaknesses might be that the length of stay for several diagnostic groups of patients is well above the provincial average, or that the nosocomial infection rate is higher than average. Opportunities might be that more young families are moving into the area, or that new treatments in a specialty area will allow patients to be treated in a day hospital rather than being admitted. Threats might be that provincial funding may be cut or there is a shortage of a particular group of professionals such as anesthesiologists or public health nurses.

Cost-benefit analysis

Cost-benefit analysis involves calculating all the financial costs as well as all of the financial benefits associated with a decision, a project, or a policy. The costs and benefits are calculated as financial costs to help decision makers determine which course of action has the most benefits for the least costs. An example of a cost-benefit analysis is calculating the cost of adding additional nurses to a hospital department and comparing it with the cost saving from lower patient morbidity and mortality. Other examples are comparing the financial cost of an employee wellness program with the financial benefit associated with lower employee absenteeism, or comparing the financial cost of a government policy to promote activity with the financial benefit of the associated higher levels of health. Research studies that demonstrate an outcome associated with a program or policy along with a cost-benefit analysis that shows the benefits outweigh the costs and/or are valued benefits are particularly effective tools for getting decision makers to support the program or policy.

Decision-making Tools and "Wicked Problems"

The term **"wicked problems"** was used by Churchman (1967) to describe difficult problems that have multiple causes, some of which may not be known, and are difficult to solve. Churchman looked at problems in organizations with a systems approach. Fixing or making a change in one part of a system inevitably leads to changes in other parts of the system, and this suggests that there are no simple solutions to fixing a problem within a system. Organizations are complex systems, and many problems have multiple causes making it difficult to assess the exact causes of the problem. We may not be able to identify all of the causes, and as the system changes over time the causes and potential solutions may also evolve.

Many decision-making tools may not identify all causes of a problem, but they may also suggest problems can be solved with a single solution. Further, the potential of a solution to have an impact on the rest of the system needs to be considered. In today's health care environment, many problems have multiple causes, and finding a solution is challenging. Solutions may require thinking outside the box or looking at a situation in a new way. Decision makers need to be creative and innovative, yet there will be times when a solution cannot be found, or if found, the manager is unable to implement the solution due to constraints such as organizational policies, lack of permission from the manager's supervisor, or lack of resources.

Much of a manager's role is to make decisions, yet the types of problems nurse managers are faced with in today's large, complex health care organizations make it hard to find effective solutions. Direct care nurses and senior managers may judge a nurse manager by the quality of his or her decisions, and in the case of multiple wicked problems it can be difficult or impossible for nurse managers to find good solutions or to be able to implement them. Consequently, staff and senior managers may blame a nurse manager for unsolved problems when the nurse manager is caught between a rock and a hard place.

Compounding the nurse manager's difficulty in finding or implementing good solutions is the fact that most nurses managers have a large **span of control**, or a large number of employees who report directly to them. This large span of control contributes to the heavy workload of nurse managers and leaves little time to think about problems. Difficult decisions, a large span of control, and a heavy workload are all sources of stress for nurse managers. In addition, the trend to close management positions when there are budget constraints leads to job insecurity and further adds to the nurse managers' stress. A nurse manager may wish to return to his or her direct care position but is unable to because these positions are assigned by seniority among union members.

Direct care nurses who see the stresses, including the job insecurity that nurse managers are faced with may hesitate to apply for nurse management positions. Unfortunately, this potentially leaves nurses who would become good managers and leaders in direct care positions, resulting in a lack of strong nurse managers. Direct care nurses who understand the wicked problems their managers are faced with along with stresses will try to work with their managers to find innovative solutions rather than blaming the managers and not the context for problems that persist. Nurses' demonstration of support for their managers may go a long way in the recruitment and retention of nurse leaders who develop their leadership skills through management positions and who are able to work with senior administrators and policy makers to promote the needs of clients and nurses.

Strategic Planning

Strategic planning refers to the process of determining long-term plans that form the organization's strategy. A **strategic plan** documents the decisions made during the strategic planning process, and generally includes the organization's **mission statement** (which is a description of focus or purpose), values, **vision statement,** (which is a description of where the organization would like to be in the future), and goals and objectives and how these can be attained. These long-term plans serve to guide daily decisions, as employees work to meet the goals and objectives set out in them. In small organizations, it may be possible for everyone in the building to be involved in the organization's strategic plan. In large organizations, the senior executive group may do most of the strategic planning, with input from managers and from all employees. In these large organizations, after the overall strategic plan is developed, each department may form its own strategic plan that flows from the overall strategy.

Organizations may find a variety of procedures useful in helping them to develop a strategic plan. Some may use an external consultant to chair one or more days of meetings to work on the plan. Others may have the senior executive team develop the plan and then consult with different groups of employees. Some may do a SWOT analysis at the start of the strategic planning process (Johnson, Scholes, & Sexty, 1989), while others may not use this or may use another tool.

In general, however, the first step is to develop the organization's mission statement and identify its values. Next, the vision statement is developed (JOP, 2009). A vision statement describes what the organization would like to be doing in the future. Goals and objectives are developed that are consistent with the mission and values and will help the organization attain its objective.

The strategic activities should be linked with the organization's financial and human resource plans (Ruder & O'Connor, 2007). If an area is prioritized in the strategic plan, it needs to have the financial and human resources required for it to be successful. Developing a plan that cannot be funded means the plan won't be achieved and those who worked on it will feel discouraged.

Performance improvement activities should flow from the strategic priorities (Lazarus, 2011). As well, the strategic activities should be consistent with the mission and values of the organization. Following the development of an organization's overall strategic plan, each department can develop its own strategic plan. The departmental strategic plans need to be consistent with the organization's mission, vision, and values as well as with the organization's strategic plan. Moreover, when departmental or program level employees develop their strategic plan, they should be realistic about what financial and human resources will be available; failure to do this will not only set them up for failure, but for disappointment when their plans cannot be initiated.

In the past, long-term strategic planning was done for a period of five years or longer. Today, the health care environment is changing so rapidly that, if we plan for the next five years, in all likelihood the plan will not be relevant before the end of this time. Instead, strategic plans for health care organizations should be made for around three years (JOP, 2009). Given the rapid change in both the internal and external environments of Canadian health care organizations, we recommend that strategic plans be reviewed annually and either revised or redeveloped if they are no longer relevant.

What does a strategic plan look like? It does not need to be a long document, although we are aware that many health care organizations' strategic plans are over a hundred pages. There will be a lot of discussion when developing or revising the

Mount Sinai's Mission, Vision, and Values

Mission

Discover and deliver the best patient care, research and education with the heart and values true to our heritage.

Vision

To be Canada's highest quality academic health science centre, providing the best medicine and best patient experience.

Values

Excellence and Innovation in Clinical Care, Teaching and Research

Pursue excellence in everything we do with continuous improvements in quality, service and cost-effectiveness.

Patient-Centred Care

Prioritize safety, quality and the patient experience in everything we do.

Teamwork

Embrace a collaborative and interdisciplinary approach to clinical care, teaching and research.

Collaboration

Establish internal and external partnerships to integrate and coordinate patient services effectively.

Respect and Diversity

Value and respect the differences of the patients and families who seek our care as well as those who provide that care.

Leadership

Promote the development and growth of leaders throughout the organization and continue to allow our leading programs to export our knowledge nationally and internationally.

Retrieved from www.mountsinai.on.ca/about_us/corporate-information/strat-plan-2012.pdf. "Mount Sinai's Mission, Vision & Values," Mount Sinai Hospital Strategic Plan 2010–2013. Reprinted with permission.

Saskatoon Health Region's Vision, Mission, and Values

Our Vision

Healthiest People, Healthiest Communities, Exceptional Service

Our Mission

We improve health through excellence and innovation in service, education and research, building on the strengths of our people and partnerships.

Our Values

- Respect
- Compassion
- Excellence
- Stewardship
- Collaboration

Retrieved from www.saskatoonhealthre-gion.ca/about_us/goals.htm. Reprinted with permission of Saskatoon Health Region.

Stages of Strategic Planning

Mission and values
Vision statement
Goals and objectives

Action plan with target dates and
person(s) accountable

organization's mission, values, and vision, or when using a tool such as SWOT analysis. However, we suggest that after presenting a brief mission, value, and vision statement, the actual plan be written in the form of a table, with columns for goals, objectives, specific actions, target dates, and person(s) accountable. This way, the plan is readily accessible and can be referred to periodically by all employees to make sure they are still on track, working to meet the goals. A strategic plan that is clear, accessible, and has specific actions with target dates and the person(s) accountable is more apt to be actively used to help the organization move towards its vision. The mission and vision statements may be very brief. For example, a number of organizations, including Mount Sinai Hospital in Toronto and Saskatoon Health Region have a one-sentence mission statement (see Box 5.3 and Box 5.4).

While mission statements may be very brief, they should be useful. Many mission statements tell us little about an organization, and for that reason Ackoff (1986) developed five characteristics of what a good mission statement should do:

1. State the organization's objectives in a way that allows progress towards these objectives to be measured

2. State how the organization differs from other organizations

3. Identify the business the organization wants to be doing (not what it is doing)

4. Be relevant to all stakeholders of the organization, and

5. Be exciting and inspiring.

Although Ackoff developed his characteristics of what a good mission statement should do for business organizations in any sector, they are useful when developing the mission statements for health care organizations.

DELEGATION AND ASSIGNMENT

In management, **to delegate** is defined as giving another person authority to have the autonomy to make a decision without first verifying the decision with the person who delegated the authority (Tourigny & Pulich, 2006). Delegation is related to decentralization, because with decentralization, decision-making authority is moved to the manager at a lower level in the organization's hierarchy. The advantages of delegation include:

1. decisions are made by persons who have the best information and thus the quality of decisions should be improved,

2. decisions are not delayed by the need to take them to a higher level of managers in the organization, and

3. lower-level managers have the opportunity to develop their decision-making skills. (Tourigny & Pulich, 2006)

When a manager delegates, the manager loses control over the situation, while retaining responsibility for outcomes. This is difficult for managers who like to maintain control, or who are insecure or micromanagers. It can also be difficult for a manager to delegate if the organization's culture is one where mistakes are not tolerated well; delegating to someone with less experience is not without risk.

In nursing, we often use the word *delegate* loosely to describe assigning tasks or procedures to another health care provider. We need to be aware that when we refer to delegating patient care, we are *not* delegating total decision-making authority for the patient's care, but rather decision-making authority within the scope of practice of the person we delegated to. And we need to ensure that the person we delegated to is aware of his or her scope of practice. For example, if we delegate the care of a patient to a licensed practical nurse, we must be certain that he or she is aware that if the patient's status changes, the LPN is responsible for informing the nurse of this change. In other words, when assigning work to other health care personnel, the nurse needs to decide if the person has the skills to do this work, as well as deciding what level of supervision is required to ensure this work is satisfactory. There is a dual responsibility when nursing care is assigned: while the nurse who does the assignment should be aware of the skills of the person being assigned to, the person who accepts the assignment has the responsibility to say whether he or she has adequate experience to carry out the activities.

The College of Nursing of Ontario (CNO) (and other regulatory bodies) defines delegation from the perspective of controlled acts and the professional group that has the legal authority for the act (CNO, 2011). From this perspective, delegation is giving the authority for a procedure that is a controlled act to someone who does not have the legal authority for this procedure. For example, an act that is a legally a medical act may be delegated to nurses by the medical association, and be referred to as a medically delegated act. In contrast to how CNO uses the term delegation, they define assignment as giving the responsibility for aspect(s) of patient care to another person (CNO, 2011).

With the shortage of registered nurses, more health care organizations are hiring licensed practical nurses and unregulated health personnel to provide nursing care. Delegating to unregulated health care providers is a decision that is challenging for direct practice nurses. Unregulated providers may have some training, but this can vary from a short orientation provided at the work setting to a program lasting a number of months provided by an educational institution. In addition, unregulated providers may have varying experiences, and while they may perform some skills expertly, there may be other skills they have never exercised. To help nurses make decisions about delegation to unregulated health care providers, CNO developed a decision tree (see Figure 5.4). Whether you are delegating or assigning a task to another health care provider, you should be aware of your provincial nursing association's regulations and guidelines for delegation, as well as your employer's policies.

Decision Tree: Making Decisions About Activities Performed by UCPs

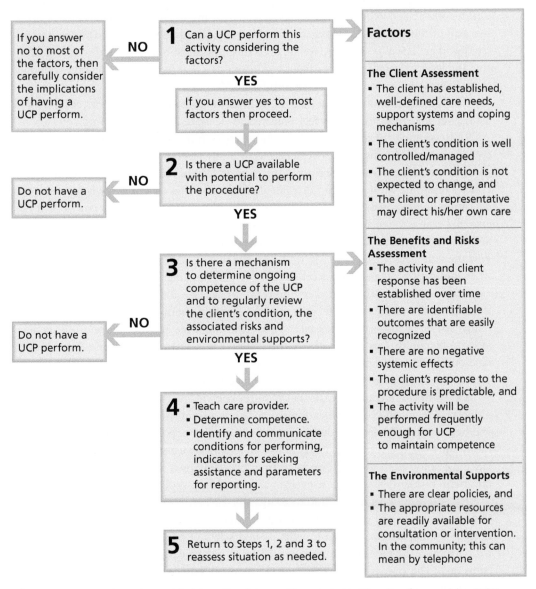

Factors

1 Can a UCP perform this activity considering the factors?

NO → If you answer no to most of the factors, then carefully consider the implications of having a UCP perform.

YES

If you answer yes to most factors then proceed.

2 Is there a UCP available with potential to perform the procedure?

NO → Do not have a UCP perform.

YES

3 Is there a mechanism to determine ongoing competence of the UCP and to regularly review the client's condition, the associated risks and environmental supports?

NO → Do not have a UCP perform.

YES

4
- Teach care provider.
- Determine competence.
- Identify and communicate conditions for performing, indicators for seeking assistance and parameters for reporting.

5 Return to Steps 1, 2 and 3 to reassess situation as needed.

The Client Assessment
- The client has established, well-defined care needs, support systems and coping mechanisms
- The client's condition is well controlled/managed
- The client's condition is not expected to change, and
- The client or representative may direct his/her own care

The Benefits and Risks Assessment
- The activity and client response has been established over time
- There are identifiable outcomes that are easily recognized
- There are no negative systemic effects
- The client's response to the procedure is predictable, and
- The activity will be performed frequently enough for UCP to maintain competence

The Environmental Supports
- There are clear policies, and
- The appropriate resources are readily available for consultation or intervention. In the community; this can mean by telephone

Figure 5.4 Decision Tree: Making Decisions About Activities Performed by UCPs

Source: "Decision Tree: Making Decisions About Activities Performed by UCPs," from page 8 of CNO's Working With Unregulated Care Providers, Revised 2011. http://www.cno.org/Global/docs/prac/41014_workingucp.pdf. Reprinted with permission.

When a nurse delegates (or assigns) patient care, he or she must first decide what can safely be delegated to a specific employee. Delegating to unregulated nursing personnel challenges nurses to find work that can be delegated safely. The introduction into nursing units, including acute care areas such as intensive care units, of unregulated workers with little training is a growing trend. On the one hand, this is not something we would like to promote, given the research evidence of better patient outcomes associated with registered nurses providing care (for some examples of research findings, see CNA, 2010). On the other hand, when no nurses are available, it might help a nurse to manage his or her workload if we can find tasks that can be safely delegated (or assigned) to an unregulated worker. The slippery slope we are on is that administrators will see this as cost effective and ignore research findings about staffing models that have better outcomes not only for patients, clients, or residents, but also for nurses.

Charge nurses and nurses in management positions are required to both delegate and assign, yet many nurses do not feel prepared to delegate or assign (McInnis & Parsons, 2009). Regrettably, nurses who are busy and stressed in the workplace often do work they could delegate (Murphy, Ruch, Pepicello, & Murphy, 1997). Delegation and assignment require knowledge of the practice act in the province where you are working, organizational policies regarding whom you can delegate different activities to, and knowledge about the education and experience of the staff member involved. However, this knowledge is not enough because the relationship that the nurse has built with a staff member and his or her ability to work on a team may influence whether a nurse requests a staff member to help and how the staff member responds. As well, how the nurse communicates with a staff member when delegating or assigning work can leave the staff member feeling anything from engaged, respected, and included on the team, to disrespected, or antagonized. Clarifying the roles of all nursing personnel as well as the **chain of command** (Hudson, 2008), or the formal system of authority to delegate to a specific employee at a lower level in the organizational hierarchy, can help with the delegation (or assignment) process. According to Hudson (2008), communicating clearly about what is required helps, as does allowing the person who is delegated an opportunity to ask questions or make suggestions.

Delegation is a complex skill that requires knowledge, the ability to work well with others on a team, and communication skills. This is a complex skill, but schools of nursing and health care settings provide minimal education and opportunities to practise it, with the result that new nurses find themselves in situations where they should delegate but lacking comfort with and skill in delegating. Encouraging a nurse to be in charge of the unit helps him or her develop delegation and leadership skills.

Kalisch (2011) conducted a study to identify the barriers to RNs and unlicensed assistive personnel (UAP) (unregulated health workers) working as a team and their perceptions of the impact this has on the quality and safety of patient care. Nine focus groups with a total of 81 registered nurses and 12 focus groups with a total of 118 UAPs were convened. The participants worked on 15 medical surgical units in 3 hospitals in an American state. As well, 10 direct care nurses, 6 UAPs, and 3 managers were interviewed individually. The groups identified seven themes:

1. lack of role clarity,
2. lack of working together as a team,
3. inability to deal with conflict,
4. not engaging UAP in decision making,
5. deficient delegation,

6. more than one boss, and

7. "It's not my job" syndrome.

In turn, the theme of not engaging UAP in decision making had three subthemes: UAP don't attend report with RNs, UAP aren't being listened to by RNs, and RNs command rather than asking in a respectful manner. The theme of deficient delegation had three subthemes: RNs don't obtain buy-in of UAP, RNs don't retain accountability and follow through, and directions by RNs are unclear. Examples of how each of the seven themes was related to quality and safety issues were presented, highlighting the importance of RNs and UAPs working together.

Kalisch's study has a number of important implications for delegating and assigning work to unregulated health workers. From the perspective of an unregulated health worker, it is difficult if all the nurses and licensed practical nurses on a unit can delegate to this person. One suggested way to avoid this is to create small teams, such as two nurses working with one unregulated health worker with responsibility for the same group of patients, and with the unregulated health worker participating in change of shift report and included as a team member (Kalisch, 2011). Nurses and unregulated health workers should have clear roles and should be oriented to the potential quality and safety problems of not working well together. The type of respect and communication that direct care nurses expect from nurse managers, physicians, and other health care professionals is the type of respect and communication that nurses should use with unregulated health workers.

MANAGEMENT OF WORKFLOW

An important function of managers is to organize how the accountability for what work, functions, and/or decisions will be organized. The following sections identify different types of reporting structures.

Reporting Structures

Everyone in a health care organization is accountable to someone. The chief executive officer is accountable to the chair of the board of directors, who in turn is accountable to the organization's funder, which in the case of Canadian hospitals is the provincial government. In the case of Canadian residential centres or community health centres, it can be the provincial government or a private owner. Reporting relationships can be drawn on an organizational chart, such as the one shown in Figure 5.5, and show the chain of command.

A **job description** is a document that includes who the person in the job reports to as well as any positions that may report to this person. The job description also includes the functions this person fulfils, including decision making. A well-written job description should promote **role clarity**, or a clear understanding of the responsibilities and functions associated with the position. Without role clarity, employees can be confused about what work they are responsible for. As well, conflict between employees might occur either because employees in different positions feel they are responsible for an area and they want the associated decision-making authority for this role, or because they feel the person in another role should assume responsibility for these functions.

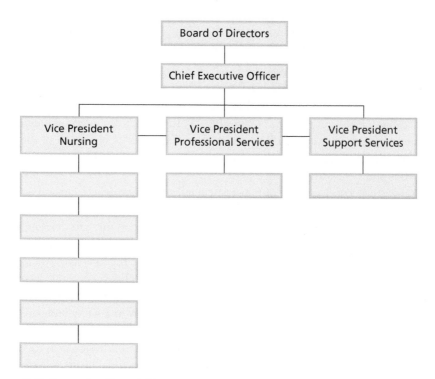

Figure 5.5 Organizational Chart

Before you accept a nursing position, it is a good idea to ask for a copy of the job description and see if the organizational structure and the role functions are clear and acceptable.

Despite having a clear job description, the management style of the person you report to can make a tremendous difference in how you are able to work. **Micromanagement** refers to the management style of frequently overseeing work and possibly controlling decisions related to this work, when this work is in the job description of a subordinate. This management style does not empower employees, but an employee who wants frequent input and does not wish to be accountable for decisions may appreciate this style. **Macromanagement** refers to management through managing aspects of the system so that the system leads to the desired work outcomes. For example, a macromanager may identify policies or job roles that are needed.

Centralized and Decentralized Structures

In an organization with a **centralized structure**, decision making is carried out by top managers. Managers on lower levels are accountable for implementing decisions and providing senior managers with information. If you are a nurse in an organization with centralized decision-making, there may be decisions you believe your manager should make with the department's staff. However, if your manager is unable to make the decision, but organizes a staff meeting that gives group members the feeling *they* can make a decision, this may set the group up for disappointment. In such a situation, the manager could state that senior administration will be making a decision, but the purpose of the meeting is to gather information and possibly identify recommendations and outcomes for senior administrators to consider. The advantage of centralized decision-making is that the organization has a consistent strategy and senior administrators know and control how the organization operates.

In a **decentralized structure**, decision-making authority is given to managers at lower levels of the organization and perhaps even to staff members. This is advantageous when quick decisions are needed, or when decisions need to be tailored to unique circumstances. In health care, decisions related to patient care are almost always delegated to the professionals caring for the patient.

New graduates may have to recognize that health care organizations are not democracies. Learning which decisions one has control over and will be held accountable for, and which decisions others are held accountable for, is part of the transition to your role as a health care employee. Direct care nurses are accountable for decisions including patient care and assignment of work to support staff. Direct care nurses are not accountable for decisions regarding budget allocations and strategic planning for the organization. However, their insights into the work of the organization are such that the wise decision maker will consult them.

Flat and tall structures

A **flat organizational structure** is one with no or very few layers of managers between staff and senior administrators, while a **tall organizational structure** (also referred to as a hierarchical structure) has a number of layers of managers. A hierarchical structure includes more opportunities for promotion and more managers to deal with work and employee concerns. However, it can also lead to communication problems between senior administration and front line staff, as well as to the higher costs associated with more managers.

With budgetary cuts in the 1990s, many Canadian health care organizations reduced the number of nurse managers. This has left the remaining front line managers (also known as first line managers) with many persons reporting to them (high span of control) and a heavy workload. These front line managers no longer have time to spend their day developing their staff members by discussing patient care with them.

Structures in Canadian Health Care Organizations

Persons within Canadian health care organizations determine which governing structures to use. However, some provinces have legislation that requires structures such as Nursing Councils with a representative on the board, and/or interprofessional councils.

Shared Governance

Professionals are responsible for monitoring their own standards of practice. In Canadian hospitals, traditionally the director of nursing played the major role in setting and monitoring standards of nursing practice within the hospital. She or he was in charge of all decision making within the nursing departments, including all decisions related to hiring and termination of nurses as well as functions such as maintaining nurses' personnel files. As health care organizations grew larger and more administrators were needed, human resource departments were formed. Over time, these departments took over some of the decisions and functions that had been under the director of nursing, such as maintaining personnel files, obtaining references, and being the first contact for the nurses' union representatives.

In contrast, traditionally, physicians who worked in hospitals in Canada were not employees of the hospital. While today a limited number of physicians are employed by hospitals, most are still not and they bill the government for their services. There are physicians with administrative responsibilities who receive a stipend from the hospital for their administrative functions, for example, a physician in charge of each medical specialty and a physician with overall administrative responsibility. While these physicians discharge some administrative responsibilities, physicians govern themselves through a council of physicians (which may also include dentists and pharmacists), which may be known as a medical advisory committee. Through their committee, physicians make decisions related to standards of professional practice, as well as exerting influence on much decision making that is outside of medical practice. The council of physicians or medical advisory committee is often a powerful group in health care organizations, particularly in hospitals.

Shared governance refers to shared decision making among different roles in an organization and is used in many types of organizations (Porter-O'Grady & Malloch, 2009) including universities. Porter-O'Grady's (1984) landmark book *Shared Governance for Nursing: A Creative Approach to Professional Accountability* applied shared governance to the governance of nurses in hospital settings, thereby starting a model of decision making that was very different from the traditional, hierarchical structure of hospital nursing departments. Shared governance allows all nurses within an organization to be involved in decision making related to their professional practice. Rather than nurse managers making all decisions, nurses within the organization, including direct care nurses and nurse managers, participate in councils.

The number and function of these councils depend on the size of the organization and its needs. For example, there may be separate councils for clinical practice, nursing education, nursing leadership, and nursing research with an overall executive council that the other councils report to (see Figure 5.6). An American hospital reported that, prior to implementing shared governance, it had spent several months determining its council structure and decided on three councils, Quality and Research, Practice, and Education and Professional Development, which reported to a fourth council, the Coordinating Council (Newman, 2011). However, several years later it divided the Quality and Research Council into two councils.

Not every nurse in the organization actually sits on all of these councils to discuss issues and develop policies and procedures. Rather, nurses elect representatives. Ideally, council members communicate with all nurses through mechanisms such as newsletters or internal websites, and consult all nurses through mechanisms such as unit representatives, polls, or votes on specific issues.

Shared governance has become a popular structure for nursing in health care organizations. Most hospitals in the United States adopted it during the 1980s

Councillor Model

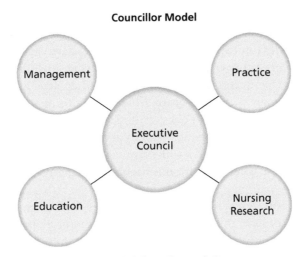

Figure 5.6 A Sample Council Model for Shared Governance

(Porter-O'Grady, 1992) as well as many Canadian hospitals, for example, St. Michael's in Toronto (2013). Shared governance allows all nurses in an organization with the opportunity to participate in decision making. This is important in part for nurses' job satisfaction because nurses want to be involved in decision making, and in part because as professionals, nurses should govern the professional aspects of their practice.

There are some major advantages for nurses working in a structure with shared governance. Younger nurses expect to be involved in decision making, which empowers them. Shared governance is also consistent with the values of transparency, trust, and accountability. Administrators share information related to budgets, safety reports, and so on, and thus exhibit transparency about issues. This sharing of information with nurses shows they trust nurses. Trust in an organization needs to work both ways, and when nursing councils openly share their rationales for policies they develop and are open with information with administration, they demonstrate trust in the administration. For shared governance to work, nurses need to be accountable by participating in the council and assuming ownership for the quality of decisions made.

Nurses at an American hospital wrote about their experience with shared governance over 16 years (Baker et al., 2009). They identified two items key for nurses to feel connected and engaged with the hospital: information sharing and meaningful voice. They found that information sharing helps nurses understand the "big picture" (p. 149) where they work. For example, information such as the budget, strategic plans, and quality and safety reports are shared with nurses, and while this helps direct care nurses to understand the big picture, it also helps them with decision making related to their professional practice. Meaningful voice comes from "having a seat at the table" (p. 149) or by having a representative at meetings where decisions are made.

While shared governance has advantages, there are some huge challenges associated with implementing and maintaining this structure (for example, Hess, 2004;

Hibberd, Storoz, & Andrews, 1992). It can be a challenge for both nurse managers and nurses familiar with working in a hierarchical structure to learn to work in a shared governance structure. In a traditional hierarchy, nurse managers control and direct nurses. In contrast, nurse managers practising in an organization with shared governance help provide nurses with the information they need and focus on developing staff. Nurse managers need to learn which issues to direct to which nursing council rather than determining a policy or directive themselves. Similarly, nurses need to learn to bring issues to nursing councils and to assume responsibility for this rather than assuming nurse managers will eventually deal with a situation. This can be difficult or impossible when a decision is needed immediately or an organization is large.

When implementing shared governance, all nurses need to know the boundaries of the areas where they have the mandate to make decisions. Shared governance does not mean that every decision made in the organization is shared with nurses. Rather, governance within the organization is shared, with nurses having the responsibility and accountability for decisions related to the professional practice of nursing and administrators having the responsibility and accountability for decisions outside of the professional.

The size of many health care organizations presents another challenge for implementing and maintaining shared governance. In such large organizations with a thousand or more nurses, communication with all nurses is difficult and many may not know what their elected council representatives are working on. In health care organizations that rely on nurses who are not their employees but are provided by an outside agency, employees have additional communication challenges. Communication tools such as a newsletter and website, and participation in a unit-based council are strategies that can help all nurses to feel involved or at least aware. Unit-based councils supplement the central councils and provide a place to discuss unit level issues in professional practice (Newman, 2011; Porter-O'Grady, 1992), for example, how care is organized on the unit, and how the work and vacation schedules are developed.

To help everyone in the organization understand the purpose and the boundaries of the shared governance councils, **terms of reference** that describe the purpose, membership, reporting relationship, quorum required for a vote, and any guidelines for how meetings are conducted should be worked out for each council. The purpose of the council provides the boundaries for which decisions it is responsible. In an organization, even the chief executive officer reports to someone, typically the chair of the board of directors. In shared governance, the chairs of councils might report to the chair of the executive council who in turn reports to the administrator in charge of nursing.

Program Management

In the 1980s and 1990s many Canadian health care organizations changed from a hierarchical organization (with the exception of the director of nursing who reported to the CEO) to a matrix style, wherein employees report to two managers (Manzano & Bufe, 2011). This matrix-style reporting structure is used in **program management,** which is a way of organizing health care organizations by groups of patients rather than by a department for each profession. In program management, direct care nurses report to a professional practice manager, who is a nurse, for professional issues, but also report to an operational manager, who may or may not be a nurse, for their work within the program. Further, the chief nurse in the hospital has a title such as chief nursing officer or professional practice director, rather than director of nursing. The operational manager for a nurse may be a nurse or a member of another professional group.

The operational manager has the responsibility for the day-to-day operations of the program, including budgets, as well as long-term planning for the program. Programs consist of an operational area of the health care organization such as obstetrics, medicine, long-term care, or community services. Since the operational program manager is responsible for a budget, this manager has the power to implement decisions that have a financial cost. In contrast, the professional practice manager has a relatively small budget for professional practice costs (such as workshops) and manages by influencing other managers and direct care nurses. The professional practice manager might be responsible for the professional practice of nurses working in many programs, and therefore there might be nurses in the organization who do not have individual contact with this manager. This huge span of control makes it challenging for the professional practice manager to communicate a vision for nursing throughout one or more sites of a multisite organization.

Program management was introduced to health care organizations because it was believed to have a number of advantages. For example, rather than members of different disciplines reporting to their own discipline, members of different disciplines who care for the same group of patients report to the same operational manager. This type of organization should foster interprofessional care rather than each discipline providing care and not knowing what the other discipline is doing.

In practice, program management can have a negative impact on nurses. Nurses, like other professional groups, develop commitment to their profession during their years of educational preparation. In the traditional hierarchical structure, direct care nurses felt connected with the nursing department, which fostered their commitment to the profession. While research evidence is needed, we believe that program management is a factor in decreasing nurses' commitment to the profession and the organization, and through this, their retention in the profession. Nurses who report to a program manager who is not a nurse may find that, although the manager wants to understand their workload or safety concerns, the manager has difficulty understanding nursing issues. Nurses may also find that without a nurse manager at the unit level, they lose a sense of what nursing is and what their unique contribution to patient care is. As well, because program manager positions can be held by persons from many professional backgrounds, including but not limited to nursing, social work, psychology, pharmacy, medicine, and administration, there are fewer management positions for nurses and thus, fewer opportunities for promotion.

Program management may also have a negative impact on the nursing profession because the word "nurse" is removed from management titles. Typically, managers in hospitals, nursing homes and community settings had job titles such as head nurse, assistant (and associate) director of nursing, and director of nursing. In program management,

The Ottawa Hospital was formed from the merger of six health care organizations and employs approximately 4,700 nurses in over 100 departments or services. The Ottawa Hospital has developed three models: the Nursing Professional Practice Model to engage nurses in decision making about nursing practice and patient care, and the models of Nursing Clinical Practice and Interprofessional Model of Patient Care to structure roles, responsibilities, teamwork, and collaboration.

The Nursing Professional Practice Model was developed from 2000 to 2002. This model includes a network of committees and groups, some unit-based, that allow nurses to participate in decisions related to nursing practice and patient care. As such, The Ottawa Hospital's Nursing Professional Practice Model is similar in purpose and structure to shared governance (Porter O'Grady, 1992).

The Model of Nursing Clinical Practice guides how work is delivered by different categories of nursing employees including registered nurses (RNs), registered practical nurses (RPNs), and unregulated care providers. Prior to implementing this model, different units used different structures for delivering nursing care, which is the case in many Canadian health care organizations. For example, units used primary nursing, total patient care, team nursing, functional nursing, or case management. This made it difficult for both non-nursing professionals and patients and families to understand who was responsible for a patient's care, as things differed throughout the hospital. As well, patients in some areas received care from a number of nursing personnel on any one shift.

With the implementation of the Model of Nursing Clinical Practice, each patient is assigned solely to either an RN or RPN, depending on the patient's needs and the RN's and RPN's expertise. Unregulated care providers are accountable to the RN or RPN for the care they give to the RN's or RPN's patients. The Model of Nursing Clinical Practice was developed to flow from the organization's beliefs and values, and in reviewing the guiding principles of this model (The Ottawa Hospital, 2009) it is evident that the intent includes respect for the skills of different levels of workers, promotes teamwork and continuity of care, and support from managers and educators for nursing employees, The model emphasizes "direct" nursing care, continuity of care for clients, and the availability of nursing experts (managers and educators) to nurses.

The Interprofessional Model of Patient Care (Health Force Ontario, 2007) guides the organization of collaborative patient care from different professional groups. Patients and members of several professions worked out this model to be used by different types of health care teams. It is believed to be the first model for interprofessional delivery of patient care.

The three models in use at The Ottawa Hospital demonstrate that nurses, members of other professional groups, and patients have done much work to cultivate structures for organization work. These structures should promote role clarity, communication among health care providers and with patients and families, and teamwork.

For more information, please see www.ottawahospital.on.ca/wps/portal/Base/TheHospital/OurModelofCare/ProfessionalModels

References

Health Force Ontario. (2007).
Interprofessional Care: A Blueprint for
Action in Ontario. Located at www.
ottawahospital.on.ca/wps/wcm/connect/
5bf2db804b25b26391b3d51faf30e8c1/
ipc+blueprint+final.pdf?MOD=AJPERES

The Ottawa Hospital. (2009), The Ottawa
Hospital/L'Hôpital d'Ottawa Model of
Nursing Clinical Practice © Guiding
Principles. Located at www.ottawahos-
pital.on.ca/wps/wcm/connect/6831658
04b25b270923cd71faf30e8c1/MONCP_
GuidingPrinciples-e.pdf?MOD=AJPERES

Discussion Questions

1. How is the Model of Nursing Clinical Practice developed at The Ottawa Hospital similar or different to the model used in settings where you have done clinical work?

2. Do you think the settings where you have done clinical work would benefit from adapting any of the three models discussed in this Leading Health Care Example? If so, how would you initiate planning for this change as a direct care nurse? As a nurse manager?

position titles for operational roles may be program manager, division manager, and vice-president of patient care. These changes have been criticized not only because the incumbent does not need to be a nurse, but also because by not including the word "nurse" in the title, nursing becomes invisible.

Horizontal and Vertical Integration

Many health care organizations, particularly in urban areas of Canada, no longer consist of one hospital but are more accurately described as health care systems. As discussed in Chapter 2, Health Care Management and the Canadian Context, these organizations have grown in size by both horizontal and vertical integration of other hospitals, community centres, long-term care centres, and nursing homes. **Horizontal integration** refers to an organization becoming larger by joining with a similar organization(s). In the case of hospitals, horizontal integration occurs when a hospital joins with another hospital(s) (Fottler, Malvey, & Rooney, 2011). **Vertical integration** refers to an organization becoming larger by joining with another organization(s) that is a supplier or purchaser of products or services of the organization. In the case of hospitals, vertical integration refers to a hospital becoming larger by joining with health care organizations that refer patients to the hospital, or where they go after hospitalization, such as community health centres and long-term care centres (Fottler, Malvey, & Rooney, 2011).

When health care organizations grow through horizontal and/or vertical integration, their governance structure may change to an overall corporate management, as well as a CEO and a management structure for each institution. Different organizations have adapted different management structures as they try to meet their needs (Fottler, Malvey, & Rooney, 2011), and the management of these evolving health care organizations has been and continues to be a challenge for managers.

A Study to Examine the Impact of a Nursing Clinical Practice Mode on Patients, Nurses, and the Organization

The Model of Nursing Clinical Practice was developed by nursing employees at The Ottawa Hospital, a large university teaching hospital formed by the merger of six hospitals. This practice model is described in the Leading Health Care Example in this chapter. Researchers aware that this model was to be implemented saw the opportunity to measure its impact on patients, nurses, and the organization. The research questions for this study were:

1. What are the effects of introducing the new nursing care model on quality of patient care?

2. What are the effects of introducing a new model for nursing care on nurse work stress and nurse well-being?

3. What are the effects of introducing the new nursing care model on organizational climate, at both the unit and hospital (site) levels? (p. 3)

Focus groups were held with nurses prior to implementing the change to obtain qualitative data about where the change was implemented as well as to help them develop items for the surveys.

The longitudinal study also included surveys that were administered to the nurses prior to the implementation of the Model of Nursing Clinical Practice on their unit, and one and two years later. While 730 nurses participated in the study, only 224 completed all three surveys. The surveys included measures of outcomes for nurses such as work stress, health, and burnout. The surveys also included measures specific to health and care organizations such as safety climate and nurse work environment.

The nurses' surveys were supplemented with surveys from 1,672 patients about the quality of their care. These surveys were also administered to patients prior to the implementation of the model and one and two years later.

One survey finding was that nurses were generally satisfied with the way they provided care *before* the model was implemented and did not feel the model improved their job satisfaction or the quality of patient care.

When asked specifically about the impact of the model, nurses did not report a change. However, 10 measures, such as nurse burnout and empowerment, showed improvement one year following the implementation (see Table 5.1). As can be seen in the table, a number of outcomes showed significant improvement at year one after implementation but not at year two. Also, the patient data surveys did not indicate improvement.

There are a number of possible reasons for these findings, some of which are identified by the researchers. One reason is that fewer nurses completed the surveys at year two, and this smaller sample size makes it harder to show a statistical difference even if all measures were below baseline two years after implementation. The patients rated their satisfaction high, 93 percent at the beginning of the study, making it hard for their scores to be even higher after the intervention. When people rate items so high on a measure, it is hard to show that an intervention improves things because the items cannot be rated any or much higher. This is known as a ceiling effect. Another reason may be that other things happened in the organization that had a negative impact on the nurse and organizational outcomes. The quasi-experimental design of one intervention group without a control did not allow comparison at year two of a group that received the intervention with a group that did not receive this intervention. However, it was not the intent of the researchers to have a control group. Rather, their intent was to examine a naturally occurring phenomenon and, because of the uniqueness of each unit, they chose a longitudinal study.

Of course, another possible reason for no significant differences for most out-come measures at year two is that the intervention was not strong enough to have an impact on these outcomes. Even if this is the case, the fact the intervention did not have a *negative* impact on the outcomes, while allowing a consistent model throughout a multi-site organization, is an important finding.

Reference: Kerr, M. et al. (2011). *Adopting a common nursing practice model across a recently merged multi-site hospital*. Ottawa: Canadian Health Services Research Foundation.

Table 5.1   Summary of Main Change Analysis Results

Factor	Change in scores from Baseline to Year 1	Change in scores from Baseline to Year 2
Patient outcomes		
patient-rated quality of care	NC	NC
Nurse outcomes		
burnout	+	NC
work stress (ERI)	+	NC
physical health	-	-
mental health	NC	NC
back/neck pain	NC	NC
work-family conflict	+	+
nurse empowerment	+	NC
Organizational outcomes		
nurse-MD relations	+	NC
nurse autonomy	+	NC
nurse control over practice	+	NC
organizational support	+	NC
safety climate	+	+
organizational justice	+	+

NOTE: ' + ' = improvement (p < 0.05); ' - ' = worse (p < 0.05); ' NC ' = no statistically significant change.

Interprofessional Teams

The importance of an interprofessional team for quality and safe patient care is a current topic in Canadian health care. Projects have been started in many nursing, medical, and other health care professional schools in which students work on interprofessional projects, with the goal that this will help them learn the knowledge and skills of other professional groups as well as how to work as a team member.

An important aspect of interprofessional care (as opposed to multidisciplinary care) is that not all members of the team may need to be involved with the patient and family after the initial assessment. Rather, the interprofessional team works together to assess the client's needs and care is provided by the professional(s) whose expertise will benefit the patient. While this seems like an effective way to provide care, there have been few examples of models of how this works in practice. One exception is the interprofessional model of patient care at the Ottawa Hospital (see the Leading Health Care Example in this chapter).

Nursing Care Delivery Models

Nursing care delivery models are the structures that determine how patients and work is assigned to nursing personnel within a department. Nursing care delivery models include primary care nursing, total patient care, team nursing, case management, and functional nursing. The Leading Health Care Example box in this chapter describes a new nursing care delivery model that was developed by nurses at the Ottawa Hospital, and the Related Research box summarizes an evaluation of this model.

Research has shown that staffing with more registered nurses is associated with better patient outcomes in both acute care and long-term care settings, that more registered nurse-worked hours is associated with higher client survival in community and long-term care, and that having more licensed practical nurses is associated with better outcomes in long-term care (CNA, 2010). Unfortunately, Canadian decision makers at the health care organization and government levels have been slow to acknowledge these findings in policy decisions.

Virtually no research on licensed practical nurse and registered practical nurse practice and outcomes, nor on models of care delivery in the community and client outcomes exists (CNA, 2010). We need research to examine client outcomes when there is respect and collaboration among all health care members (including physicians, nursing personnel with different educational preparation included unregulated health care workers, pharmacists, and so on) working with different care delivery models in different settings.

Interview

Interview with Dr. Ginette Rodger, RN

Dr. Ginette Rodger is the Senior VP, Professional Practice, and Chief Nursing Executive at The Ottawa Hospital. She has experience in clinical, research, education, and management nursing and has held many leadership positions including President of the Canadian Nurses Association and Executive Director of the Canadian Nurses Association. She is a recipient of an Order of Canada and an Award of Excellence in Nursing Leadership from the Ontario Hospital Association.

Q: How is The Ottawa Hospital's Nursing Professional Practice Model similar and different from shared governance as described by Porter-O'Grady?

A: The Ottawa Hospital (TOH) has two models that guide nursing; one is the Professional Practice Model and the other the Model of Nursing Clinical Practice (MONCP).

The Ottawa Hospital's Professional Practice Model is different from shared governance and is a model that manages four domains of nursing practice—clinical, research, education, and management. These four domains are guided by the organization's strategic plan and values. The Ottawa model is based on the organization of work in the 21st century. One part of the model is *committees* as well as *unit councils* and *interprofessional councils*, but there are also *work groups* that come together to improve any of the four domains of nursing practice, and *reflective groups* that come together because members have a kindred spirit and want to stay at the leading edge of knowledge on a topic such as nursing informatics.

Porter-O'Grady noted in an article recently that the unit councils in shared governance were not working 30 years after he developed this model. A major difference between shared governance and The Ottawa Hospital's Nursing Professional Practice Model is the locus of control. The unit councils in the Professional Practice Model are co-chaired by two clinical nurses, and the clinical nurses have the responsibility and authority to make decisions. This is very different than just consulting with clinical nurses. The Ottawa Hospital's Nursing Professional Practice Model includes a decision tree to guide nurses in what decisions they can make and what decisions may need to be referred to or discussed by others. For example, decisions that have implications for other departments are corporate issues and need to be referred to that level, or decisions such as the need to replace all mattresses have cost implications and need to be referred.

Q: From your observations, can you describe how The Ottawa Hospital's Nursing Professional Practice Model has helped the typical nurse at The Ottawa Hospital feel more involved in decisions about nursing practice and patient care?

A: We have evidence that the model has helped nurses feel more in control. For example, we surveyed nurses one year prior to implementing the model, and then one and two years later. There was a significant difference for nurses on the measure for organizational justice, meaning increased control by nurses over their work environment. As well, job satisfaction was 18% higher. Our vacancy rate changed from 13% to only 2.9%, evidence of our ability to both recruit and retain nurses.

Q: How is this different than when nurse managers held weekly staff meetings, unit staff were involved in quality assurance projects, and nurses sat on committees such as the Policy and Procedure Committee and Hospital Ethics Committee?

A: It is very different from weekly staff meetings. Clinical nurses have the responsibility for clinical practice and for the work environment. At the unit level, the meetings are co-chaired by two clinical nurses. A nurse manager is present for support, but the clinical nurses run the meeting and set the agenda. Managers have the responsibility for the infrastructure and organizational elements, but clinical nurses have the responsibility for clinical practice. In the old days, the manager covered some clinical and some organizational issues in staff meetings. Clinical nurses were present on other committees but most of the members were nurse managers, educators with token clinical nurses representation.

Q: How is The Ottawa Hospital's Model of Nursing Clinical Practice different from total patient care, with RPNs replacing diploma nurses? With total patient care, the assignment was done based on patient complexity and the nurse's expertise.

A: The issue of RPNs has nothing to do with the model. The model is similar to total patient care in that the person who is assigned to the patient, whether this is a RN or a RPN, does everything for the patient. There is a *single accountability* with *whoever* is assigned to the patient accountable for the patient's care.

The model has a number of tools and one of these tools is a staff mix model. Based on the complexity, the unpredictability, and so on of the patients, the percentage of patients on a unit that can receive care by a RPN and by a RN is determined. For example, it may be determined that 20% of the patients can receive care from a RPN. If your question is "What is the difference between a RPN and a RN?" then the RN has the responsibility of the initial patient assessment, the first care plan, and the decision if a RPN can be assigned a patient. However, if the patient is assigned to a RPN, the RPN does everything for the patient including rounds with the MD. A RN is not assigned to do some activities for that patient. It is a single accountability. If the patient's status changes, the RPN is accountable for reporting back to the RN.

Q: There is some concern within the profession that RPNs now carry out essentially the same role as RNs and are in fact, replacing them in hospitals. How does your Model of Nursing Clinical Practice differentiate the roles?

A: At times the RPN and RN do the same tasks, and also others professionals such as MDs, for example taking vital signs. It is possible for RPNs to have complex patients, which is often the case in long-term care centers. However, it is the *unpredictability component* that requires a RN to be assigned to a patient. At an acute care centre such as The Ottawa Hospital there are 4 700 nurses including 400 RPNs.

Q: The Ottawa Hospital's Model of Nursing Clinical Practice notes nurses have access to nurse managers and clinical experts. Is this 24/7?

A: The clinical experts are available 24/7. In most cases, the clinical expert is also assigned a reduced patient load but this depends on the unit's decision. If a unit has a lot of novice nurses, they may decide it is better for the clinical expert to have no patients and to work with the novice nurses, and for the other nurses to take an extra patient.

The nurse managers work mostly on the day shift but there is always a charge nurse on the unit for the other shifts and a site clinical coordinator 24/7.

Q: Was there a trade-off in ensuring this access to nurse managers and clinical experts by adopting a model that has proportionately fewer RNs with more RPNs?

A: The Ottawa Hospital's Model of Nursing Clinical Practice does not cost more, and in fact, there are 4 700 nurses including 400 RPNs at The Ottawa Hospital because most of the care is unpredictable. This model is a way of organizing care that is based in *guiding principles*. An important guiding principle is a *single accountability* for a patient, whether it is a RN or RPN who is given this accountability. Another guiding principle came from the fact that patients want *continuity of care*—they want one nurse.

The principles are simple, but it can be challenging for the nurses at the unit level to reorganize how they give care. For example, the nurses in an emergency department were fighting against implementing the continuity principle, saying it is not possible in their specialty. But the guiding principles are essential for quality care and after around six weeks the nurses in the emergency department came up with their own solution so they could provide continuity of care. It is also challenging for the nurses to develop continuity of care with 12-hour shifts and part-time nurses. Another component of the Ottawa model is that there is a *safety net* for clinical nurses by enabling them to have *access to a clinical expert or manager* whenever they practice.

The Ottawa Hospital's Model of Nursing Clinical Practice is being implemented in a number of hospitals in Ontario, Saskatchewan, Quebec, and Newfoundland and Labrador. It is the first nursing management model in Canada, the first one of the 21st century and a leading practice in Canada for Accreditation. It is not a prescriptive model as models such as Primary Care Nursing or Total Patient Care are, but it is a model based in guiding principles that the nurses on each unit must custom design its application. It is a realistic and simple model and we have research evidence that it improves patient care and nurses' satisfaction, retention, and recruitment.

Source: Interview with Dr. Ginette Rodger. Reprinted by permission.

SUMMARY

Canadian health care organizations continue to grow in complexity.

Organizational structures such as vertical and horizontal integration, program management, and shared governance are more complicated than the traditional, one-site, hierarchical structure. Further, health care treatments and technologies continue to grow in complexity. Health care organizational structures and the associated reporting structures and flow of work are in a state of flux, as managers and employees try to find systems that will work in their organization and promote patient safety, quality care, and staff retention and satisfaction. This is a huge challenge, and one that you will work toward when you enter the nursing workforce.

We need to cultivate nurses with good decision-making and delegation skills, as these are crucial for leadership and direct care positions. In this chapter we have summarized some models and tools for decision making. We have also discussed the importance of not only knowledge about delegation, but also the importance of communication and teamwork when delegating or assigning work and strategies to improve these. Nursing education programs have provided relatively few opportunities to practice delegation, and therefore we encourage you to practise these skills in a simulated environment (for example, see Critical Thinking questions and activities #5).

Glossary of Terms

Brainstorming is a technique to generate innovative ideas by encouraging everyone to generate ideas about the issue. To encourage everyone to give their ideas, others are asked not to evaluate the ideas when they are presented. The idea is to generate a number of ideas, which in turn may stimulate others to build on these ideas.

Centralized structure refers to the structure of an organization where decision making is by top managers.

Chain of command refers to the formal system of authority in which one position links to increasingly higher positions within an organizational hierarchy. In traditional organizational structure, one must "follow the chain of command" in sending directives down the hierarchy or requests up the hierarchy and not break this orderly sequence of communication and authority.

Consensus decision making refers to the decision-making process wherein the

group makes the decision, and there is general agreement about the decision. Further, efforts are made to work through opposing positions, to try and lesson the number or intensity of upset of those who remain in disagreement with the decision.

Cost-benefit analysis involves calculating all the financial costs as well as all of the financial benefits associated with a decision, a project, or a policy.

Decentralized structure refers to the structure of an organization where decision-making authority is given to managers at lower levels of the organization and perhaps even to staff members.

Decision trees A decision tree shows a tree-like path with branches showing the implications of making a certain decision.

Delegate In management, is defined as giving authority to another person to have the autonomy to make a decision without first verifying the decision with the person who delegated the authority. In nursing, the term *delegate* is often used to mean assigning tasks or procedures to another health care provider, and may not include the transfer of decision-making authority. In nursing, the term delegation may also refer to giving the authority for a procedure that is a controlled act to someone who does not have the legal authority for this procedure.

Flat organizational structure is one with no or very few layers of managers between staff and senior administrators.

Groupthink Term used to describe the decision-making process that occurs when group members do not bring up dissenting points of view, and support a course of action without critical evaluation.

Horizontal integration refers to an organization becoming larger by joining with a similar organization(s). In the case of hospitals, horizontal integration is when a hospital joins with another hospital(s).

Job description is a document that includes who the person in the job reports to as well as any positions that may report to this position. The job description also includes the functions of the person in the job, including the areas in which this person may make decisions.

Macromanagement refers to management through managing aspects of the system so that the system leads to the desired work outcomes. For example, a macromanager may identify policies or job roles that need to be developed.

Micromanagement refers to the management style of frequently overseeing work and possibly controlling decisions related to this work, when this work is in the job description of a subordinate.

Mission statement An organization's mission statement is a brief description of the focus or purpose of the organization.

Nursing care delivery models are the structures that determine how patients and work is assigned to nursing personnel within a department (for example, primary care nursing, total patient care, team nursing, case management, functional nursing, and so on).

Pareto chart A bar and line diagram with the bars indicating the approximate percentage of the problem associated with each cause as well as a line to shore the cumulative total of the causes.

Pareto Principle The Pareto Principle is also known as the 80–20 rule, and refers to the idea that 80 percent of the results come from 20 percent of the efforts, and that 80 percent of the problems come from 20 percent of the causes.

Program management is a way of organizing health care organizations by groups of patients rather than by departments with members of one professional group

Role clarity A person with role clarity has a clear understanding of the responsibilities and functions associated with his or her position.

Satisficing The term used by Herbert Simon to describe how decisions are made—by selecting an alternative that is satisfactory without spending additional time identifying the pros and cons of all possible solutions.

Shared governance Shared Governance refers to an organizational structure where decision making is shared with staff. Porter-O'Grady (1992) applied shared governance to nursing, involving nurses within an organization in decision making related to their professional practice. Depending on the organization, there may be several councils, such as one each for clinical practice, for nursing education, for nursing leadership, and for nursing research with an overall executive council that the other councils report to.

Span of control A term used to refer to the number of employees who report directly to a manager.

Strategic plan Documents the decisions made during the strategic planning process, and generally include the organization's mission, values, vision, goals, objectives, and how these can be obtained.

SWOT analysis SWOT (Strengths, Weaknesses, Opportunities, Threats) analysis is the assessment of *internal* factors, the strengths and weaknesses of their organization, and the assessment of *external* factors, the opportunities for and threats to their organization.

Tall organizational structure is also referred to as a hierarchical structure, and has a number of layers of managers.

Terms of reference describe the purpose, membership, reporting relationship, quorum required for a vote, and any guidelines for how meetings are conducted, for a committee or work group.

Vertical integration refers to an organization becoming larger by joining with another organization(s) that is a supplier or purchaser of products or services of the organization. In the case of hospitals, vertical integration refers to a hospital becoming larger by joining with health care organizations where patients may be referred to the hospital or go to after hospitalization, such as community health centres and long-term care centres.

Vision statement An organization's vision statement is a description of where the organization would like to be in the future.

Wicked problems An expression to describe difficult problems that have multiple causes, some of which may not be known and are difficult to solve.

CASE

Susan had worked for over five years in an ICU at Hospital A and was much respected for her competence by patients, their family members, nurses, and physicians. She was offered a clinical educator position at the ICU at Hospital B, and while she was deciding if she wanted to work as a nurse educator, she was offered a position at Hospital C. Susan decided she wanted to be a nurse educator, but her next decision was at which hospital. In the end, she decided on Hospital B because she knew Beth, the person who would be her nurse manager, and trusted her. Susan discussed the job description with Beth, who assured her that as decisions needed to be made about the specifics of the job, they would be made in collaboration with Susan because that was the style of the organization. Beth assured Susan that administrators at this hospital wanted their employees to be happy, because they knew if they were not, other potential employees would hear about this and Hospital B would have more difficulty in hiring.

Shortly after Susan started working at Hospital B, Beth was promoted to another position, and Susan had a new nurse manager, Joanne. Susan discussed with Joanne that, while her job description said she would do general orientation to the hospital, she had not done this yet and felt educators in central staff development department could do this better. Joanne agreed and told her she did not need to do this. In less than a year, Joanne left Hospital B, and Carol became Susan's third manger since she started. Carol asked why Susan was not involved in general orientation, and Susan replied that it had been agreed with Joanne that she would not do this. A few days later, Carol emailed Susan and wrote the previous manager had left detailed notes for her about all the decisions she had made, and this had not been noted. Since general orientation was in her job description, she had to do this.

1. What type of decision making did each of Susan's managers use related to this issue?

2. Discuss the reason Carol's decision may be seen as fair or unfair, from both Carol and Susan's perspectives.

3. Susan was insulted when she read Carol's email. Discuss possible reasons for why.

4. Susan took this position because she liked and trusted Beth, and Beth had told her that her management style mirrored the values of the organization. A psychological contract refers to the beliefs an employer and employee have about their mutual obligations. Discuss how Susan's psychological contract with Hospital B was broken.

5. Instead of emailing a directive to Susan, is there another way she could have handled this situation that may have led to less anger from Susan?

6. Several months later, Carol asked Susan if she would provide some in-services to the nurses on medical units. This is not in Susan's job description. Will Susan agree? What are the long-term outcomes for Susan and for the hospital if she agrees or disagrees?

Critical Thinking Questions and Activities

1. Obtain a copy of your school of nursing's mission, values, and vision statements.
   a. Discuss examples of how you see the mission, values, and vision implemented.
   b. From your observations, do you agree that the mission, values, and vision statements accurately reflect the actions of faculty and staff members at your school of nursing?

2. a. Using Ackoff's five characteristics of what a good mission statement should do, can you develop a mission statement for the health setting where you are doing clinical work?
   b. If the developers of the mission statements shown in Box 5.3 and Box 5.4 had used Ackoff's five characteristics, would their mission statements include different information?

3. a. Identify a "wicked problem" where you do clinical work and discuss what makes this a wicked problem.
   b. What types of information would be useful to work on improving the wicked problem?

4. This statement is made in this chapter: "New graduates may have to recognize that health care organizations are not democracies."
   a. In what way(s) are health care organizations not democracies?
   b. Thinking outside the box, do you believe that health care organizations could be run as democracies?
   c. Canada is a democracy, yet in many contexts decisions are made that individuals may not agree with. Given this, is there a structure that could be developed and communicated so

that health care organizations could be considered democracies?

5. **a.** To what degree do you believe today's patient safety problems are related to fewer front-line nursing managers?

   b. How would you structure the health care organization where you are currently doing clinical work to improve patient, client, or resident safety?

6. In groups of three, role play delegating or assigning an activity to another person. One member of the group acts as the nurse who is delegating or assigning an activity, the second member acts as the person who is being delegated or assigned an activity (a licensed practical nurse, an unregulated health care provider, or another nurse), and the third member observes. After the role play, each member can discuss what he or she observed and felt.

Self-Quiz

1. The strategic planning process:

   a. Includes a number of steps that should be followed in order
   b. Is part of a SWOT analysis
   c. Includes developing the organization's mission, values, and vision
   d. Should not be done at a departmental level

2. A typical mission statement for a health care organization:

   a. States the values of the organization
   b. States and describes the values of the organization
   c. Is part of SWOT analysis
   d. Is brief

3. A difficulty that usually occurs when a nurse manager has a large span of control is:

   a. Little time to spend with each individual nurse who reports to you
   b. The need to write a more detailed strategic plan for the nursing department
   c. An increase in "wicked problems"
   d. Shared governance is less likely to be supported by senior nurse managers

4. Which of the following illustrates a nurse manager's behaviour that is consistent with the value of transparency?

   a. A nurse manager consults with nurses in his/her department
   b. A nurse manager initiates a quality improvement project
   c. A nurse manager works with his/her door open and tries to minimize the number of meetings he/she attends outside of the department
   d. A nurse manager explains his/her rationale for making a particular decision

Useful Websites

Alberta Health Services Strategic Plan
http://www.albertahealthservices.ca/190.asp

Mount Sinai Hospital, Toronto, Ontario, Strategic Plan
http://www.mountsinai.on.ca/about_us

Ontario Hospital Association Strategic Plan 2010–2013
http://www.oha.com/AboutUs/StrategicPlan/Documents/StrategicBrochure_Large_Aug6%20-%20FINAL.pdf

References

Ackoff, R. (1986). *Management in small doses.* New York: Wiley.

Baker, C., Beglinger, J., DeRosa, J., Griffin, C., Leonard, M., Vanderkolk, C. (2009). On the scene St. Mary's Hospital, Madison, Wisconsin. *Nursing Administration Quarterly, 33*(2), 148–158.

Benner, P. (1984). *From novice to expert: Excellence and power in clinical nursing practice.* Menlo Park, CA: Addison-Wesley.

Churchman, C. (1967). Guest editorial. *Management Science, 14*(4). B141–142.

CNA (Canadian Nurses Association). (2010). Invitational round table. *Nursing care delivery models and staff mix: Using evidence in decision-making.* Ottawa: Canadian Nurses Association. Retrieved from www2.cna-aiic.ca/CNA/documents/pdf/publications/Roundtable_Report_Evidence_Decision_e.pdf

CNO (College of Nurses of Ontario). (2011). *Working with uneducated care providers.* Retrieved from www.ona.org/documents/File/professionalpractice/CNOPracticeGuideline_WorkingWith UnregulatedCareProviders_2011_41014.pdf

Diehl, M., & Stroebe, W. (1991). Productivity loss in idea-generating groups: Tracking down the blocking effect. *Journal of Personality and Social Psychology, 61*(3), 392–403.

Dressler, L. (2006). *Consensus through conversation. How to achieve high-commitment decisions.* Berkeley, CA:Berrett-Koehler.

Fottler, M., Malvey, D., & Rooney, K. (2011). Organized delivery systems. In: Wolper, L., *Health care administration. Managing organized delivery systems,* 5th ed. (pp. 67–106). Boston: Jones and Bartlett Publishers.

Hess, R. (2004). From bedside to boardroom – Nursing shared governance. *The Online Journal of Issues in Nursing, 9.* Retrieved from www.nursingworld.org/MainMenuCategories/ANAMarketplace/ANAPeriodicals/OJIN/TableofContents/Volume92004/No1Jan04/FromBedsidetoBoardroom.aspx

Hibberd, J., Storoz, C., & Andrews, H. (1992). Implementing shared governance: A false start. *Nursing Clinics of North America, 27*(1), 11–22.

Hudson, T. (2008). Delegation: Building a foundation for our future nurse leaders. *MEDSURG Nursing, 17*(6), 398–412

Janis, I. 1982. *Groupthink: Psychological studies of policy decisions and fiascos,* 2nd ed. Boston: Houghton Mifflin.

JOP. (2009). Strategic planning: why it makes a difference, and how to do it. *Journal of Oncology Practice, 5*(3), 139–143.

Johnson, G., Scholes, K., & Sexty, R. (1989). *Exploring strategic management.* Scarborough, Ontario: Prentice Hall.

Kalisch, B. (2011). The impact of RN-UAP relationships on quality and safety. *Nursing Management, 42*(9), 16–22.

Kerr, M. et al. (2011). *Adopting a common nursing practice model across a recently merged multi-site hospital.* Ottawa: Canadian Health Services Research Foundation.

Klein, G. (1998) *Sources of power: How people make decisions.* Cambridge, Mass: MIT Press.

Klein, G. (2003). *The power of intuition: How to use your gut feelings to make better decisions at work.* New York: Crown Publishing Group.

Lazarus, I. (2011). What will it take: Exploiting trends in strategic planning to prepare for reform. *Journal of Healthcare Management, 56*(2), 89–93.

Newman, K. (2011). Transforming organizational culture through nursing shared governance. *Nursing Clinics of North America, 46,* 45–58.

Manzano, W., & Bufe, G. (2011). The management of nursing services. In: Wolper, L., *Health care administration. Managing organized delivery systems,* 5th ed. (pp. 307–324). Boston: Jones and Bartlett Publishers.

McInnis, L., & Parsons, L. (2009). Thoughtful nursing practice: Reflections on nurse delegation decision-making. *Nursing Clinics of North America, 44,* 461–470.

Murphy, E., Ruch, S., Pepicello, J., & Murphy, M. (1997). Managing an increasingly complex system. *Nursing Management, 28*(10), 33–38.

Porter-O'Grady, T. (1992). *Implementing shared governance*. St. Louis MO: Mosby Year Book.

Porter-O'Grady, T., & Finnigan, S. (1984). *Shared governance for nursing: A creative approach to professional accountability*. Gaithersburg, MD: Aspen Publishers, Inc.

Porter-O'Grady, T., & Malloch, K. (2009). Leaders of innovation: Transforming postindustrial healthcare. *Journal of Nursing Administration, 39*(6), 245–248.

Probst, T.M. (2005). Countering the negative effects of job insecurity through participative decision-making: Lessons from the demand–control model. *Journal of Occupational Health Psychology, 10,* 320–329.

Ruder, S., & O'Connor, D. (2007). Strategic planning: What's your role? *Nursing Management, December,* 54–56.

St. Michael's Hospital. (2013). *Nursing. Shared governance.* Retrieved from www.stmichaelshospital.com/nursing/governance.php

Simon, H. (1956). Rational choice and the structure of the environment. *Psychological Review, 63*(2), 129–138.

Tourigny, L., & Pulich, M. (2006). Delegating decision making in health care organizations. *The Health Care Manager, 25*(2), 101–113.

Chapter 6

Nursing Workforce Issues:
Recruitment and Retention, Selection, Socialization and Transitioning

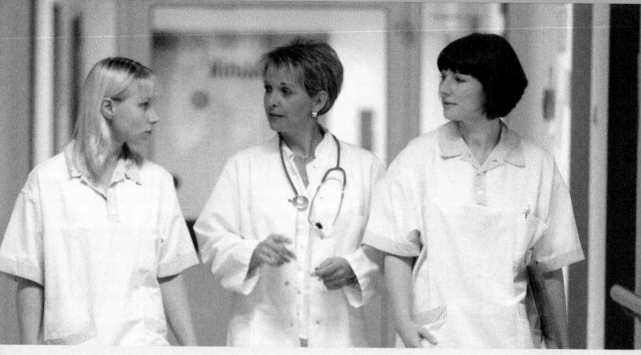

Jochen Tack/Alamy

Learning Objectives

After reading, studying, and reflecting on this chapter's content, you will be able to:

1. Suggest ways health care employers can recruit nurses
2. Identify how direct care nurses play a role in recruiting nurses
3. Propose how your work setting could select new nurses
4. Develop an interview guide to hire nurses for your work setting using behaviour-based questions
5. Debate the pros and cons of socializing nurses to a work setting
6. Discuss issues related to transitioning from the role of nursing student to direct care nurse
7. Recommend how nurse educators, nurse managers, experienced nurses, and transitioning nurses themselves can foster the transitioning of nurses to the workplace

INTRODUCTION

An employer who can recruit nurses has the advantage of being able to choose new nurses from a pool of applicants. This is always beneficial because the employer can screen individuals to select one who is a good fit for a particular department. An employer who can attract nurses not only attracts new applicants but also is able to retain nurses after they are employed. When there is a shortage of nurses, it is particularly beneficial to be able to recruit and retain nurses because this means the nursing positions at the health care setting can be kept filled. Nurses working in a setting where all of the nursing positions are filled may have a more manageable workload and feel more satisfied than nurses employed in a setting with unfilled positions. As nurses' satisfaction with a work setting gets known within a region, new nurses may be even more likely to apply for a position at this setting.

The decision to hire a nurse is an important one. Hiring a nurse who is a good fit for the position and the organization can contribute to the quality of patient care and team functioning. In contrast, a nurse who is not a good fit for the position and/or the organization might contribute to problems in delivering competent patient care; poor team functioning; the manager's time being spent to deal with problems related to the nurse's patient care or interpersonal relationships; or costs associated with a grievance, arbitration, lawsuit, or termination of employment. Whether or not you become or are a manger or member of a selection committee, the section on hiring and selecting a nurse should provide you with information that will help you when you apply for a nursing position.

When nurses start employment at a new organization, they begin to be socialized to this organization. If this is the nurse's first job, he or she also starts the process of transitioning from a student to a graduate nurse role. Nurses who are successfully socialized or who make a good transition to the workplace are more likely to be satisfied with their job and stay in their position and their profession. But if the work setting is undesirable, do you want nurses to be socialized or transition well to this setting, or do you want the new nurses to be able to change the setting? If managers hope that new nurses will change the way a team works, how can they help facilitate this?

In this chapter we discuss what attracts nurses to a work setting and how we can recruit nurses. Next, we discuss ways to select a nurse that help increase the likelihood that the nurse will be a good fit for the position and the organization. As well, we present an interview with Dr. Janice Waddell to suggest strategies for career planning and for doing well during a job interview. The processes of professional socialization, socialization to a new nursing role, and transitioning from the role of nursing student to an employee are described. Recruitment, retention, selection, socialization, and transitioning are important topics for ensuring a work setting has adequate numbers of nurses who provide quality patient care, work well with colleagues and supervisors, and adapt to their role and place of employment.

Relevance of Recruitment, Retention, and Selection Topics for All Nurses

Recruitment and retention are activities that management nurses have typically been responsible for. Nurses at all stages of their career have occasions when they use leadership skills, and nurses at any stage of their career have occasion to use management skills. In management structures such as shared governance and councils of nursing, direct care nurses may be included in activities that were traditionally management functions. For example, nurses may participate on a committee that advises or makes decisions in areas such as recruitment and retention. Therefore, all nurses should learn not only about leadership but also about management skills. As well, most nurses are employed in organizations and benefit from learning about issues and realities related to being a manager or being an employee in health care organizations.

Much of this text focuses on issues related to leadership and life in health care organizations; however some topics, including recruitment, retention, and selection, which are covered in this chapter, as well as topics in other chapters such as budgeting, staffing, and management theories are more related to the functions of managers. Although the majority of nurses are not employed in management positions, these topics are included because it is helpful for all nurses to understand the work that managers do and to consider how their own work can support and be supported by the work of managers. In addition, there are some management functions, including recruitment and selection, that nurses who are not managers may still be involved with. Finally, learning about management issues is important for all nurses because it helps them to understand aspects of the organization that are outside their own work, and may also help them learn if they would be interested in a position as a nurse manager.

RECRUITMENT AND RETENTION

A key way that health care organizations can recruit nurses is to be known for their excellence in nurses' work life, including how nurses are treated and how they are able to make decisions and provide quality nursing care. During a shortage of nurses in the United States it was found that one hospital could fill all of its nursing positions while another hospital in the same city had vacancies (McClure, Poulin, Wandelt, & Wandelt, 1983). The hospitals that were able to attract and retain nurses despite a shortage of nurses in nearby hospitals became known as **magnet hospitals** (Kramer, 1990). Chapter 9, Quality of Work Life Issues, provides an in depth description of magnet hospitals including their characteristics. In this section, we focus on recruitment and retention strategies related to generational differences, visible minorities focusing on gender, rural nurses, community and primary care nurses, and internationally educated nurses. We also discuss some innovative ways that have been used to recruit and retain nurses and suggest how direct care nurses can foster the recruitment and retention of nurses.

Generational Diversity

To fill nursing positions, health care employers need to know how to recruit, attract, and retain nurses aged from their early 20s to mid 60s and older. Nurses in different age groups may have different needs, and therefore employers who wish to employ nurses of all ages may need to develop different incentives for different nurses. Generational cohort theory suggests that people born during a specific period experience similar things, and this results in differences between generations (Inglehart 1977; Strauss & Howe, 1991).

We caution you to interpret generalizations about different generations the same way you would interpret generalizations about any group; variations exist within any group because individual members are influenced by other factors such as individual characteristics, culture, and socio-economic status. That having been said, three distinct generations that have been described and are currently in the workforce are **baby boomers**, **generation X**, and **nexters**. Nexters are also referred to as generation Y, the millennial generation, millennials, generation next, the net generation, or the echo boomers. Baby boomers were born from 1946 to 1964, generation X from 1965 to 1981, and nexters from 1982 to 2000 (Reynolds, Bush, & Geist, 2008 cited in Lester, Standifer, Schultz, & Windsor, 2012). Today's practising nurses are primarily baby boomers or members of generation X, with nexters gradually increasing in numbers in the workplace.

Baby boomers are service oriented, enjoy material success, and may prioritize work before their non-work life (Zemke, Raines, & Filipczak, 2000). In contrast, members of generations X and nexters appreciate balance between their work and non-work lives (Hart, 2006). Members of generation X adapt well to change and their values include informality (Hart, 2006). Nexters "want immediate authority, independence and a voice in major decisions. They are technologically savvy…" (Jennings, 2000, p. 55 quoted in Hart, 2006, p. 11).

Incentives to attract and retain nurses can be tailored to generational diversity. For example, baby boomers may be motivated by salary while members of generation X and nexters appreciate time off (Hart, 2006). In a review of the literature on attracting and maintaining generation Y (nexters) in nursing, the authors conclude that while there are descriptions of this generation in the nursing literature, research is needed to determine what has attracted them into nursing and what will keep them there (Hutchinson, Brown, & Longworth, 2012).

If nursing is to attract nexters, we recommend nursing informatics systems that are current and widely available to support their work. Student nexters may have used a personal digital assistant (PDA) to look up information about nursing care while in a clinical setting. This is a skill they can teach baby boomers and members of generation X, along with helping them and members of the public learn that they are working and not texting friends when using their PDAs.

Nexters' desire for decision-making ability may mean we need to change our typical organizational structures and how patient care decisions, decisions about how the department is administered, and decisions about the organization's strategic plan are made. This means baby boom managers need to learn a different way of thinking. They were drilled with the importance of bringing issues up through the chain of command, which involved a direct care nurse discussing an issue with his or her manager, who would then discuss it with his or her manager, and so on. In recent years the number of layers of managers has been reduced in part because of budgetary cutbacks and in part because of the recognition that direct care nurses want to be involved in decision making. Organizational structures such as shared governance and professional practice committees are in place in many work settings but more innovative structures may be needed to retain nexters (see Chapter 5, Decision Making and Management of Workflow, for a discussion of shared governance). The need for baby boomers who currently hold most of the nursing management positions to manage differently suggests a paradigm shift is needed in the leadership, management, and administrative practices of nursing departments and health care organizations.

Limitations to Generational Cohort Theory

While there has been much discussion about differences between generations, research is needed to examine if these differences actually exist. One study examined if the differences between generations were actual differences or if they reflected the way different generations perceived other generations (Lester et al., 2012). They found some actual and some perceived differences between generations. Their findings highlight the importance of using caution when considering the characteristics of individuals; although individuals may be members of groups, they may not have all the characteristics of these groups.

Relevance of Diversity For Nurses

Not only managers need to understand the needs of different generations if nurses are to be recruited and retained in direct practice settings; all nurses have a role to play. Nurses who are members of different age cohorts may benefit from learning about the needs and values of other age cohorts and recognize these may clash with their own needs and values. For example, members of generation X and nexters value leisure time and informality and baby boomers may be interested in retirement plans and be more accepting of management making certain decisions. Learning about the values of another age cohort can help nurses understand that the other cohort is not unmotivated, disrespectful, or resistant to change.

Canadians are becoming increasingly diverse and if the nursing profession is going to be able to recruit new members and retain practising nurses, we suggest this diversity needs to be understood and translated into work life. Generational differences are one source of diversity, but there are many other sources of diversity, including gender, rural or urban dwellers, sexuality, religion, and ethnic background. As with all types of diversity, the characteristics of a particular group are generalizations, and individuals within the group may vary. Therefore, while it is important to learn about different groups, it is important that each individual be approached as an individual who may or may not share characteristics with a group we think they belong to.

The need to attract excellent candidates into nursing and keep them in the profession means we can no longer insist that new nurses change to meet the expectations of the organization. Instead, we need to work toward understanding each individual employee and translating our respect for each individual into flexible incentives and new ways of making decisions and organizing work.

Recruiting and Retaining Members of Visible Minorities and Men Who Are Nurses

We want to be able to select good applicants for entry into the nursing profession and for any nursing position. Members of visible minorities not considering nursing as a career choice has a serious impact on the potential applicant pool. In this section, we focus on nurses who are men as a visible minority in nursing; however, a similar discussion could be had about other visible minority groups that are underrepresented in nursing.

If men who select a career in nursing experience discrimination, exclusion, or being singled out, they may resign from their department or leave the profession. In 2009, only

6.2 percent of registered nurses registered in Canada were men (Canadian Nurses Association, 2011), reflecting the profession's lack of attraction to men.

Evans (2004), a Canadian nurse historian, published an interesting paper about the history of men who are nurses. She notes that there were men in nursing at the time of the crusades, such as the Knights of St. John of Jerusalem who housed and cared for sick pilgrims. This order is known today as the St. John Ambulance Association and now trains people in first aid. It was Florence Nightingale who developed nursing into a profession for women in the late nineteenth century. The patriarchal values of society segregated women's and men's work, and men were discouraged from doing women's work. Nightingale believed that nursing was an extension of the role of women and her establishment of schools of nursing with female residences, excluded men from many schools of nursing. As late as 1961, only 25 of the 170 Canadian schools of nursing permitted male students (Hunter, 1974, cited in Evans, 2004).

In a Canadian study, Meadus and Twomey (2011) looked at male nursing students' experiences in a bachelor of nursing program. Participants were 27 male nursing students from three sites of a collaborative nursing program in Atlantic Canada. The researchers used qualitative, phenomenological methodology and identified five themes that described the male nursing students' experiences:

1. choosing nursing,
2. becoming a nurse,
3. caring within the nursing role,
4. gender-based stereotypes, and
5. visible/invisible.

Choosing nursing contains the reasons the students gave for entering nursing school, specifically "job security, demand for nurses, career mobility and opportunities, nurse role models, and the wish to help others" (p. 273). *Becoming a nurse* describes their increased attraction to nursing as they progressed in their program. *Caring within the nursing role* reflects some of the ambivalence the students had in demonstrating the caring behaviours associated with nursing, and the challenges they faced when doing clinical work in women's health. *Gender-based stereotyping* refers to the prevalent view that nurses are female and the tendency for female nurses to ask the male students to help with lifting or with aggressive patients. *Visible/invisible* portrays the realization the male students are easily recognized in a group of women students and therefore singled out. Meadus and Twomey (2011) note a number of implications for recruiting male students into nursing programs, including having male nurses visible in recruitment advertisements and in nursing textbooks.

Meadus and Twomey's (2011) findings suggest issues we can consider for recruiting and retaining nurses who are men to the profession and to a health care setting. Men may go into nursing because they wish to help, but nursing instructors, preceptors, and mentors may need to learn about masculine ways of demonstrating caring in order to coach novice nurses who are men. Male students may be less visible and feel they fit in more if, at a multi-site collaborative program, one site specializes in educating nurses who are men and looking at men's health issues. Similarly, a lone male nurse may feel less connected to a nursing department than if several nurses who are men worked in the department. We all need to avoid gender bias in our language and not refer to a nurse only as "she."

The male nursing students in Meadus and Twomey's (2011) study spoke of the challenges they experienced in clinical rotations in women's health. Since these male students may never work in women's health settings, should nursing instructors find ways of developing their competence in this area without direct practice, in cases where the men students request not to go to certain areas? Since the time of Florence Nightingale nursing programs have required clinical practice in medical, surgical, pediatric, obstetric, and psychiatric hospital departments, but can clinical competence be learned if not all of these departments are used and other clinical learning activities become part of students' practice? For example, clinical expertise can be gained in simulated patient centres or in well-baby clinics instead of post-partum units. However, if a male student wants experience in providing direct care with women, including in maternity units, as Meadus and Twomey suggest, nurse educators should work with nurses in these settings and with the male students to make this a positive experience. Some men do practise in maternal child departments, including in labour and delivery. In May 2012, the first man to graduate in Canada from a midwifery program received his Bachelor of Sciences in Midwifery from McMaster University (Perdomo, 2012).

Recruiting and Retaining Nurses in Rural Areas

The recruitment and retention of nurses in rural areas of Canada has unique challenges. Most schools of nursing are in urban centres, and upon graduation, even nurses from rural areas may feel attracted to remaining in the health care settings where they practised as students, or in tertiary care settings where they will be able to use complex medical technology. Rural settings offer unique benefits including the satisfaction of living in a community where the nurse is from (Penz, Stewart, D'Arcy, & Morgan, 2008), managerial support and autonomy (Teasley et al., 2007), and workplace social networks (MacPhee & Scott, 2002).

Much of Canadian research has focused on nurses in urban hospitals. One study explored the experiences of rural Newfoundland and Labrador (NL) healthcare managers related to the recruitment and retention of nurses. Eight rural NL managers were interviewed to explore their experiences and the data were analyzed to identify categories of barriers and facilitators to recruiting and retaining nurses. Three main categories of barriers were found: personal factors, rural NL characteristics, and the limiting nature of rural nursing structure. These three main categories of barriers and examples of each are shown in Figure 6.1. Figure 6.2 shows the two main categories of facilitators: connection to the community and a supportive work environment, with examples of these categories. While this study interviewed a small number of managers and did not ask the rural direct care nurses themselves what attracted them to and kept them in a rural setting, the findings do suggest barriers that can be reduced and facilitators that can be highlighted to recruit and retain nurses. The rotation of nursing students to a rural setting is one strategy that may lead to the students seeing the positive aspects of the rural setting and rural life.

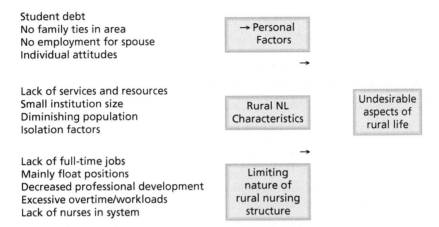

Figure 6.1 Barriers to Nurse Recruitment and Retention in Rural NL

Source: From the *Journal of Rural Nursing and Health Care*. Reprinted by permission of the Rural Nursing Organization.

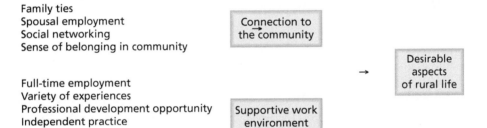

Figure 6.2 Categories of Facilitators

Source: From the *Journal of Rural Nursing and Health Care*. Reprinted by permission of the Rural Nursing Organization.

Recruiting and Retaining Community and Primary Health Care Nurses

Much of the focus of recruitment efforts and research about quality of work life that may help retain nurses has focused on hospitals. Shorter patient length of stays in hospitals, more acutely ill patients cared for in the community, more frail elderly persons assisted to remain in their homes, and increased emphasis on health promotion and prevention of illness means there is an increased need for nurses in community and primary care settings.

One project looked at strategies to attract and retain nurses in primary care by meeting with groups of primary care workers in England (Drennan, Andrews, Sidhu, & Peacock, 2006).

The researchers developed a framework of strategies to attract and retain nurses at four different points in their careers:

1. prior to completing their nursing program,
2. upon graduation from nursing or transition to primary care position,
3. nurses experienced in primary care, and
4. nurses at times of transition such as maternity leave or retirement.

At different points in their careers, different strategies attract and retain nurses. For example, prior to completing their nursing program, strategies include helping nursing students learn about nursing roles in primary care and allowing them to provide nursing care in primary care settings. Strategies for nurses who have just graduated or are new to primary care include rotating new employees through different roles for nurses in primary care settings. Strategies for nurses experienced in primary care include providing career progression opportunities. Strategies for nurses at transition points include providing education to help nurses enter primary care roles. These strategies may be useful for other clinical areas seeking to recruit and retain nurses.

Recruiting International Nurses

Canada, like other countries, including the United States and Great Britain, has historically relied on international recruitment to fill nursing vacancies, and this practice is continuing. Nurses who were educated in other countries and moved to Canada have made many positive contributions to the health care of Canadians (RNAO, 2008). York University School of Nursing in Toronto offers a Bachelor of Science in Nursing for internationally educated nurses. Nurses educated outside of Canada can apply for this 20-month program that is designed to help them meet Canadian standards of nursing practice and write the Canadian registration exam.

In recent years, concerns have been raised about the ethics of recruiting nurses from developing countries where there may be a shortage of nurses (for example, Cho, Masselink, Jones, & Mark, 2011; ICN, 2007; RNAO, 2008).

The International Council of Nurses (ICN) developed a position statement about nurse migration that includes the following statements:

> ICN believes that nurses in all countries have the right to migrate as a function of choice, regardless of their motivation.
>
> ICN acknowledges the potential benefits of migration, including learning opportunities and the rewards of multicultural practice. At the same time, ICN acknowledges that international migration may negatively affect health care quality in regions or countries seriously depleted of their nursing workforce.
>
> ICN believes that migration is a symptom of dysfunctional health systems and condemns the practice of recruiting nurses to countries where authorities have not engaged in human resources planning or addressed problems which cause nurses to leave the profession and discourage them from returning. (ICN, 2007, p. 1)

The Registered Nurses' Association of Ontario's (RNAO) (2008) policy brief entitled *Recruitment of Internationally Educated Nurses* comments on the ICN's condemnation of international recruitment by a country that has done inadequate planning to educate the number of nurses it requires or made efforts to keep nurses in nursing. They note Canadian policies support the need for human resource planning for the nursing workforce, but the implementation of plans is inadequate.

If Canadian human resource planning for the nursing workforce and efforts to keep nurses in the profession fall short, then our recruitment of nurses from developing countries is condemned by the ICN. This does not mean that nurses from any country, including developing countries, do not have the right to migrate to Canada, nor does it mean that when these nurses move to Canada their contribution is not valuable. However when recruitment efforts target a developing country, the needs of the targeted country for nurses may not be met, as in the case in the Philippines (RNAO, 2008) and India (Khadria, 2007), two countries where Canada has recruited nurses.

Similarly, the United States also recruits from the Philippines and India. In a study that examined the hiring of internationally educated nurses in the United States, the highest number came from the Philippines, followed by Canada and then India (Cho et al., 2011). The migration of Canadian nurses to the United States probably reflects in part the desire of nurses to travel and experience life in another country. As well, it may reflect the disconnect in human resource planning in Canada, where nursing programs are funded to graduate nurses to meet an anticipated nursing shortage, and yet these graduates are unable to find full-time positions here because of budget cuts.

Countries such as India have developed businesses to educate nurses and prepare them to meet the registration requirements of other countries (Khadria, 2007). While on one hand nurses from developing countries may be needed in their own country, on the other hand they have the right to migrate, often send funds home to support their families, and add to the richness and diversity of our health care system.

Innovative Approaches to Recruitment and Retention

Innovative approaches to recruitment and retention may be required to fill vacancies during a nursing shortage while preserving the ability to choose among many applicants. If nurses at a health care organizations work together to generate ideas for recruitment and retention, they may come up with an innovative strategy(s) that helps them attract nurses. Some recruitment strategies may require going "downstream" to create interest among high school or younger students in becoming a nurse. Changing the image of the nurse to a desirable career option; and/or to an option where minorities such as men, Aboriginal persons, mature students; and members of ethnic, racial, or religious minority groups feel welcome are other recruitment and retention strategies. Schools of nursing as well as health care settings have a role to play in changing the image of the nurse and making members of minorities feel included.

One strategy to attract and retain nurses that is within the control of the work group is good interactions among colleagues. One study that looked at the effects of a team-building intervention found increases in group cohesion, nurse–nurse interactions, and job enjoyment, and a reduction in turnover (DiMeglio, Padula, Piatek, et al., 2005).

Nursing departments where horizontal violence has become endemic may develop a reputation and have difficulty recruiting as well as retaining nurses (see Chapter 10, Team Building and Managing Conflict).

Another strategy for recruiting new graduates that is within the control of direct care nurses is to recognize the work of nursing students and help them feel part of the nursing team when they come to the department. A nursing team that compliments and treats students with respect goes a long way in making students feel this would be a good team to join. Nursing departments could link with a nursing school or class, and together work on a study of interest and benefit to both groups. This has the potential of students getting to know nurses in a department and feeling valued for their work on the project. Ultimately, the students may be attracted to apply for a job on this unit, in addition to the study's findings that would enrich patient care.

Another strategy that is within the control of nurse managers is flexible scheduling, including shifts of several hours to 12 hours that might start and end at times that are different from the majority of nurses in the department. Such flexible shifts can be a win for the organization, which gains nursing hours, and for the nurse who may only be able to work at specific times due to other commitments.

Involving nexters in decision making and nurses of all generations in continuing education and opportunities to rotate to other areas of nursing and be promoted while remaining in direct patient care are other strategies that can help with recruitment and retention. See Chapter 7, Motivation and Performance, for more information about promotions while remaining in direct patient care positions (career ladders).

Huckabay (2009) describes an innovative partnership designed to increase the number of graduates in California between a university school of nursing and a hospital. The partners developed a two-year (six-semester) bachelor's program at a time when the university school of nursing was experiencing budget cuts. They did this through increasing the size of theory classes and having clinical faculty members employed by the hospital teach clinical courses. Further, the hospital subsidized the students' tuition and books for those who agreed to be employed by the hospital for two years. Of the eight classes that had graduated at the time Huckabay's article was published, 95 percent of the graduates had been retained by the hospital.

One suggestion for retaining nexters is to recruit a cohort of this age group to a particular department, rather than dispersing one or two nexters in each department of an organization. Of course, you might want to have some baby boomer and generation X nurses also on the unit to share their experience and expertise to help ensure quality patient care. The cohort of nexters would be able to support each other and explore different ways of organizing work and using technology to support their care. Ultimately, the goal would be to share lessons learned from new ways of making clinical and administrative decisions and new ways of using technology and working with other departments within the organization and with other organizations.

The Leading Health Care Example in this chapter discusses initiatives to retain older workers. The retention of older nurses is an issue of importance in many Canadian health care organizations because many have a high percentage of employees nearing retirement at a time when there may be a shortage of nurses to hire.

In 2008, the Seven Oaks General Hospital in Winnipeg, Manitoba, had a high percentage of nurses and other health professionals who were older. As these professionals retired, the hospital would experience a large loss of expertise as well as many positions to fill at a time when there might be a shortage of persons to recruit. Employees at the Seven Oaks General Hospital initiated a *Retention of Older Workers* project that started by identifying what would keep older health professionals working. A survey of nurses and health professionals who were 45 years of age and older was performed and led to the findings that these professionals valued being respected and recognized for their work, flexible work hours and schedules, and sharing their knowledge with newer staff.

Based on the survey findings, a number of initiatives were piloted and evaluated. An Older Worker Leave initiative allowed older workers to have unpaid leave, to help them reduce fatigue and manage stress. The Older Worker Leave pilot was evaluated by interviews with the nurses who took leaves and their replacements, by focus groups of nurse managers, and surveys of both nurses who took leaves and the older nurses who decided not to take leaves. The findings showed the nurses who took the leaves were more rested and energetic when they returned to work. As well, they said it helped them prepare for retirement. Managers reported the nurses returned from leave feeling motivated; however they also reported some problems in covering their work while on leave and in those who were not allowed leaves feeling some resentment. Regrettably, for financial reasons, the Seven Oaks General Hospital was unable to continue the Older Worker Leave program.

Other initiatives included education about retirement and work–life balance and a nurse mentorship program. Participants in the education programs were satisfied with these programs. The nurse mentorship program continues to be used for all new nurses who are hired at Seven Oaks General Hospital.

Discussion Questions

1. What strategies can you identify to help keep older nurses in direct care positions?

2. Are there additional financial costs associated with the strategies that you identified to keep older nurses in the workplace? Are there other costs associated with these strategies such as their impact on the job satisfaction of younger nurses?

3. Are any of the strategies that you identified to keep older nurses in the workplace the same or different than those to keep new graduates in direct care positions?

Source: A new approach to reta-ining older workers. *The Canadian Nurse, 108*(6), 18–20. Reprinted by permission of the Canadian Nurses' Association.

Cost of a Nurse's Resignation

The financial cost of replacing a nurse includes advertising costs, time spent recruiting and selecting a replacement, orientation costs, and overtime costs while the position is vacant or the new nurse is being oriented. One estimate for the costs associated with the resignation of a nurse in the United States was US $82,000 (Jones, 2008). Estimates of the cost of replacing a nurse vary greatly, but even low estimates indicate this is costly for an organization, particularly when there is a high turnover rate (HSM Group, 2002). When a nurse resigns, a department may not be able to immediately replace the nurse. Lower registered nurse worked hours have been found to be associated with higher patient mortality (for example, Aiken et al., 2002; Needleman et al., 2011) and patient morbidity and adverse (events for example, Cho, Ketefian, Barkauskas, & Smith, 2003) that are associated with longer stays, and thus additional costs.

When health care administrators are approached with innovative ideas to retain nurses (or reduce turnover) they consider how much the innovation will cost. Studies are needed that look at the implementation of retention strategies along with an economic analysis of the costs incurred by the retention strategy and saved by reduced nurse replacement costs and patient morbidity, patient mortality, and longer stays associated with a vacant nurse position. Such studies may require the use of multi-sites and research teams that include an economist. However their findings may be powerful in convincing policy makers in health departments and administrators in health care organizations of the importance of a nurse retention strategy.

SUMMARY ON RECRUITMENT AND RETENTION

Hospitals with magnet characteristics have become known among the nursing community for their quality of work life and patient care, and will attract nurses to apply for a position and to remain there (McClure et al., 1983, Kramer, 1990). Many of the strategies for recruiting and retaining nurses that we have discussed in this chapter focus on implementing a characteristic of a magnet hospital. For example, nexters' desire to make decisions in the workplace is consistent with how magnet hospitals include nurses in nursing governance. Flexible scheduling and continuing education are other aspects related to quality of nurses' work life. More research is needed on what will help with recruitment and retention of nurses in non-hospital settings, including rural, community, primary care, and long-term care settings. This research should include an economic analysis to help convince policy makers and health care administrators of the cost benefits of recruitment and retention strategies.

SELECTING AND HIRING NURSES

The process of selecting a new nurse to be hired includes reviewing the applicant's application letter, resume, and possibly an application form, and interviewing the nurse. The process also includes checking references and obtaining a copy of the nurse's license to practise (Brooke, 2008), degrees and/or diplomas, and often a certificate of conduct. In most health care organizations, the hiring process is supported by the human resources department, which provides valuable information about laws related to hiring, such as those related to human rights and privacy.

The best predictor of future behaviour is generally considered to be past behaviour, and with that in mind it is important to obtain references when you are hiring. If the nurse is not a new graduate, it is good to obtain a reference from the nurse's previous manager(s). Ideally, you would obtain as many references as you can and from persons who have worked with the applicant in different capacities, sometimes referred to as 360-degree references. Persons who have worked with a nurse in different ways may have a different view of this nurse. For example, there are nurses who do well in university clinical and theory courses and are perceived positively by a nurse educator. However, this nurse may not enjoy working in teams and therefore be seen less positively by colleagues. A nurse may be viewed by his or her immediate supervisor or educator as someone who works well with them and possesses leadership skills. This same nurse may be seen as condescending and non consultative with support staff, and if given a management position, may be unpopular with his or her staff. However, this does not mean this nurse should not be hired, just that the type of position he or she would do best in needs to be considered.

While it is important to obtain references, a less-than-favourable reference does not necessarily mean that the person should not be hired. There are possible reasons why even good applicants may have a poor reference. For example, the applicant may not have been a good fit for another position or the person providing the reference may be problematic and not the applicant. Potential issues raised by a referee can be explored with other referees and with the applicant.

In many large health care organizations, human resources staff will telephone for a nurse's references. The questions asked by the human resources staff member may be standardized questions from a form and may not be the best questions to ask in relationship to the position. As well, the person who is providing the reference may be more forthcoming if he or she is talking with a nurse colleague. If in your organization the human resources department obtains references, we suggest that a nurse manager also contact at least one of the persons who agreed to provide a reference.

With both written letters and verbal references, it is important to look for what is not said as well as what is said. Many individuals are reluctant to provide negative information, perhaps fearing they could be sued if the person is not employed. Also, because of information laws it is possible the applicant may have access to his or her references. If any statements seem suggestive of a problem or if information appears to be missing, contact the person providing the reference again with follow-up questions.

As health care employers realize the importance of obtaining a large number of references and 360-degree references, nurses in direct care positions may be asked to provide a reference about a colleague. In most cases you will be happy to do this, with your only hesitation being that you will lose a valuable co-worker. If you are aware of an issue related to the nurse's competency at work such as the nurse's clinical judgment or substance use, there may be legal (Brooke, 2008) as well as ethical issues associated with withholding this information. For example, if the nurse is hired and later harms a patient while under the influence of a substance and the new employer learns you were aware this could happen, the employer could say your withholding of information led to this situation.

Interviewing Applicants

As nurses, we have developed our interviewing skills. Perhaps that is why we feel so confident about our ability to accurately select staff based on interview data. Yet job interviews do not always provide a valid assessment of the applicant (McDaniel et al., 1994).

A number of perceptual biases, such as stereotyping, can lead to not choosing the best applicant for the job. Another perceptual bias that can lead to inaccurate assessments about interviewees is described by Bruner's (1957) perceptual model. This model suggests that when we meet a new person we look for information to help us learn more about the person in order to categorize the person. If the first information we process about the person is positive, we may look for other positive cues. Eventually, if negative information is found we may discount this information. In an interview, when we first meet the applicant we may form either a positive or negative impression and then continue to build on this rather than providing equal weight to contrary information. This indicates the importance of the first few minutes of an interview when you are applying for a job.

One way to correct for individual bias in interviewing is to have a discussion about the desired characteristics of the person to be hired and make sure you do not hire someone who lacks these characteristics (Hader, 2009). Preparing interview questions in advance and sticking with these questions also improves the possibility of selecting the best applicant (McDaniel et al., 1994). One strategy used by many organizations is the group interview. A pitfall of a group interview for a new nursing position is that the group may put undue weight on the interview, rather than on other sources of information, such as references, previous experience, and education. Another difficulty with this approach occurs when the group does not obtain a consensus—how should the final decision be made? When someone who is not a good fit for a job is hired, it can consume much of management's time for months (or years) to come.

When a committee consisting of the manager and nursing representatives from the department interviews a nurse, the manager may have concerns that an applicant would not do well in a position but the other committee members feel positively about the applicant. This is a challenging situation for the manager, particularly those who are members of generation X and nexters who have less acceptance of a hierarchy in organizations than baby boomers. Nexters in particular expect to be able to make workplace decisions. In such a situation the manager may successfully have committee members understand his or her concerns. Committee members themselves may realize that for the success of a new nurse in the department, it is important that the manager and the new nurse be able to work together.

You can construct an interview guide based on the characteristics that you want the nurse hired to have. Obviously, when hiring a direct care nurse you will want to learn about the quality of nursing care a nurse provides. Most nurses work in both nursing and interdisciplinary teams, and therefore you need to know how they work with team members, managers, and support staff. You will also learn more about applicants by asking what work they would like to be doing five years from now (Hader, 2009). An interview can start by asking applicants to summarize their work experience, or clinical experiences during their educational program in the case of new graduates. Nurses who have worked in other positions can be asked why they left these positions (Hader, 2009). If the best predictor of future behaviour is past behaviour, previous unhappiness with managers or co-workers may indicate future unhappiness with their next manager or coworkers.

The Related Research box that discusses "The Gap Between Education Preferences and Hiring Practices" (Weinberg, et al., 2011) reflects a disconnect between what has been reported in the literature and managers' use of literature in making decisions. Clinical decisions are based on available evidence, but management decisions should also be based on evidence. This study's findings are limited in that only 27 managers in New York State were interviewed, and their views may differ from nurse managers in countries such as Canada. Nevertheless, the findings have implications for nurses applying for a position and may help all members of the nursing profession understand that nursing is a knowledge profession as well as a caring profession where work attitudes and personal characteristics are important.

RELATED RESEARCH

Nurse Managers' Hiring Preferences

The purpose of Weinberg and colleagues' (2011) study was to describe nurse managers' perceptions of diploma and bachelor of nursing graduates and how these perceptions influenced whom they hired. Their study was part of a larger study on nurses' education and patient outcomes. For the part of the larger study that investigated nurse managers' perceptions of graduates and hiring practices, they conducted telephone interviews with 27 nurse managers from eight hospitals (including university hospitals and small rural hospitals) in New York State. In this state, educational programs for registered nurses include both associate degree programs (often referred to as diploma-prepared nurses in Canada) and bachelor of nursing programs.

While a number of questions were asked during the telephone interviews, in this article the authors reported the nurse managers' responses to two questions:

1. What do you look for in hiring a new nurse?

2. How important is baccalaureate preparation for RN staff in your opinion? (p. 24)

Our summary of their article focuses on their findings for the first question.

The data were analyzed by forming categories of the responses. Only seven of the 27 nurse managers interviewed mentioned they looked for skills, education, and experience, while 23 stressed personality or attitude. Five nurse managers said they hired nurses more on their personality than on their education because this is what made someone a good nurse. A number of personality traits and attitudes were identified as important when hiring a nurse, including being hard working, dependable, flexible, interested in continuing education, and caring, and having good communication skills and a strong desire to be a nurse.

The researchers discuss how their finding that nurse managers emphasize personality traits and attitudes when hiring is contrary to the image that nursing is a knowledge profession where knowledge, judgment, and skill are needed for quality patient care.

Source: Weinberg, D., Cooney-Miner, D., Perioff, J., & Bourgoin, M. (2011). The gap between education preferences and hiring practices. *Nursing Management, 42*(9), 23–28.

Behavioural-based Interview Questions

Behavioural-based interviews are used because we know that past behaviour is a good predictor of future behaviour. A **behavioural-based interview question** asks the applicant to describe a particular type of situation he or she experienced and how he or she managed it. The interviewer then assesses how the applicant dealt with the situation (Klingner & Nalbandian, 2003). For example, if you want to know how a nurse would deal with a complaint from a family member, you could ask him or her to think of an example of this situation and describe this situation. Next, you could ask the nurse how he or she dealt with this situation. Similarly, if you want to know how a nurse might deal with receiving multiple requests, you could ask the nurse to describe a situation like this and how he or she handled it.

You may wish to learn how the applicant performs under stress. If you decide to do this by putting the applicant under stress during the interview, you will learn how he or she deals with stress in the context of a job interview. If you wish to learn how the applicant deals with stress in a clinical situation, ask a behavioural-based interview question. For example, "Can you think of a time in your clinical practice when you felt stressed, and describe it?" After the applicant describes the situation, follow up with "How did you manage this situation?" Rather than putting the applicant under even more stress than is already experienced during a job interview, you want the applicant to feel relaxed in order that he or she can share with you as much information as possible.

Behavioral-based questions may take more time than other types of interview questions. The applicant should be told that he or she can take a few minutes to think of a situation (Strausser, 2005). The goal is not that the applicant thinks of a situation immediately, but that the interviewer hears a rich description of the applicant's previous performance that will allow the interviewer to assess potential future performance.

Recruiting Nurses while Interviewing

All interviews include a component of recruitment. Even when you interview a nurse whom you suspect you will not hire, it is important to be respectful. The applicant is a colleague who has taken the time to come to your organization and be interviewed. The applicant will also share impressions of your health care setting with other nurses and therefore, his or her view will contribute to your reputation and ultimately to your future applicant pool. A good question to end an interview with is, "Is there any aspect of your education or experience that we did not ask you that you think would be useful for us to know?" This prevents the applicant from thinking that you did not provide enough opportunity to get to know him or her.

When there are a number of vacant nursing positions and few applicants, nurses conducting the interview may start talking about the positive points of their workplace and why the applicant should choose to work there. This may shorten the time available to learn about the applicant. As well, if you describe the strengths of the nursing team and the forthcoming objectives of the team prior the interview questions, the applicant may describe him- or herself in a way that is consistent with what you said, which may not be an accurate description. Discussing only the positive points of a position prior to hiring a new nurse can also lead this person to be surprised by negative aspects of the position. (All jobs and organizations have these.) To prepare an applicant for the position he or she is applying for, the interviewer can provide a **realistic job preview**, which is a description of both positive and negative features of the position that is provided to a job applicant before he or she accepts a position (Wanous, 1992).

While there are potential problems with recruiting while interviewing, Mayer and Carroll (2011) describe an innovative approach they implemented that combines recruitment with interviewing. Using this approach, they were able to fill their vacancies with the candidates they desired. They developed a vision for nursing that nursing leaders shared with applicants to help them feel as though they could be an important part of the hospital's culture. The chief nursing officer met with applicants and shared this vision and the hospital's values. Instead of the human resources department screening a few applications for the nursing selection committee to interview, all applicants were interviewed. Rather than informing the applicant the time for his or her interview, the applicant was asked to provide a good time for the interview. Applicants were greeted warmly and enthusiastically and were interviewed using behavioural interview questions.

The strategy discussed by Mayer and Carroll (2011) was designed to help inform the nursing community about the hospital's nursing vision. Approaches such as meeting with the chief nursing officer and asking the applicant what time would be convenient for an interview convey respect for and the importance of the applicant. At the same time, we caution that, if you can tell from their applications there are applicants whom you would not hire, taking their time for an interview in order that you can inform the community about your nursing department is not an ethical managerial practice. Also, we suggest informing the applicant not only about your vision for the future and positive aspects of the position but also any less-than-positive aspects. It is preferable that applicants have an accurate view of the position in order to make an informed decision when accepting the position, rather than being shocked when they start work, and later resigning. To assist with this, applicants can be invited to spend time in a department and to meet members of the work team during their application process.

SOCIALIZATION AND TRANSITIONING

Socialization

Professional socialization for nurses is the process whereby new nurses learn and internalize the knowledge, skills, values, attitudes, and norms of their profession that guide their behaviour in their professional role (Howskins & Ewens, 1999). For example, socialization to the nursing profession involves learning the importance of respecting all persons, therapeutic communication skills, and being caring with clients. Thus, professional socialization provides members of the nursing profession with the characteristics of the profession that clients recognize and expect from nurses. Regrettably, professional socialization may also involve learning less-than-desirable knowledge, skills, values, and norms. For example, nursing students in the clinical setting may experience nurses who do not support them, and after graduating they may treat students similarly.

Professional socialization starts when students enter their professional education program and continues after they graduate. In addition to being socialized to the profession, when nurses begin a new position they are also socialized to this role. **Role socialization** is the process whereby an employee learns the work setting's policies, procedures, norms, and role expectations associated with a job. For example, role socialization for a nursing position might include learning the norm of what clothes to wear in the health setting, the norm related to taking sick days, and the norm related to bullying other nurses. (Chapter 10, Team Building and Managing Conflict, discusses bullying other nurses or horizontal violence in more detail). Depending on the norms, the socialization of new nurses to existing practices will have positive or negative outcomes for the setting, to clients, and/or to the nurses themselves.

Socialization to Nursing

Price, a Canadian researcher, did a qualitative meta-synthesis of ten qualitative studies that examined why people entered nursing and how they then became socialized to the profession (to being a nurse) (Price, 2008). A qualitative meta-synthesis is a review procedure that involves analyzing findings from a number of qualitative studies to find a higher level of themes. Of the ten studies in this meta-synthesis, three of the studies were done in Canada, two in the United Kingdom, two in the United States, one in Australia, one in Japan, and one in Sweden. Three main themes were found in this meta-synthesis: *influence of ideals*, *paradox of caring*, and *role of others*.

Price found that, in all of the studies, the process of becoming socialized to nursing involved nurses reconstructing their view of what nursing was to help them adjust to the difference between their original view and the reality of their nursing practice in the workplace. *Influence of ideals* refers to the nurses' original ideals about nursing, such as the desire to care for others and make a difference, that often led them to choose nursing as a career. *Paradox of caring* reflects how the nurses' view of their profession as caring was challenged by seeing nurses who were uncaring. This theme also reflects the nurses' ambivalence about being viewed only as caring and their desire to be seen as knowledgeable and competent. *Role of others* reflects how the desire to be accepted by others influenced nurses' socialization. The nurses assumed the values and behaviours of other nurses but also behaved in ways the public expected of their profession.

The importance of the role of others in the socialization of new nurses is supported by an ethnographic study in Sweden designed to study the socialization of new nurses in hospitals (Bisholt, 2012). Ethnographic research is a type of qualitative research where people are studied in their own environment to understand their behaviour and culture. Eighteen new nurses on four hospital medical or surgical units were observed as well as interviewed to ask about some of the observations. The researcher found one main theme, *being formed into the profession*, and five categories for this theme:

1. being accepted in the profession,
2. being questioned in the profession,
3. being integrated into a hierarchical organization,
4. finding oneself in alienation, and
5. developing through taking responsibility.

The theme *being formed in the profession* captures how the new nurse is formed through open and hidden norms and social rules. *Being accepted in the profession* captures the importance of being accepted by other nurses, which in part requires that the new nurses accept the unit's culture. *Being questioned in the profession* captures the new nurses' awareness that other professionals questioned their education and whether they would be able to meet the requirements of a practising nurse. *Being integrated into a hierarchical organization* reflects new nurses learning what their role was and how they should behave in relationship to the roles of others in the organization. *Finding oneself in alienation* reflects the idea that new nurses who do not assume the norms and behaviours expected by the other nurses became outsiders on the unit. New nurses who became outsiders were ignored, spoken to negatively, blamed for things, and/or talked about in negative terms when they weren't present. While the researcher does not use the term violence to describe these behaviours, they do reflect inter-colleague or horizontal violence. *Developing through taking responsibility* captures how the new nurses developed when they made patient care decisions themselves rather than with more senior nurses.

Implications of Socialization for Nursing Research

That nurses' desire to be accepted by others influences their socialization to the profession is supported by the evidence. Therefore, positive role models are crucial not only when nurses begin their career but also throughout their careers. Professional socialization is most intense for new nurses; however, it continues throughout their career. Nursing educators, preceptors, and mentors play an important role in determining how new nurses will internalize their profession and interact with clients. In particular, it is important when new nurses are hired by a health setting to assign them to preceptors or mentors who set positive examples of caring and to nursing departments where there is a culture of caring and respect for others.

As well, if new nurses who resist adapting undesirable norms or behaviours are treated as outsiders, a cycle of violence within the nursing profession may start. Nurses who are treated badly may later behave similarly with others. We need to figure out how to stop this cycle in nursing. The cycle can start early if, when students, they observe a nurse providing poor care or being unhelpful with a student and the approach of the nursing instructor is to discuss with students that this is not right but to not discuss this with the nurse. Nursing instructors may be concerned that if they address problems with unit staff or managers then they will not be welcomed on the unit or be treated even less favourably in the future. Indeed, most nursing instructors can probably give a few examples to illustrate this. What may be needed are efforts at a higher level within both schools of nursing and health care settings. Administrators should discuss what is happening between staff and students on a unit and how conflicts can be resolved. Efforts such as these may be required as part of the plan to foster successful transitioning of new nurses to the workplace.

There are some realities of nursing practice that nursing students need to come to terms with, such as shift work and the need to shift priorities to deal with the workload on a particular day. There are also professional care and interpersonal issues that practising nurses may need to change to ensure new nurses are treated ethically and are retained in the profession. One way might be to create awareness among nurses of the importance of a positive socialization process for new nurses for retaining these nurses in the profession and for decreasing the cycle of violence in the profession. Another way might be to ensure new nurses are in a supportive environment. These areas need more work to develop and evaluate innovative approaches. It is indeed a paradox that people go into nursing because they want to help others and are caring with their clients, yet can be hurtful toward other nurses. All nurses need to be aware of the existence of this paradox and the need to care about their colleagues the same way they do their clients—as persons worthy of respect and support.

Transitioning

Reality Shock

If new nursing graduates find the knowledge, skills, values, attitudes, or norms in the workplace vary much from those they learned in their nursing program, they find the transition difficult. In 1974, Kramer coined the term **reality shock** to describe the reactions of nursing graduates to the realities of what was expected of them in their first job. In her landmark study, Kramer (1974) noted that the new nurses found the values they had learned during their nursing education conflicted with the type of care they were able to provide in the workplace. She identified four phases that nurses move through over this transition period: honeymoon, shock, recovery, and resolution. Ultimately, if the new nurses were unable to work through the recovery and resolution phases, they either remained unhappy with their nursing role or left the profession.

Kramer's (1974) identification of the reality shock experienced by new nurses has resulted in nurse educators and nurse leaders in health care organizations working to make the transition from the role of student nurse to the workplace easier. Despite almost four decades of efforts to reduce reality shock, new nurses still find the transition difficult. This may be partly because patients are more acutely ill, not only in hospital settings but also in community and residential settings. Partly, this may be because to help nursing students learn what holistic, quality patient care is, nurse educators use tools such as nursing care plans wherein students identify every possible client issue and client strength. When students graduate, they find that not only are nursing care plans not used, but also the job they are hired to do does not allow time to consider all client issues. In addition, during their nursing program students may be assigned to community settings where there are no nursing jobs to help them identify what nurses could do in such a setting. When students are later employed, they are not able to focus on every possible client issue as they did when students. In community settings, new graduates may be assigned a high load of clients or programs and not have time to develop innovative programs.

Nursing students may wonder why educators employ nursing care plans and clinical practice in community settings that do not hire nurses, when these strategies differ from the work they will be hired to do after graduation. These educational methods help students learn what holistic, quality nursing care is and what nursing could do in unstructured settings. This helps to graduate nurses who know what excellence in care is and who are able to identify innovative interventions and roles for nurses in novel situations. Perhaps nurse educators could inform nursing students why they use these teaching strategies: that they may differ from what is experienced in the workplace, but that there will be opportunities

Novice Nurses and Quality of Work Life

Ten novice nurses who had graduated less than two years ago were interviewed to answer the research question "What are the factors influencing the quality of work life for novice nurses?" Eight of the novice nurses worked in an acute care hospital, one in long-term care, and one in mental health, all in St. John's, Newfoundland and Labrador.

The research findings included that this was both an exciting and a stressful time for the novice nurses who felt very motivated to provide quality care. Their greatest reward came from connecting with patients and family members. The researchers identified four themes: *human resources issues, workload and work life, relationships,* and *support and mentoring issues.*

Human resources issues captured the novice nurses' comments that if they had been on the unit as a student and this had been a good experience, or had a good preceptor, their transition to the workplace was easier. In contrast, if they did not feel valued during the hiring process or were hired for float or part-time positions, their transition was more difficult.

Workload and work life captured that, as with experienced nurses, workload and work life issues have a negative impact on nurses. As well, the novice nurses noted that they were expected to carry the same workload as experienced nurses, and this made them feel stressed and be concerned for patient safety. *Relationships* is related to the novice nurses' anxiety from experiencing or observing difficult personalities (other nurses, health care professionals, managers, and so on) and included the experience of verbal abuse, bullying, and intimidation. *Support and mentoring issues* describes how the novice nurses found support or lack of support from other nurses and nurse managers had an impact on their transition, including how valued they felt.

The researchers presented a list of suggestions made by the novice nurses, about how health settings could help them transition to the workplace.

Source: Based on Weinberg, D., Cooney-Miner, D., Perioff, J., & Bourgoin, M. (2011). The gap between education preferences and hiring practices. *Nursing Management,* 42(9), 23–28.

when what the students have learned will come in useful, particularly after they develop expertise in a clinical setting and it becomes less time consuming to provide required care.

Career Planning and Successful Transitioning

Many nursing students assume career planning should start in their final year of nursing education, when they start to look for a job (Waddell, Donner, & Wheeler, 2009). However, when you enter nursing school you have already started to plan your career by selecting the profession of nursing (Waddell et al., 2009). As well, by the time you graduate, you should have a vision for your career. Rather than looking for a job in your final year of nursing studies, you can look for a nursing position where you will be able to develop the skills you need for the positions you would like to hold in 5, 10, and 25 years time. The interview with Janice Waddell RN, PhD, at the end of this chapter provides useful advice about successful transition planning including how to prepare for obtaining a nursing position.

Unsuccessful Transitioning

A number of studies have looked at resignation rates for new graduates during their first year of practice and found them to be high, for example, "30% (Bowles & Candela, 2005), 36% (Beecroft, Kunzman, & Krozek, 2001), and 47% (Nelson, Godfrey, & Purdy, 2004)" (Hoffart, Waddell, & Young, 2011, p. 335). To a certain extent, the high rate of resignation among new graduates is due to them wanting to experience different types of nursing and continue learning by rotating through departments or organizations, something they learned to do as a student. Further, many of these resignations may be associated with new nurses taking a position in an area where they would prefer to work; for example a nurse may start working in a general medical or surgical department and then accept a position in a medical or surgical specialty department or in the community. Other resignations may be associated with new nurses temporarily leaving the profession but returning later. Nevertheless, the high rates of resignation of nurses during their first year of employment are shocking and suggest their first work setting is unattractive to them and/or they find the transition to the workplace difficult.

Programs to Ease Transition

In an article that reviewed research on the effectiveness of programs to ease the transition of new graduates to the role of the nurse, the authors note that decades after Kramer (1974) identified reality shock, new nurses still have difficulty in transitioning to the workplace (Hoffart et al., 2011). One strategy that many schools of nursing have used to ease the transition is a preceptored clinical course, yet in their review of the literature Hoffart et al. found relatively few studies to assess the effectiveness of these preceptored courses. Other strategies are summer externships, or the employment of nursing students by health agencies during the summer, and cooperative education, or the integration of paid work terms into the nursing program. While Canadian schools of nursing have not historically used work terms, other countries have. For example, an Irish university includes a 47-week period during the fourth year of the nursing program when students are supported by the health setting and their university, are assigned patient care, and are paid by the health setting (Deasy, Doody, & Tuohy, 2011).

While a limited number of studies have evaluated approaches to ease the transition of new nurses to the workplace and found some positive outcomes, in general the studies are limited in that the approach is only offered by one school or one health setting and to a limited number of students. For more conclusive knowledge about the effectiveness of these programs, it would be useful to study a strategy that was implemented across schools and included all students at these schools (Hoffart et al., 2011). Similarly, strategies to ease transition that are offered by health care organizations include orientation programs, mentorship programs, internships or residencies, and clinical experiences either using patient simulation or on a special education unit. Hoffart et al. note that findings were mixed in studies that have looked at the effectiveness of these programs on outcomes for the new nurses, such as job stress, job satisfaction, support from nurses on the unit. Studies that have looked at the effectiveness of these programs on outcomes for the employers, such as turnover intent, turnover (or the reverse, retention), and return on investment (ROI) or the savings from reduced turnover compared with the cost of the program, suggest the programs are beneficial. As with the studies that have evaluated programs offered by schools of nursing to ease transition, the studies that evaluated the programs offered by health agencies are limited in that often only one site is evaluated, the number of new nurses may be small, there is no control group or, if there is a control group, new nurses were not randomly assigned.

Hoffart et al. (2011) recommend that, to learn more about how we can ease transition to the workplace or reduce reality shock, we need longitudinal studies, which look at outcomes over time, and are multi-institutional, which look at outcomes from a program offered at different sites. Longitudinal studies could examine the effects of programs offered by schools of nursing, such as preceptored courses not only on outcomes for students at the time of their graduation but during their first years of work. Multi-institutional programs could look at the effect of a program offered at a number of schools of nursing and/or a number of health settings. They also suggest that rather than schools of nursing and health settings working separately to develop separate programs to ease transition to the workplace, they could work together to develop a program that starts at schools of nursing and continues into the workplace.

A study in Alberta examined the expectations of new nurses, direct care nurses, nurse educators, and employers for the performance of new nurses, as well as recommendations to ease the transition of new nurses to the workplace (Romyn et al., 2009). This study is summarized in Related Research.

RELATED RESEARCH

The Transition of New Nurses to the Workplace

Romyn and colleagues, researchers in Alberta, designed a qualitative, descriptive study to increase understanding of the expectations of persons in educational settings and in practice settings for the performance of new graduate nurses. An additional purpose of the study was to identify innovative strategies for helping new nurses transition to the practice setting. The researchers were interested in the transition of registered nurses, licensed practical nurses, and registered psychiatric nurses (a category of nursing staff who are educated and registered in Manitoba, Saskatchewan, Alberta, and British Columbia).

The researchers reviewed literature that found that employers want new nurses to be able function as a nurse when they are employed (Ellerton & Gregor, 2003, cited in Romyn et al.) and that new nurses are often expected to function at the same level as experienced nurses in the setting even though they are just learning the setting's policies and procedures (Romyn et al.). They note this expectation contrasts with Benner's (1984) findings that nurses' expertise goes through five phases of development: *novice, advanced beginner, competent, proficient,* and *expert* and that new nurses are likely to be at the phase of *advanced beginner.*

To learn more about the transition of nursing graduates to the workplace, the researchers held discussion groups with participants from eight different Alberta health regions. Participants were 14 new nurses and 133 staff nurses, employers, or educators. In addition, 5 new nurses and 34 staff nurses, employers, or educators emailed or faxed input. The majority of participants were employed in hospitals (95%) with the minority employed in the community (5%). Very few licensed practical nurses (1%) or

(Continued)

registered psychiatric nurses (< 4%) participated, with registered nurses making up the majority of the participants (95%).

After obtaining research ethics approval, 15 discussion groups were held, 6 of which were with only new nurses. The discussion questions included:

- How would you describe the gap between new graduates' knowledge and skills and the expectations placed on them in employment settings?

- What strategies would you suggest to help narrow the gap?

- How would you describe a successful transition to practice?

- What have you either observed or experienced that assists in a successful transition?

- What would fundamentally change for the better the transition of the new graduate to the workplace? (p. 5)

The data were analyzed using content analysis to identify themes. The findings were combined with those from a literature review to develop recommendations.

The researchers found that there was a gap between new graduates' performance and the expectations in the workplace. The participants recognized this gap but believed that it was unrealistic to expect new graduates to function as experienced nurses. Suggestions to help new nurses function better in hospital settings included changing nurse education programs from generalist preparation by eliminating some community rotations, reducing the number of different placement settings a student is rotated to, and having a senior practicum experience in the area they will work.

Participants also suggested more "hands-on" experience during educational programs and a stronger emphasis on anatomy, physiology, pathophysiology, normal lab values, physical assessment skills, and nursing procedures. Other suggestions included having nurses work as paid employees during their educational experience for course credit, and instituting an internship year either as the final year of a four-year program or as an additional, fifth year. Participants also spoke of the urgent nursing care needs in health care settings. New nurses spoke of their fear of making a mistake and their reluctance to burden other nurses when they needed help, as well as the nurses' responses if they felt the new nurses should not require help. The importance of mentoring and the need to protect some of nurses' time to allow for mentoring was discussed. Another suggestion was that nurse educators and clinical nurses should work together to support new nurses. Participants spoke of how clinical educator positions in nursing departments had been cut, but these positions were important for supporting new nurses. Generational differences were also identified as a potential source of misunderstandings.

Romyn and colleagues present recommendations to improve new nurses' transition to health care settings. Some of the recommendations were for policy makers, such as the recommendation for a funded, provincial strategy for the transition of new nurses. Other recommendations were for schools of nursing, such as ensuring curricula evolve with the changing needs of health care settings. Recommendations for workplaces included helping registered nurses, licensed practical nurses, and registered psychiatric nurses work to their scope of practice; employing nursing students; supporting new nurses in the workplace; and resolving scheduling, workload, and absenteeism problems. Recommendations such as an internship program and receiving university credit for paid employment require nurse educators and practice leaders to work together.

This is a summary of the research article by Romyn, D., Linton, N., Giblin, C., Hendrickson, B., Limacher, L., Murray, C., Zimmel, C. (2009). Successful transition of the new graduate nurse. *International Journal of Nursing Education Scholarship,* 6(1). (17p)

Literature cited in Romyn et al. (2009):

Benner, P. (1984). *From novice to expert. Excellence and power in clinical nursing practice.* Menlo Park, CA: Addison-Wesley.

Ellerton, M., & Gregor, F. (2003). A study of transition: The new nurse graduate at three months. *The Journal of Continuing Education in Nursing, 34,* 102–107.

Source: Romyn, D., Linton, N., Giblin, C., Hendrickson, B., Limacher, L., Murray, C., Zimmel, C. (2009). Successful transition of the new graduate nurse. *International Journal of Nursing Education Scholarship*, 6,(1), p.17.

RELATED RESEARCH

The Effectiveness of a Career Planning Intervention for Nursing Students

Janice Waddell, a nurse researcher at Ryerson University has recently conducted a study with Dr. Karen Spalding, Dr. Jennifer Stinson, Dr. Linda McGillis Hall, and Michelle Connell entitled *Building a Career Resilient Nursing Workforce: A Curriculum-Based Career Planning and Development Program*. The objectives of this study were to:

1. Examine the effect of a career planning and development (CPD) program compared to standard curriculum (without CPD) on the development of career resilience in baccalaureate nursing students using a single blind randomized controlled study design, and

2. Examine the impact of a faculty career intervention on nursing faculty outcomes of confidence in providing student career coaching and education.

A randomized control trial design (with repeated measures) (pre- and post-test and at 12-month follow-up) was used to evaluate the CPD intervention in undergraduate nursing students in a collaborative baccalaureate program. Eligible undergraduate nursing students were randomly assigned to one of two conditions: a) 4-year CPD group (intervention group), or b) 4-year standard undergraduate curriculum without the intervention (control group). Faculty participants were randomly assigned to the CPD educator/ coach intervention or control group. The study was conducted at three academic sites of an urban collaborative nursing degree program. The collaborative nursing degree program shares a common curriculum across one university and two community college sites, with the BScN degree granted to all students by the university site. Student participants were drawn from

(Continued)

a target population of first-year under-graduate nursing students across the collaborative program. Faculty participants were drawn from across the collaborative program sites.

Student Intervention: The Career Planning and Development Program used in this study was a standardized, multi--component CPD model developed by Donner and Wheeler (2001). The design of the CPD program intervention was slightly modified to respond to the student context, based on findings from a CPD pilot study conducted at one collaborative program academic site (Waddell & Bauer, 2005). All participants were introduced to the CPD model in a 3-hour workshop. Following the introduction to the model, the program was designed as year-specific working sessions wherein the model was used to guide and structure intervention discussions across all years of the curriculum. Year-specific working sessions were held per term for each year group. Application of the model was consistent across all years of the program and is responsive to unique curricular foci and unique student experiences within the context of their program year. Two faculty educators with expertise in career coaching facilitated workshops for each year. The faculty intervention trained faculty educators to lead the student groups as beginning career coaches. The control group did not receive the CPD intervention during the 4 years of the program but were offered the intervention after the 12-month follow-up.

Quantitative and qualitative data were collected from student participants in both intervention and control study groups at the outset of the study and at the conclusion of each academic year, as well as at 12 months post graduation. Questionnaires measured perceived career resilience and career decision-making self-efficacy. Semi-structured focus groups explored participants' perception of their sense of career resilience and career decision-making self-efficacy.

Faculty Intervention: In order to build capacity and sustainability of this intervention, faculty needed to enhance their knowledge and comfort level in providing CPD education and coaching to undergraduate students. Intervention group faculty participated in a training program that provided them with the knowledge and skills to a) facilitate student career planning development workshops and b) be beginning career coaches. Each faculty coach had the experience of observing workshops across program years, providing supervised workshops to intervention student groups, and supervised career coaching.

Qualitative data, through semi-structured focus groups, were collected from faculty participants in both intervention and control study groups. Focus group discussions were held at the outset and conclusion of the study to explore faculty members' perceived sense of confidence in their role as career educators/coaches and their sense of career satisfaction.

Acknowledgement: This summary was written by Dr. Janice Waddell. Please see the interview in this chapter for a brief biography of Janice Waddell.

Literature cited: Donner, G. & Wheeler, M. (2001). *International Nursing Review, 48*(2), 79–85.

Waddell, J. & Bauer, M. (2005). Career planning and development for students: Building a career in a professional practice discipline. *Canadian Journal of Career Development, 4*(2), 4–13.

Source: From Dr. Janice Waddell, Professor at Ryerson University. Reprinted with permission.

Janice Waddell RN, PhD

Dr. Janice Waddell is Associate Dean, Faculty of Community Services at Ryerson University and Associate Professor of the Daphne Cockwell School of Nursing. In these roles, as well as her past role as Associate Director of the Ryerson, Centennial, George Brown Collaborative Nursing Degree Program, she has been engaged in undergraduate and graduate program curriculum development, coaching and mentoring faculty colleagues and providing guidance and support to students.

Janice has worked for the last several years with the Canadian Nursing Student Association to provide career development workshops at the local, provincial, and national levels and has been awarded a CNSA Honorary Life Membership for her contributions to the professional development of student nurses across Canada. Janice has had a long-standing commitment to advancing the professional development and career success of student, new graduate, and early to mid-career nurses.

Q: What suggestions do you have for graduate nurses when they apply for their first job?

A: First, create a career vision which describes where you want to go in your nursing career. Your vision is kind of like your professional fantasy. Ask yourself what are your hopes and dreams for your future. Who do you wish to be as a person and as a nurse, how would you like colleagues to describe you, what kind of work do you hope to be doing, and what type of organization will help you attain your career vision?

Know yourself and what you can offer to the success of the organization and what you need from the organization to be happy and successful in your role as a registered nurse. You can do this by completing a self-assessment that focuses on your values, interests, knowledge, and skills related to your unique career vision. Reflect on the strengths that you have that will help you achieve your vision and the areas of development that you would need to address to "live" your vision. If you don't have one area of interest, your self-assessment can consolidate your overall professional interests, skills, and knowledge base. Obtain a copy of the job description to determine how your skills, knowledge, and interests fit with the job requirements. With each specific job you apply for, you can refine your assessment to respond to the particular position—that is, streamline the self-assessment to help you articulate how your strengths will contribute to your success in the position and how the position would help you to develop in key areas. The position should also allow you to continue to advance toward your career vision.

Identify what you would seek from the organization to continue your development as a nurse. Research the organization's philosophy, mandate, and the resources of the nursing department and assess how well these fit with the values and interests in your career vision. As a new graduate, you have unique needs as you transition to the role of graduate nurse. How does the organization respond to your unique transition needs?

Consider how you can shape your work in any position you take on in such a way that you are building your nursing career—rather than getting a job.

Take time before going for a job interview to learn the current trends and issues in your area of interest, health care in general, and the organization in particular.

Get a business card. You can make your own card by going to websites designed for this person. As a student, you can include your university email address and the name of your nursing program and university. Use your business card as an attachment to your resume, and a marketing tool to give to colleagues and employers you meet at career fairs. It can be an effective tool to help you market yourself across many situations!

(Continued)

Finally, it is never too early to start planning your career. Your career does not begin at graduation; you began your nursing career the day you sat in your first nursing class. With each course you take, and each assignment you do, think about how you can shape your learning so that you are progressing toward being the kind of nurse you describe in your career vision.

Q: Are there tips for having a good job interview?

A: There are many things I can suggest, and many of them seem little, but they can make a difference!

- Find out if you will be interviewed by an individual manager or a panel, who the persons interviewing you are and their roles. Knowing what to expect will give you a chance to think about how to prepare for your interview and respond to questions. Different persons are interested in different information about you.
- Confirm the place of the interview and the site. Don't assume that, if you are being interviewed by a large, multi-site organization, that your interview will be at the main site.
- Visit the site of the interview prior to your interview, learn how to get there and where there is parking or the nearest public transit station. Take into consideration that there may be traffic or other delays on the way to the interview, so give yourself plenty of time to get there so you are not feeling stressed when you arrive.
- Do not schedule another meeting following your interview. If your interview goes longer than you anticipated, you don't want to be feeling pressure about whether you will get to your next appointment on time. You want to be able to focus on the interview so that you can market yourself in the best way possible.
- Research the values, mission, philosophy, and strategic plan of the organization. Be able to articulate your own career goals related to the organization's goals. Also think about your strengths and how these can help the organization meet their goals. Be enthusiastic about how the work in the organization can help you to build your nursing career.
- Prepare questions to ask that are aligned with the key values from your career vision. Interviewers will get a sense of who you are and you will gain information to help you determine if this organization is a good fit with who you are and how you wish to develop as a nurse. Also, prepare questions related to your self-development plan to learn if this organization is one where you can work toward your goals. You may end up not asking these questions if they are covered during the interview, but it is good to have them prepared.
- You may be asked about your weaknesses and therefore be prepared to discuss these in relation to your self-development plan.
- If you are asked where you would like to be in 5 years, do not think of your response in terms of which organization or region you would like to be working in. Talk about where you see yourself as a professional in 5 years' time. The work you will have done to create your career vision will help you to articulate your response.
- Do a practice interview.
- Bring extra copies of your resume in case the interviewers do not have one at hand. Be polite and respectful of everyone in the organization. Remember that everyone you encounter from the time you enter the building may give their impression to the person in charge of hiring.
- Choose who you will use as referees carefully, and you may wish to use different referees, as the positions to which you are applying may require different competencies. You may choose to request references from referees who can best speak to how your strengths fit with the requirements of the nursing positions to which you are applying.

- As a new graduate, at least one of your referees will be one of your nursing professors. When considering faculty referees for specific positions, consider how well the professor can speak to the fit between your strengths and the competencies required for the position. You may wish to meet with the professor and update him or her on your achievements and objectives so that they can provide a strong reference; bring your updated resume to the meeting and let the professor know what you would like them to focus on for their reference.
- When you ask someone if he or she will provide you with a reference, be direct and ask if they will provide you with a *positive* reference. If they hesitate, you may wish to consider asking someone else.
- The organization is interested in what you can contribute to patient care and in your enthusiasm for learning, the profession, and how you see your potential as a positive and contributing team member.
- During the interview, try and be yourself. Remember that the interview is a mutual process with you and the interviewers having an interest in learning about one other in order to make a decision that will be the right one for all.

Q: What recommendations do you have for writing a job application letter or preparing a resume?

A: Whether you are a first-, second-, third-, or fourth-year nursing student, begin to build your resume now. Create your career vision as early as possible and re-visit regularly as you progress through your nursing program. Develop headings for each component of your resume (career objective, education, clinical placements completed within each year of your program); focus on competencies you developed and your unique accomplishments within each placement setting; recent employment; extracurricular activities; volunteer work; awards; and professional memberships. Early in your nursing program, you may not have a

great deal of activity to include in some of these components. However, you can use these components as prompts to seek opportunities to help build a rich resume. Review your resume regularly, and add your activities and accomplishments on an ongoing basis. This version of your resume is generic. You can then customize your generic resume in your applications to various positions—including those experiences and accomplishments that best fit with the requirements of the position. You may wish to provide additional details about your strengths and achievements that you believe will be of most relevance for the position.

In your cover letter, you do not need to repeat everything that is in your resume. Instead, highlight what you think you can contribute to the role and organization and how you believe you can further your professional development within the role. Remember to attach your business card!

Q: Are there questions a nurse should ask at the end of the job interview to help ensure the job will be a good fit?

A: Prepare one question for each of the key values you have identified in your self-assessment. Ask about what you might expect in terms of your orientation, if you will be working with a preceptor, and, if so, how that relationship is structured. You may wish to know about the skill mix on the unit you would be working on and what other health care professionals you would be collaborating with in your day-to-day work. Ask your interviewers how they would describe the ideal candidate for this position and what they believe are the major challenges of this position.

Q: What advice would you give a new graduate who is transitioning to his or her new role as a graduate nurse?

A: As a new graduate you need to be confident about your strengths. You have graduated with a bachelor's degree in nursing and passed the national exam, and therefore you have demonstrated that you possess the entry-level competencies for your professional practice.

(Continued)

Remember that as a student, you have experienced many different clinical settings across diverse health care organizations. The breadth of your experiences can illustrate your current level of knowledge and practice competencies and your demonstrated ability to adapt to new situations and change.

Get involved, both in your professional association and in your organization.

Seek out a potential mentor and ask this person to be your mentor. A nursing professor is often a good choice because they know your background, are aware of some of the issues you will be facing, and have an interest in graduates of their program doing well. However, select someone who you feel comfortable with, is accessible, and who you can talk to during your transition, because challenges during this time are inevitable and part of the process. Do not get discouraged during your early career; it is important to continue to reflect on your career vision and keep it alive. Having a mentor to talk with about your career may help you to do this.

It may happen, particularly if there is not a nursing shortage in the region where you wish to work, that you have to take a job in an area that is not your first choice. For example, you may wish to work with acutely ill children but the only position you can find is with the elderly in a long-term care centre. In this case, go back and look at the competencies you wish to develop in order to be successful in pediatric nursing practice and think about how you can develop these competencies in your new position. For example, you may wish to develop competencies in family-centred care, physical and psychosocial assessment, developmental care, and interprofessional teamwork. You can develop each of these competencies in long-term care, and your knowledge and skills in working with the elderly will position you to be successful in your work with children and families. Try to avoid framing your job in long-term care as a position you had to take but do not want; rather, frame it as an opportunity to develop competencies that span the care of the elderly and children. It can be "freeing" to realize that, regardless of where you are, you can focus on developing competencies and experience that relate to who and what you wish to be.

Source: From Dr. Janice Waddell, Professor at Ryerson University. Reprinted with permission.

SUMMARY

There is quite a contrast between a nursing department where nurses who are hired are a good fit for their position, staff are retained, and new nurses are supported; and a nursing department with even one nurse who is a poor fit for his or her position, a high rate of turnover, and low support for new nurses. The former department in all likelihood is one where quality care is provided, has a core of experienced nurses with expertise in dealing with complex situations, and helps makes the next generation of nurses feel respected. The latter department is probably one where nurses become dissatisfied and stressed and resign from their positions, which in turn may lead to a loss of expertise on the unit, unfilled positions, and a continuing and worsening cycle of nurses leaving the department.

We can assume that nurses want to work in well-functioning, well-staffed departments where they are able to provide quality care to clients. This speaks to the importance of the topics addressed in this chapter: recruiting the right person for the job, making good hiring or selection decisions, socializing new nurses as well as nurses who are new to a department in ways that contribute to well functioning departments and quality care, and helping new nurses transition to the role of the nurse in order that the next generation of nurses is there to contribute to health care and to the profession.

Baby boomers   Baby boomers were born from approximately 1946 to 1964.

Behavioural-based interview questions   Questions that ask the applicant to describe a particular type of situation experienced and how he or she managed it. They are used because we know that past behaviour is a good predictor of future behaviour.

Generation X   Born from approximately 1965 to 1981. They are more informal and place more importance on their non-work life than baby boomers.

Magnet hospitals   are hospitals that attract and retain nurses despite a shortage of nurses in nearby hospitals.

Nexters   Nexters are also referred to as generation Y, the millennial generation, millennials, generation next, the net generation, or the echo boomers. Nexters were born from approximately from 1982 to 2000 and are the generation who are currently entering the workforce. They are comfortable with computer technology and want a voice in decision making as new employees, and like generation X they place more emphasis on their non–work life than baby boomers.

Professional socialization   is the process whereby new professionals learn and internalize the knowledge, skills, values, attitudes, and norms of their profession that guide their behaviour in their professional role.

Realistic job preview   is a description of both positive and negative features of the position that is provided to a job applicant before he or she accepts a position.

Reality shock   is the term used by Kramer (1974) to describe the reactions of nursing students to the reality of what was expected of them in their first job.

Role socialization   is the process whereby an employee learns the work setting's policies, procedures, norms, and role expectations associated with a job.

CASE

Since graduating two years ago, Elizabeth has worked on a neurosurgical unit. Her first months on the unit had been difficult, not only because she had to learn a lot about the type of care provided on the unit and the organization's policies and procedures, but also because she had a stressful relationship with the preceptor she was assigned to, Krista. Krista was one of the most senior nurses on the floor and was a very competent neurosurgical nurse. When she went to Krista with a question, Krista would often roll her eyes and say she was surprised Elizabeth did not know the answer. At times, Krista was abrupt with Elizabeth as well as with other nurses on the unit. Elizabeth did not say anything to the other nurses or her manager about her relationship with her preceptor because she wanted to fit in and did not know how they would react. Elizabeth now feels comfortable with her knowledge and skills for this client population and loves her work. In fact, if not for the ongoing negative relationship she has with Krista, it would be her perfect job.

This morning, Elizabeth was shocked when she read her email and received an email with a request for a reference for Krista, saying Krista had given her name. Elizabeth went to her nurse manager and told her Krista had not asked her for a reference, and because of Krista's interpersonal relationships with other nurses and the way she treats new nurses, she would have trouble giving a reference. Her nurse manager replied that she had also been asked for a reference and gave a good one because if she did not, Krista would work there forever. The nurse manager said if Krista gets this other job, the nursing team would be really cohesive.

Questions

1. Should Elizabeth provide a reference? If so, what should she say in this reference?

2. Do you agree with the nurse manager's response to Elizabeth? How could the nurse manager work with this situation differently?

3. If Elizabeth had complained about her preceptor during her orientation, how do you think Elizabeth would have been perceived by the other nurses and the nurse manager?

4. How could Elizabeth have given Krista feedback during the preceptor period? Practise role-playing this in groups of three, with one person playing the role of Elizabeth, a second person playing Krista, and one an observer.

5. If Elizabeth had brought the issue of her preceptor forward to her manager, what could she have said?

6. Elizabeth had known that the other nurses sometimes found Krista abrupt, but when she discussed the reference request with her nurse manager, she was surprised to learn that her manager knew Krista was difficult to work with, yet had assigned Krista to be her preceptor. In fact, it made Elizabeth feel that her manager did not care about her success on the unit. Discuss what you think about the manager's assignment of Krista as a preceptor. What could the manager have discussed with Krista when making this assignment? What could she have discussed with Elizabeth? Keep issues of confidentiality and privacy laws in mind.

Critical Thinking Questions and Activities

1. Discuss why recruiting and selecting nurses is a key function of nurse managers and/or nursing recruitment and selection committee members.

2. Do you feel the characteristics of health care settings that attract nurses have changed over time? Why or why not?

3. Suggest strategies for recruiting nurses. Discuss your rational, for the effectiveness of these strategies.

4. Identify limitations of the job interview and discuss strategies to help compensate for the limitations of the job interview.

5. Identify a competency that you believe a nurse should have for a particular nursing department. Develop a behavioural-based question that you could use to assess the nurse's competency in this area.

6. Reflect on what helped or hindered your transition to a nursing student role when you entered your nursing program. How could you use this knowledge about your past adaptation to help you with your transition to a graduate nurse role?

7. Socialization to the nursing profession or to a nursing role can have benefits as well as negative outcomes. Provide some examples of benefits and negative outcomes to socialization to nursing and to socialization to a nursing role.

Self-Quiz

1. A behavioural-based interview question
   a. Is designed to provide a realistic job preview
   b. Helps determine level of motivation
   c. Focuses on nursing skills
   d. Helps determine previous behaviour

2. The international recruitment of nurses
   a. Is a relatively new practice in Canada that started with the shortage of nurses in the 1980s
   b. In Canada, focuses on the recruitment of nurses from developed countries
   c. Has ethical issues because nurses in developing countries should not have the right to migrate
   d. Has contributed to the Canadian health care system for many years

3. A example of a recruitment strategy is
   a. Improving the image of the nurse
   b. Having high school students spend a day with a community health nurse
   c. Displaying posters that include nurses of different genders and visible minority groups
   d. All of the above

4. In preparing to be interviewed for a job, it is useful to do all of the following *except*:
   a. Think of a few jokes that you can say at the beginning of the interview, to help you and the interviewer get to know each other
   b. Go the location of the interview a day or so prior to the interview, to ensure you know the location
   c. Prepare questions you would like to ask
   d. Think about what you would like to be doing in 5 and 10 years, time

Useful Websites

Alliance for Ethical International Recruitment Practices
www.fairinternationalrecruitment.org/

Canadian Nurses Association position statement on Pan-Canadian Health Human Resources planning
www2.cna-aiic.ca/CNA/documents/pdf/publications/PS118_Pan_Canadian_HHR_Planning_2012_e.pdf

International Council of Nurses (ICN). (2007). Nurse Retention and Migration. Position statement. Geneva. Retrieved from
www.icn.ch/images/stories/documents/publications/position_statements/C06_Nurse_Retention_Migration.pdf

Nursing Health Services Research Unit (A collaboration of the University of Toronto, McMaster University, and the Province of Ontario). This website lists studies in the area of international nursing including recruitment and retention of nurses from other countries to Canada.
www.nhsru.com/category/publications/international-nursing

Recruitment and Retention of Inuit Nurses in Nunavut. Prepared for Nunavut Tunngavik Incorporated, March 2009.
www.tunngavik.com/wp-content/uploads/2010/03/2010-02-nti-recruitment-retention-inuit-nurses-report_english.pdf

Registered Nurses' Association of Ontario policy brief about recruitment of nurses from other countries. November 2008.
rnao.ca/sites/rnao-ca/files/storage/related/4083_Recruitment_of_Internationally_Educated_Nurses_(IENs)._November_10_2008.pdf

This website provides sample behavioural-based interview questions.
www.quintcareers.com/sample_behavioral.html

YouTube video Generational Differences (starts with Traditionalists or Veterans who were born prior to 1946 and are largely no longer in the nursing workforce) shows typical experiences of each generation during their childhood and early adult years
www.youtube.com/watch?v=i4JxRqWkNIQ

YouTube video Behavior Based Interview Questions shows an example of a behaviour-based interview question with a good response
www.youtube.com/watch?v=4sKhOETBSIE&feature=related

References

Aiken, L., Clarke, S., Sloane, D., Sochalski, J., & Silber, J. (2002). Hospital nurse staffing and patient mortality, nurse burnout, and job dissatisfaction. *JAMA, 288*, 1987–1993.

Aylward, M., Gaudine, A., & Bennett, L. (2011). Nurse recruitment and retention in rural Newfoundland and Labrador communities: The experiences of healthcare managers. *Online Journal of Rural Nursing and Health Care, 11*(1), 54–69.

Beecroft, P., Kunzman, L., & Krozek, C. (2001). RN internship: Outcomes of a one-year pilot program. *Journal of Nursing Administration, 31*, 575–582.

Bisholt, B. (2012). The professional socialization of recently graduated nurses—Experiences of an introduction program. *Nurse Education Today, 32*, 278–282.

Bowles, C., & Candela, L. (2005). First job experiences of recent RN graduates: Improving the work environment. *Journal of Nursing Administration, 35*, 130–137,

Brooke, P. (2008). Hiring and firing: Know the consequences. *Nursing Management, 39*(9), 50–52.

Bruner, J. (1957). On perceptual readiness. *Psychological Review, 64*, 123–152.

Canadian Nurses Association. (2011). 2009 Workforce Profile of Registered Nurses in Canada. Retrieved from www2.cna-aiic.ca/CNA/documents/pdf/publications/2009_RN_Snapshot_e.pdf

Cho, S., Ketefian, S., Barkauskas, V., & Smith, D. (2003). The effects of nurse staffing on adverse events, morbidity, mortality, and medical costs. *Nursing Research, 52*, 71–79.

Cho, S., Masselink, L., Jones, C., & Mark, B. (2011). Internationally educated nurse hiring: Geographic distribution, community and hospital characteristics. *Nursing Economic$, 29*, 308–316.

Deasy, C., Doody, O., & Tuohy, D. (2011). An exploratory study of role transition from student to registered nurse (general, mental health and intellectual disability) in Ireland. *Nurse Education in Practice, 11*, 109–113.

DiMeglio, K., Padula, C., Piatek, C., Korber, S., Barrett, A., Ducharme, M., Lucas, S., Piermont, N., Joyal, E., DeNicola, V., & Corry, K. (2005). Group cohesion and nurse satisfaction. Examination of a team-building approach. *Journal of Nursing Administration, 35*, 110–120.

Drennan, V., Andrews, S., Sidhu, R., & Peacock, R. (2006). Attracting and retaining nurses in primary care. *British Journal of Community Nursing, 11*, 242–246.

Dziadekwich, R., Andrushko, K., & Klassen, K. (2012). A new approach to retaining older workers. *The Canadian Nurse, 108*(6), 18–20.

Evans, J. (2004). Men nurses: A historical and feminist perspective. *Journal of Advanced Nursing, 47*, 321–328.

Hader, R. (2009). Hiring? Be picky. *Nursing Management, 40*(5), 6.

Hart, S. (2006). Generational diversity. Impact on recruitment and retention of registered nurses. *JONA, 36*, 10–12.

Hill, R. (2002). Managing across generations in the 21st century: Important lessons from the ivory trenches. *Journal Management Inquiry, 11*, 60–66.

Hoffart, N., Waddell, A., & Young, M. (2011). A model of new nurse transition. *Journal of Professional Nursing, 27*, 334–343.

Howskins, E., & Ewens, A. (1999). How students experience professional socialization. *International Journal of Nursing Studies, 35.* 41–49.

HSM Group, Ltd., The (2002). Acute care hospital survey of RN vacancy and turnover rates in 2000. *Journal of Nursing Administration, 32*, 437–439.

Huckabay, L. (2009). Partnership between an educational institution and a healthcare agency—Lessons learned: Part I. *Nursing Forum, 44*, 154–164.

Hutchinson, D., Brown, J., & Longworth, K. (2012). Attracting and maintaining the Y generation in nursing: A literature review. *Journal of Nursing Management, 20*, 444–450.

Hunter, D. (1974). Men in nursing. *The Canadian Journal of Psychiatric Nursing, 15*(4), 12–14.

ICN (International Council of Nurses). (2007). Nurse Retention and Migration. Position statement. Geneva. Retrieved from www.icn.ch/images/stories/documents/publications/position_statements/C06_Nurse_Retention_Migration.pdf

Inglehart, R. (1977). *The silent revolution. Changing values and political styles among western publics.* Princeton, NJ: Princeton University Press.

Jennings, A. (2000). Hiring generation-X: The apple doesn't fall anywhere near the tree any more. *Journal of Accountancy, 189*(2), 55–58.

Jones, C. (2008). Revisiting nurse turnover costs: Adjusting for inflation. *Journal of Nursing Administration, 38*, 11–18.

Khadria, B. (2007). International nurse recruitment in India. *Health Research and Educational Trust, 42*, 1429–1436.

Klingne, D., & Nalbandian, J. (2003). *Public personnel management contexts and strategies,* 5th ed. Upper Saddle River, NJ: Prentice Hall.

Kolawole, B. (2010). International nurse migration to Canada: Are we missing the bigger picture? *Nursing Leadership, 23*(2), 16–20. Retrieved from www.longwoods.com/content/21829

Kramer, M. (1974). *Reality shock: Why nurses leave nursing.* St. Louis: C.V. Mosby.

Kramer, M. (1990). The Magnet hospitals: Excellence revisited. *The Journal of Nursing Administration, 20*, 35–44.

Lester, S., Standifer, R., Schultz, N., & Windsor, J. (2012). Actual versus perceived generational differences at work: An empirical examination. *Journal of Leadership & Organizational studies, 19*, 341–354.

MacPhee, M., & Scott, J. (2002). The role of social support networks for rural hospital nurses. *Journal of Nursing Administration, 32*, 264–271.

Maddalena, V., Kearney, A., & Adams, L. (2012). Quality of work life of novice nurses. *Journal for Nurses in Staff Development, 28*(2), 74–79.

Mayer, K., & Carroll, V.S. (2011). Visioning as a hiring strategy for quality outcomes. *The Journal of Nursing Administration, 41*, 369–373.

McClure, M.M., Poulin, M., Wandelt, S.M., & Wandelt, M. (1983). *Magnet hospitals: Attraction and retention of professional nurses.* American Academy of Nursing Task Force on Nursing Practice in Hospitals. Kansas City, MO: American Nurses Association.

McDaniel, M., Whetzel, D., Schmidt, F., & Maurer, S. (1994). The validity of employment interviews: a comprehensive review and meta-analysis. *Journal of Applied Psychology, 79*, 599–616.

Meadus, R., & Twomey, C. (2011). Men student nurses: The nursing education experience. *Nursing Forum, 46,* 269–279.

Needleman, J., Buerhaus, P., Pankratz, V.S., Leibson, C., Stevens, S., & Harris, M. (2011). Nursing staffing and inpatient hospital mortality. *The New England Journal of Medicine, 364,* 1037–1045.

Nelson, D., Godfrey, L., & Purdy, J. (2004). Using a mentorship program to recruit and retain student nurses. *Journal of Nursing Administration, 34,* 551–553.

Penz, K., Stewart, N., D'Arcy, C., & Morgan, D. (2008). Predictors of job satisfaction for rural acute care registered nurses in Canada. *Western Journal of Nursing Research, 30,* 785–800.

Perdomo, G. (May 28, 2012). The delivery man. *MacLean's Magazine, 125*(20), 62.

Price, S. (2008). Becoming a nurse: a meta-study of early professional socialization and career choice in nursing. *Journal of Advanced Nursing, 65,* 11–19.

RNAO (Registered Nurses' Association of Ontario). (November 2008). Recruitment of Internationally Educated Nurses. Retrieved from http://rnao.ca/sites/rnao-ca/files/storage/related/4083_Recruitment_of_Internationally_Educated_Nurses_(IENs)._November_10_2008.pdf

Reynolds, L., Bush, E., & Geist, R. (2008). The gen Y imperative. *Communication World, 25,* 19–22.

Romyn, D., Linton, N., Giblin, C., Hendrickson, B., Limacher, L., Murray, C., Zimmel, C. (2009). Successful transition of the new graduate nurse. *International Journal of Nursing Education Scholarship, 6*(1), 1–17.

Strasser, P. (2005). Improving applicant interviewing using a behavioral-based questioning approach. *AAOHN Journal, 53,* 149–151.

Strauss, W., & Howe, N. (1991). *Generations: The history of America's future.* New York, NY: William Morrow.

Teasley, S., Sexton, K., Carroll, C., Cox, K., Riley, M., & Ferriell, K. (2007). Improving work environment perceptions for nurses employed in a rural setting. *Journal of Rural Health, 23,* 179–182.

Waddell, J., Donner, G., & Wheeler, M. (2009). *Building your nursing career. A guide for students,* 3rd ed. Toronto: Mosby Elsevier.

Wanous, J. (1992). *Organizational entry: Recruitment, selection, orientation, and socialization of newcomers,* 2nd ed. Reading, MA: Addison-Wesley.

Weinberg, D., Cooney-Miner, D., Perioff, J., & Bourgoin, M. (2011). The gap between education preferences and hiring practices. *Nursing Management, 42*(9), 23–28.

Zemke, R., Raines, C., & Filipczak, B. (2000). *Generations at work: Managing the clash of veterans, boomers, xers, nexters in your workplace.* New York: AMACON.

Chapter 7
Motivation and Performance

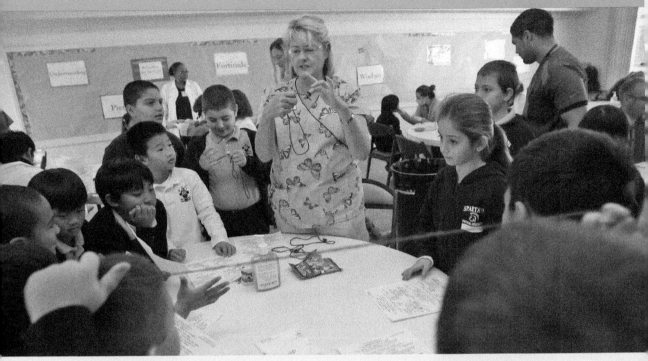

David Crane/ZUMAPRESS/Newscom

Learning Objectives

After reading, studying, and reflecting on this chapter's content, you will be able to:

1. Analyze how different theories of work motivation can be applied to the motivation of nurses in the workplace
2. Discuss how career development plans can facilitate nurses' motivation and performance
3. Debate the pros and cons of performance appraisals
4. Suggest situations when disciplinary procedures may help or hurt nurses' motivation and performance in the workplace
5. Identify how nexters, members of generation X, and nurses nearing retirement (baby boomers) may differ in what motivates them in the workplace
6. Relate issues related to motivation and performance to your practice setting(s)
7. Suggest ways nurses can foster their own motivation and performance

INTRODUCTION

Why are we concerned about nurses' motivation? We believe that nurses who are motivated about their work are more engaged in their work. This may mean that they spend more time with their patients, reflect more on how they can improve patient care, search the literature for evidence-based practice, engage in special projects on their unit, advocate more for their patients, identify clinical ethical issues, and so on. Ultimately, we anticipate that motivated nurses will perform better, and this should mean higher quality of care and patient safety. That is what we believe, but is there research evidence for this?

Are nurses motivated? What is their level of motivation? Can we improve their level of motivation, and if so, how? In this chapter we explore theories of motivation to help us identify how these may be applied to facilitating nurses' motivation in the workplace. We also explore specific strategies to improve motivation and performance, including performance appraisals, career development, and **career ladders**. It is also important to consider what may lower a nurses' motivation, and what outcomes there are for the nurse, other employees, and the organization when an event leads a nurse to no longer be motivated. The needs of **nexters** (the generation born from approximately 1982 to 2000 and who are currently entering the workforce), **generation X** (born from approximately 1965 to 1981), and **baby boomers** (born from approximately 1946 to 1964 and currently retiring) will be related to motivation and performance. Further, we discuss disciplinary procedures as a measure to deal with problems with motivation and performance. (Note: For more discussion of the different generations in the workplace please see Chapter 6, Nursing Workforce Issues: Recruitment and Retention, Selection, Socialization, and Transitioning.)

THEORIES OF MOTIVATION

A person's motivation is the individual's desire or drive to perform behaviours or reach goals. Any individual might be motivated to behave in a certain way or reach certain goals, but not motivated to behave in other ways or reach other goals. Therefore, when discussing a person's motivation it is useful to state what behaviour or goals the motivation is related to, such as **work motivation**. Work motivation is the intensity and persistence of an employee's work-related behaviour. It is "the extent to which persistent effort is directed towards a goal" that is related to work (Johns & Saks, 2011). Work motivation is important, because an employee who is not motivated to work might be present in the workplace, but will expend little effort in meeting the goals of the organization. In recent years, the concept of **work engagement** has been discussed frequently in health care settings. Work engagement sounds like it may be the same concept as work motivation, but it is not. Work engagement is the opposite of burnout and refers to positive feelings of enthusiasm, absorption, fulfillment, and dedication toward one's work (Schaufeli, Salanova, González-Romá, & Bakker, 2002).

A number of theories have been developed to explain what motivates employees in the workplace. The following sections describe selected well-known theories of motivation. Some of these theories discuss an individual's motivation for behaviour in general (for example, Bandura's social cognitive theory) while others describe an individual's motivation for work (for example, McClelland's theory). All of these theories of motivation can be applied to nurses and their work in health care settings.

Maslow's Hierarchy of Needs Theory

Maslow's (1943) hierarchy of needs theory is an early theory of motivation. We now have theories that are better explanations of motivation; however, we are providing a brief introduction to this theory because:

1. the theory has historical importance, and is still referred to in the motivation literature, and

2. although the theory has been replaced by other theories of motivation, it is a useful heuristic, or tool, for nurses in prioritizing patient needs (a purpose outside its intended purpose of explaining motivation) and is therefore widely referred to in nursing.

Maslow theorized that people have needs ranging from lower level needs to higher level needs. His most-known model of motivation has five levels of needs as shown in Figure 7.1. The lowest level of needs is physiological, the next is safety, then love and belonging, esteem, and finally self-actualization. For a person to be motivated by a need, the person's needs at lower levels must first be filled. For example, for a person to be motivated by the need for love and belonging, physiological and safety needs need to have

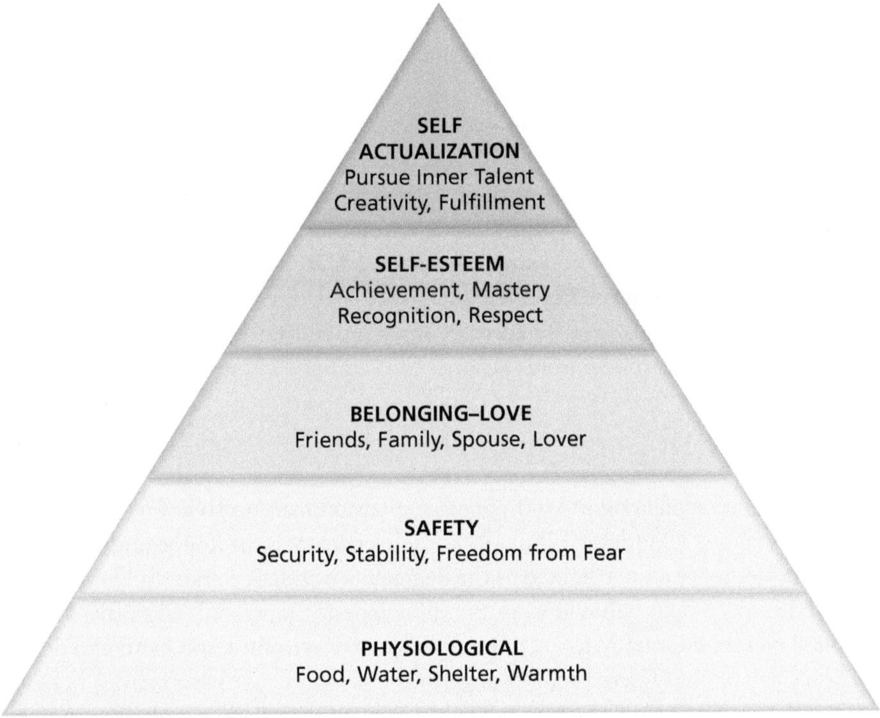

SELF ACTUALIZATION
Pursue Inner Talent
Creativity, Fulfillment

SELF-ESTEEM
Achievement, Mastery
Recognition, Respect

BELONGING–LOVE
Friends, Family, Spouse, Lover

SAFETY
Security, Stability, Freedom from Fear

PHYSIOLOGICAL
Food, Water, Shelter, Warmth

Figure 7.1 Maslow's Hierarchy of Needs

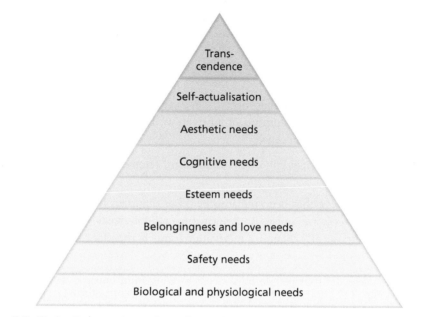

Figure 7.2 Eight-Stage Hierarchy of Needs Based on Maslow's Theory

been met. Applying this example to work motivation, an employee will not find being part of a team is motivating if the person feels his or her job is not secure, or if the person feels the work environment is not safe (safety needs not met). In later years, Maslow refined his model to include three additional levels of needs, cognitive, aesthetic, and transcendence, as shown in Figure 7.2.

Criticisms of Maslow's theory include that there is little evidence that the needs occur in this order or indeed, in any order (Wahba & Lawrence, 1974). The theory does not explain persons with unmet lower level needs who are motivated by a higher need, such as a nurse who has not had time to take a lunch break (physiological need for food and rest) and does not have a permanent position (safety need) but is motivated to provide exceptional care to his or her clients (self-actualization). As well, the placement of self-actualization as a high level need or even as a need reflects Western values rather than the values of collective cultures (Cianci & Gambrel, 2003).

Social Cognitive Theory

Bandura developed social cognitive theory to explain human motivation, as well as learning and performance (Bandura, 1986; 1997). **Self-efficacy** is an important component of social cognitive theory and is defined as the degree of confidence an individual has that he or she can do a particular behaviour. In Bandura's theory, a person's cognitive factors and behavioural factors interact with each other and with environmental factors to determine the person's behaviour. Therefore, a change in the person's cognitive factors, behavioural factors, and/or environmental factors can lead to a change in the person's other factors and behaviour. Cognitive factors are the person's knowledge, expectations, and attitudes related to a specific behaviour. Behavioural factors refer to the skill, practice, and self-efficacy of the person related to a specific behaviour. Environmental factors are social norms, access in the community, and the influence of others as these have an impact on cognitive and behavioural factors and behaviour. Figure 7.3 illustrates the interaction of cognitive factors, behavioural factors, and environmental factors.

In social cognitive theory there are two mechanisms of motivation that are cognitively based: 1. forethought, and 2. internal standards or self-evaluative reactions (Bandura, 1986; 1997). An individual has forethought about the consequences of his or her future behaviour. This forethought serves to motivate and regulate behaviour. An individual also sets internal standards or goals and evaluates his or her behaviour against these goals. When the individual's goals are met, he or she feels satisfied, but when the goals are not met, dissatisfaction occurs. It is the feeling of dissatisfaction that helps motivate the individual to strive and meet goals, or to improve performance. However, the dissatisfaction only leads to the individual being motivated to try again if the individual has high enough self-efficacy that he or she will be able to meet the goal. If the individual's self-efficacy for performing the particular behaviour is low, the result is discouragement rather than motivation.

Different individuals can have the same goals and skills but perform differently because their self-efficacy for performing the skill differs. Individuals who do not meet a goal, who have low self-efficacy for the behaviours required to meet this goal become discouraged. In contrast, individuals who do not meet their goal but who have high self-efficacy for the behaviours required to meet this goal are motivated to repeat their attempts to attain their goal. Once the goal is attained, the individual's self-efficacy increases. This leads him or her to feel confident in setting a higher goal for future performance.

Bandura (1986; 1997) identified four factors or sources of information that helped increase self-efficacy. First, actual performance has an impact on self-efficacy. After an individual is successful at a task, his or her self-efficacy for performing that task increases. Second, self-efficacy is affected by vicarious experience. In particular, observing a similar person successfully performing a behaviour helps an individual increase his or her own self-efficacy for this behaviour. Third, verbal persuasion that the individual is capable of performing a behaviour helps to increase self-efficacy. The fourth source of information

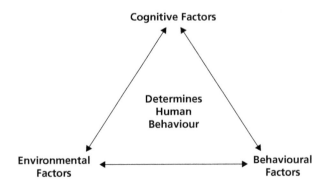

Figure 7.3 Social Cognitive Theory

that helps to increase self-efficacy is physiological feedback. An individual uses his or her physiological state to help construct feelings of self-efficacy for performing a specific task. As self-efficacy increases so does motivation for this behaviour, and therefore, altering any of the four sources of information for self-efficacy can alter self-efficacy and motivation.

Applying this theory to nursing, a nurse who has high self-efficacy for working with families will be more apt to approach family members and initiate therapeutic communication with them. Similarly, a nurse with low self-efficacy for acting as an advocate for other nurses may be less apt to bring the concerns of his or her colleagues to the attention of a nurse manager or to apply for a position as a nursing leader.

Herzberg's Motivation-Hygiene Theory

Hertzberg and colleagues (1959) identified two factors of employee needs: 1. motivating factors, and 2. hygiene factors. When motivating factor needs were met, the employee experienced either no satisfaction or a varying degree of satisfaction, but did not experience dissatisfaction. These motivating factors include personal achievement, status, recognition, challenging work, responsibility, and advancement opportunities. When hygiene factors needs were *not* met, the employee experienced dissatisfaction, but when these needs *were* met they did not cause dissatisfaction but did not motivate the employee. Hygiene factors include salaries and benefits, employer policies and administration, interpersonal relationships, supervision, job security, working conditions, and work/life balance. Thus, the presence of motivating factors leads to work motivation (and satisfaction and commitment) while the presence of hygiene factors prevents work dissatisfaction but does not lead to work motivation.

The following examples apply Herzberg's motivation-hygiene theory to nurses. A nurse who finds his or her work challenging and feels a sense of achievement may experience work satisfaction as well as work motivation. A nurse who does not have his or her needs met for working conditions, job security, and salary will experience dissatisfaction. However, if a nurse's needs for working conditions, job satisfaction, and salary are met, he or she does not experience dissatisfaction, but neither does this nurse experience motivation.

McClelland's Theory

McClelland (1955; 1975) theorized that an employee has three motivating needs in the workplace:

1. the need for achievement,
2. the need for affiliation, and
3. the need for power.

The need for achievement is the need to have visible outcomes of success, the need for affiliation is the need to be liked by others and to feel included in groups, and the need for power is the need to influence others and have control. Each employee differs in the strength they experience these three needs.

Applied to nursing work, a nurse who has a high need for power will feel motivated when he or she is able to influence others, such as through teaching others, leading others, or influencing client growth or development. A nurse who has a strong need for affiliation may be motivated by working on a team where he or she is liked and feels part of the group. A nurse with a high need for achievement will be motivated by seeing the successes of his or her work and receiving recognition for this from others.

Equity Theory

Much has been written in the management literature about equity or fairness in the workplace because situations of inequity (actual or perceived) evoke much negative emotion and dissatisfaction. John Stacey Adams (1963) developed his equity theory to explain work motivation. Adams theorized that for a person to experience equity in the workplace, his or her outcomes given his or her inputs, need to be in balance with the outcomes experienced by others, given their inputs.

Applied to nursing work, a nurse who is experienced and is assigned more challenging clients or a higher work load but also is paid at the top of the salary scale and receives much recognition from others may experience equity if a newer nurse has less challenging clients or a lower work load, but is paid less and does not receive as much recognition from others. In contrast, a nurse who believes he or she provides excellent care may experience inequity if he or she perceives another nurse brings less expertise to patient care but is the one who is given a valued promotion.

Vroom's Expectancy Theory

In his expectancy theory, Vroom (1964) describes force or effort as the product of the value (valence) an individual places on a goal or outcome and his or her expectation that this goal or outcome can be obtained (expectancy). Specifically, force (or effort) = valence × expectancy. If an individual values a goal or outcome and has a high expectancy that he or she can attain this goal, he or she will be motivated to work toward the goal. Figure 7.4 illustrates how the person's effort or motivation to obtain a goal or outcome is related to the value of the outcome/goal and how likely his or her effort will lead to performance and how likely this performance will lead to the outcome/goal.

A nurse who values family-centred care but does not believe that he or she has the skills to work with challenging families may not request this type of patient assignment. A nurse who values making a contribution to her or his quality assurance committee and who believes he or she will be able to provide valuable input to this committee will be motivated to ask to join this committee.

Application of the Theories

We have presented a number of well-known theories of work motivation or theories of motivation that can be applied to motivation to work. This overview will be useful to you because these key theories are frequently referred to in management literature. We encourage you to

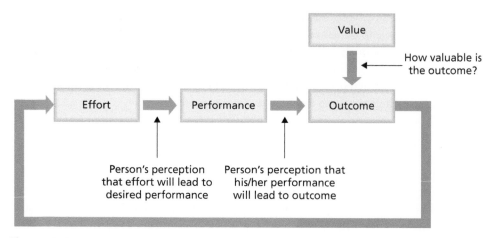

Figure 7.4 Vroom's Expectancy Theory

select the theory(ies) that you find useful when thinking of your own work motivation or the work motivation of persons for whom you may be responsible, and to read additional literature to facilitate your use of the theory(ies) in your practice.

SOURCES OF NURSES' WORK MOTIVATION

Toode and colleagues (2011) reviewed 24 nursing research studies, published between 1990 and 2009, that examined factors that had an impact on nurses' work motivation. They did a content analysis of these studies to categorize the factors associated with nurses' work motivation and identified five categories:

1. workplace characteristics
2. working conditions
3. personal characteristics
4. individual priorities
5. internal psychological states

Regarding workplace characteristics, Toode et al. (2011) identified studies that showed nurses were motivated by good collaboration with other members of the health care team, social support within the team, positive team spirit, being an equally valued member of the team, high autonomy, variety of different work-related activities, manual work, opportunities to learn, opportunities to share their knowledge with physicians, and receiving supervision.

There is some evidence to support the importance of working conditions to nurses' work motivation, for example, a manager's ability to manage the unit; working days as opposed to rotating shifts; and pay raises, rewards, and promotions.

Personal characteristics affecting nurses' motivation included age (although several studies showed work motivation increased with age while only one study found nurses under 30 years of age were more motivated). Higher college-level preparation and awareness of nursing philosophy, knowledge, and skills were also found to be associated with higher motivation.

The category of individual priorities included studies in which nurses were more motivated when certain individual values and needs were met through their work. One study found the ability to meet a nurse's needs and have control over time was associated with motivation. Other studies found the opportunity to help others, a strong sense of having chosen a profession that the nurse values, or a positive view of ethical factors in the workplace were important job motivators.

Internal psychological states studies found nursing work characteristics had an impact on nurses' work motivation because they affected the nurses' internal psychological state. For example, one study found nurses who found their work meaningful were motivated to provide care even if it risked their own health.

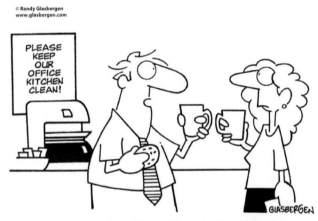

"I have a great idea that will revitalize the company, prevent bankruptcy and save hundreds of jobs. But I'm saving it for the day before my performance review."

Randy Glasbergen

Newton and colleagues (2009) interviewed nurses working in Australia to understand what motivates nurses to select nursing as a career, what keeps them motivated to continue nursing, and what type of organizational support can foster the retention of nurses in the workplace. They interviewed 29 undergraduate nursing students, 25 practising nurses, 6 unit nurse managers, and 4 directors of nursing from a variety of clinical areas and 4 sites within one organization. They found four themes that were common to the students, practising nurses and managers:

1. a desire to help
2. caring
3. sense of achievement
4. self-validation (pp. 392–400)

The theme "a desire to help" captured the nurses' motive to nurse as this was a profession where they could help others, and is supported by other research findings that helping others is a key motivator for entering the nursing profession (for example, Boughn, 2001; Meadus & Twomey, 2007). The nursing students' and nurses' desire to help was related to their intrinsic motivators of both self-fulfillment and success. Many of the nurses spoke of how helping others is a motive they had had since they were young. Closely related to the theme of a desire to help was caring. This need to care was for patients but also for other nurses and nursing students. Sense of achievement relates to nurses' feeling satisfied that they have helped a patient to recover or improve their health status. The theme of self-validation refers to the desire to feel good. Self-validation was met through activities such as being thanked by others and seeing visible outcomes of their work or learning skills.

These researchers note that three of their themes are similar to those of other researchers who have examined nurses' motivation, while their theme of self-validation is a new finding. Contrary to other researchers, this study did not find that nurses' motivation to nurse differed across age cohorts, from young student nurses through senior nurse managers. They note that De Cooman and colleagues (2008) also found that new graduates and older nurses had similar motivators to nurse, particularly as related to helping others and building relationships with others.

Newton and colleagues' (2009) research findings support the need for health care organizations to ensure nurses' work allows them to meet their desires to help others, to care, and to experience a sense of achievement. An important contribution of this study is the identification of nurses' need for self-validation. This need for self-validation has implications for nurse managers and educators because it provides evidence that they need to remember to thank nurses and help nurses to see the outcomes of their work.

While Newton and colleagues' (2009) study found similar themes of motivation to nurse across age cohorts, other studies have identified some differences. For example, McCabe and colleagues (2005) found that nurses 30 years of age and younger were more motivated by exciting and challenging work situations than nurses aged 40 to 50 years. In addition, they found the older nurses were more motivated by experiencing community respect for nurses and the prestige of the nursing profession than younger nurses.

HOW MOTIVATED ARE NURSES?

Toode et al.'s (2011) review of the literature on work motivation also looked at how motivated staff nurses are. Seventeen of the 24 studies that they reviewed included the level of nurses' work motivation and found that in general, nurses were motivated to work. One study looked at if there was a difference in work motivation of nurses in intensive care and non–intensive care units. Another looked at whether there was a difference between those in hospitals and nursing homes, with no significant differences found in either study. The Related Research summarized in this chapter examineds job motives of new graduates and compares this with what is known about older nurses. While this study was done in Belgium, we present it to point out that different generations have different needs.

Freshmen in Nursing: Job Motives and Work Values of a New Generation (2008)

This study examined the job motives and work values of new nursing graduates in Belgium. The authors note that if we want to retain young nurses in nursing, we need to know what motivates them and what they value about their work. Specifically, their research questions were:

Which work values and job motives do graduate nurses indicate as most important to them?
Are the values and motives related to each other and how are they organized and into how many groups?
Do male and female graduate nurses differ in the importance they attach to the work values and job motives? (p. 58)

A questionnaire was mailed to 1,142 Belgian nurses who had recently graduated, and 344 nurses responded for a response rate of 30.1%. The respondents were 86.4% female, with 71.5% between the ages of 21 and 24 years, 15.9% between 25 and 30, 10.2% between 30 and 40, and 2.4% over 40 years. Further, 88.1% were employed in nursing practice, 6.1% were taking a postgraduate program, 3.8% working outside nursing, and 2% unemployed.

The questionnaire included 27 items about job motives. Nurses rated their agreement with each item on a scale ranging from 1 (totally disagree) to 5 (totally agree). In addition they selected the three items that most motivated them and the three items that least motivated them. Work values were measured with the adapted Dutch version of the Work Importance Study instrument (Coetsier & Claes, 1990). Nurses were asked to rate each item from 1 (totally unimportant) to 5 (totally important).

One finding was that helping was one of the most important job motives and another that working hours was the least important. Work values that were rated highly by males and females were financial security and recognition. Males were more apt to value career opportunities, executive powers, and autonomy; and females were more apt to value interpersonal characteristics.

The authors conclude that, given this generation's job motives and the work values of helping (altruism) and interpersonal aspects of work, care must be taking when considering staffing and restructuring if these nurses are to be retained in the workplace. They compare their findings with those of Sadler's (2003) literature, which dealt mainly with the needs of baby boomers, and found nurses had entered nursing for altruistic reasons but their reasons for staying in nursing were mainly related to with extrinsic, ergonomic, and physical working conditions.

Sources: Coetsier, P., & Claes, R. (1990). *Belang van levensrollen en warden* [Importance of life roles and values]. Infoservice, Oostende, Belgium.

Sadler, J. (2003). Who wants to be a nurse: Motivation of the new generation. *Journal of Professional Nursing*, 19 (3), 173–175.

De Cooman, R., De Gieter, S., Pepermans, R., Du Bois, C., Capers, R., & Jegers, M. (2008). Freshmen in nursing: Job motives and work values of a new generation. *Journal of Nursing Management, 16*, 56–64.

Discussion Question

1. Do you think the work values and motives of Canadian and Belgian new graduates are similar? Why or why not?

THE SOURCES AND IMPACT OF NURSES' WORK MOTIVATION

Germain and Cummings (2009) reviewed eight research articles that examined nurses' perceptions of what influenced their motivation and performance. Their review of these eight research articles (four from Canada, three from the United States, and one from Singapore) was guided by these questions:

What factors do RNs perceive as influencing their motivation to nurse well?

What leadership behaviors positively correlate with high nurse performance? (p. 426)

The nurses reported 25 factors that affected their motivation or their performance. The researchers grouped these into five categories:

1. autonomy
2. work relationships
3. resource accessibility
4. individual nurse characteristics
5. leadership practices

Autonomy refers to nurses being able to make decisions and implement their decisions without approval from others. Working relationships included strong communication, trusting relationships, mentoring, and clear expectations among nurses and their managers. Resource accessibility refers to a work environment wherein nurses have the resources they need to do their job, which includes adequate supplies, equipment, and staffing. Individual nurse characteristics refers to characteristics such as a nurse's tolerance for ambiguity (ability to be comfortable with new situations and complex issues) and hardiness (commitment to self and to work, embracing challenges, and internal locus of control, which is the belief that you can affect outcomes) (Salyer, 1995). Leadership practices include modelling by doing, setting clear goals, creating a shared vision, improving work processes, helping nurses feel empowered and competent, encouraging performance, and rewarding performance.

Germain and Cummings note that this fifth category, leadership practices, can affect the first three categories, autonomy, work relationships, and resource accessibility. They also discuss the fact that nurses can take responsibility for their own motivation and performance by considering how they can have an impact on the five themes. For example, nurses can work to build trusting relationships among themselves and nurse managers. Further, nurses can inform their managers of the resources they need to do their work.

A number of studies have found nurses' work motivation is positively associated with their job satisfaction (a high level of work motivation is associated with a high level of job satisfaction) (Blegan, 1993; De Loach & Monroe, 2004; Freeman & O'Brien-Pallas, 1998). Another study found that nurses' work motivation is negatively associated with their intent to leave nursing (a low level of work motivation is associated with high level of intent to leave nursing) (Yildiz et al., 2009). This study also found that low work motivation and job satisfaction led to a decrease in service quality and patients' intent to return for further care, and to an increase in the cost of patient care. Taken together, these studies support the importance of work motivation for nurses (job satisfaction), organizations (retention of nurses, cost of patient care), and patients (quality of care).

More research is needed to examine the outcomes of nurses' motivation on their performance and on actual patient outcomes. To date, research on the effect of nurses' motivation has focused more on nurses' perceptions of how they or their patients are impacted.

FACILITATING MOTIVATION AND PERFORMANCE

In the next section we discuss tools that nurses or managers might use to facilitate motivation and performance. First we discuss career development as an approach to facilitate motivation and performance. Next we discuss performance appraisals and how they can play a role in motivation and performance. Finally, we discuss disciplinary procedures that can be used when there are problems with motivation and performance, ideally with the initial goal of helping the nurse to work effectively.

Career Development

Nurses' career commitment was significantly correlated with their job performance ($r = .457$) in a survey of Jordanian nurses ($N = 640$) (Mrayyan & Al-Faouri, 2008). Career development can be initiated by the nurse or by health care organizations.

Career Development Initiated by the Nurse

Professional purpose statements involve nurses writing their view of their own professional purpose and values. Through reflection and articulating their purpose and values, nurses can increase their motivation to fulfill their desired purposes and act in accordance with their professional values (Cooper & Cottrell, 2010).

Professional purpose is each individual nurse's unique reason that he or she has for practising nursing and is intertwined with each nurse's unique capabilities and values. The nurse's reason for choosing to become a nurse and to continue to practise are articulated, and help motivate the nurse to direct his or her practice and self-development in congruence with his or her professional purpose. In challenging clinical or workplace situations, reflecting on your professional purpose statements can help guide your decisions and behaviours, enabling you to be the type of nurse you want to be.

Career Development Initiated by Health Care Organizations

One outcome of health care budget reductions in the 1990s is that many nursing leadership positions were closed. Prior to these budget reductions, most nursing departments had their own head nurse, and many also had additional leadership positions, such as assistant head nurses, clinical nurse specialists, and nurse educators. These entry-level leadership positions helped provide nurses with the experience and skills for middle and upper leadership positions, and provided organizations with a source of leaders whom they could promote into more senior leadership jobs.

Laschinger and colleagues (2008) conducted a national study of nurse leaders in Canadian hospitals ($N = 1,164$) and found that first-line nurse managers had an average of 71 persons (range 5 to 264) reporting directly to them, middle managers an average of 12 (range 1 to 40), and senior nurse leaders an average of 12 (2 to 47). Further, they found the average age of these nurses was 49. An encouraging finding of their research was that although these nurse leaders had a wide span of persons reporting to them and of responsibilities, they were positive about their work life, felt empowered, and believed they had significant influence within their hospitals.

As noted by O'Brien-Pallas, another prominent Canadian nurse researcher, given the age of Canadian nurse leaders, human resource planning is required to ensure an adequate supply of skilled nurse leaders (O'Brien-Pallas et al., 2001). One initiative to develop nurse leaders is the British Columbia Nursing Administrative Leadership Institute for First Line Nurse Leaders (BC NLI) (McPhee & Bouthillette, 2008). This initiative is a partnership of British Columbia's Chief Nursing Officers, the Ministry of Health Nursing Directorate, and the University of British Columbia School of Nursing. Together, they offer a four-day educational program and a year-long leadership project in which the program participants work with a mentor. Emphasis is placed on evidence-based leadership practice. Nurse managers who are new to their position learn management and leadership competencies, and with the support of their mentors, apply these in their workplace.

Other Canadian leadership programs include the Dorothy M. Wylie Nursing Leadership Institute (DMW NLI) in Toronto, which provides leadership education for nurses. The Executive Training for Research Application (EXTRA) was started in 2004 by the Canadian Health Services Research Foundation (CHSRF) to increase the use of research in the practice of Canadian health care executives, including nurses, physicians, and health administrators (Kerr & Jeans, 2006). An evaluation of EXTRA has found that participants were satisfied with the program and gained knowledge. The authors of this evaluation acknowledge that future research needs to look at how participants' practice in the organization is changed, and what are the benefits for organizations (Anderson & Lavoie-Tremblay, 2008).

Clinical Ladders

One mechanism that health care organizations use to help motivate nurses is a **clinical ladder** (Buchan, 1999; Burket, Greider & Rohrer, 2010). Health care organizations that develop clinical ladders promote nurses as they gain additional expertise. This enables nurses to progress in their career while remaining in direct patient care positions. New nurses start at the first step on the ladder, and as they gain expertise, they might be promoted to the next step. Each step of the ladder might have a different job title (for example, Clinical Nurse 1, Clinical Nurse 2, Clinical Nurse 3, Clinical Specialist). Each step of the ladder might also have a different salary scale range. There is variation among health care organizations in the number of steps on the ladder, the position titles for each step, and whether there is a different salary scale for each step. Nurses at different steps may be assigned patients with different types of needs, with nurses at the top step sometimes assigned to different roles such as patient nurse educator or clinical specialist. Clinical ladders have also been used to motivate LPNs (Asselin, 2003).

Clinical ladders were started in American hospitals in the 1970s and are widely used in that country. Other countries where clinical ladders are used include Australia, New Zealand, the United Kingdom, and Norway (Buchan, 1999). For example, in Canada clinical ladders have been implemented at Fraser Health Authority in British Columbia (the Leading Health Care Example has a detailed description). The International Council of Nurses has supported the use of structures to promote nurses who work in direct care (ICN, 1995)

Leading Health Care Example

Clinical Laddering at Fraser Health Authority in British Columbia

The Fraser Health Authority serves over one-third of the population of BC across 17 municipalities, 12 acute care hospitals, and over 100 residential care, home health, public health, mental health and substance use, and primary care facilities. Fraser Health's Professional Practice & Integration service began developing clinical ladders in 2005 when they established their New Graduate Nurse Program. Pamela Thorsteinsson, the Interim Chief Nursing Officer and Director, Professional Practice – Nursing at Fraser Health Authority, says that a key component of their clinical laddering are the competencies identified for nurses practising at different levels, from "employed student nurses" in their third or fourth year of their nursing program to nurses in specialty areas of practice. The competencies are linked to the College of Registered Nurses of British Columbia's (CRNBC) standards for nursing practice.

Competency-based frameworks are also used in the Educator Pathway that was developed in partnership with the Vancouver Coastal Health Authority, Fraser Health, the University of British Columbia, and University of Victoria, and the BC Nurses Union, and initiated in Fraser Health by Barbara Mildon (President of the Canadian Nurses Association, 2012–2014). The Educator Pathway has now been expanded in Fraser Health to support allied health professionals as well and has been adopted by several other health authorities in British Columbia. Clinical educators who would like to further their development or health care providers and clinical support staff who are interested in becoming an educator or who deliver staff education can attend these workshops to help prepare them for this type of role. Furthermore, the Educator Competency Assessment Tool is being validated in a research project conducted by Angela Wolff, current executive sponsor of the Pathway in Fraser Health. The educator competencies have been used to guide job description development for clinical nurse educators, interview tools, and a Clinical Educator Orientation Pathway. According to Angela Wolff, more and more nurses are enrolling in the Educator Pathway to prepare for a career move into an educator role in the practice setting.

Competency Assessment Planning and Evaluation (CAPE) tools have been developed for many types of nursing roles including Registered Nurses in medical/surgical, home health and other specialty practices, licensed practical nurses, and registered psychiatric nurses. A Patient Care Coordinator (PCC) CAPE Tool has recently been developed as part of an overall PCC "Front Line Leader" role development initiative. The CAPE Tools are designed to support the nurse to identify their learning needs and develop a learning plan, using Benner's (1984) novice to expert framework. Additional research incorporated into the "practice transition" framework is Boychuk-Duchshers' (2008) Transition-Shock Model.

(Continued)

Fraser Health Authority offers mentorship workshops for staff supporting these nurses entering practice and/or transitioning to a new area or role. New graduate nurses attend a series of workshops to help them transition from student to nurse. The clinical programs provide additional structured education to support nurses moving to a new/different area of practice. Nurses use the CAPE tools to guide their learning and development as nurses.

Pamela Thorsteinsson says that nurses at Fraser Health Authority find career laddering has benefited them. First, the CAPE tools provide clarity of expectations to the nurse and their mentor(s). A nurse may have many years of experience in one type of nursing, but if he or she moves to another area, he or she cannot be expected to practise as an expert in that area. Second, the CAPE tool serves as a guide to mentors to help improve how they mentor. As well, the workshops and mentoring hours help nurses to develop their expertise, and attending workshops about another area of practice or role helps nurses with career planning.

References

Benner, P. (1984). *From novice to expert: Excellence and power in clinical nursing-practice*. Menlo Park, CA: Addison-Wesley. Boychuk-Duchscher, J. (2008) Transition shock: the initial stage of role adaptation for newly graduated Registered Nurses. *Journal of Advanced Nursing*, Available from www.letthelearningbegin.com/documents/pdfs/shock.pdf

Discussion Questions

1. Clinical ladders are one strategy that health care organizations can use to foster nurses' work motivation. What impact do you think clinical ladders would have on your motivation?

2. How would the clinical ladders at Frazer Health Authority be useful in promoting the quality of performance?

3. The use of clinical ladders in Canadian health care organizations is less frequent than in the United States. What reasons can you identify for the less frequent use of clinical ladders in Canada?

Source: Interview with Pamela Thorsteinsson. Reprinted with permission.

Health care organizations have developed and implemented clinical ladders to motivate nurses as well as for other benefits seen to arise from career ladders, which include keeping nurses in direct care positions, promoting the professional development of nurses, and rewarding nurses' performance and competency (Zimmer, 1972). It is believed that clinical ladders can help keep nurses motivated because they are recognized for their expertise. As a result, nurses may continue working in direct patient care roles (Buchan, 1999). Clinical ladders promote nurses' self-development, as nurses engage in self-learning or participate in education programs within the health care organization and at university to help meet the requirements for promotion.

Most of the literature about clinical ladders describes the use of clinical ladders at a particular health care organization. Buchan (1999) reviewed the few evaluations of clinical evaluations available at that time. He noted that Patricia Benner's research (Benner, 1982, 1984) that describes the progress of nurses from novice to advanced beginner, competent, proficient, and expert has been used to provide a theoretical rationale for the importance of clinical ladders. Buchan (1999) also noted that there have been few evaluations of clinical ladders. Of the research studies that did examine clinical ladders, some support was found for an increase in nurses' satisfaction, the retention of nurses, and their work performance, while other studies did not find evidence for these improvements. In the decade following Buchan's publication, there has been a paucity of research.

Performance Appraisals

Many health care organizations use performance appraisals to provide health care workers with feedback about their performance, to help them set their performance objectives, and to identify their development needs. Typically, performance appraisals are done once a year. However some systems include additional meetings between the manager and employee throughout the year. Providing ongoing feedback is one strategy that has been suggested to improve the effectiveness of performance appraisals (Martin and Bartol, 1998; Schraeder, Becton, and Portis, 2007). Another is using feedback from different persons, a method that is referred to as **360-degree feedback** (Kubicek, 2004). Related to 360-degree feedback are **peer appraisals**, where the appraisal is done by coworkers, and **upward appraisals**, where employees evaluate their manager (Milliman et al., 1994).

In a survey of current practice of performance appraisals, 41 health care organizations in Northern Ireland identified the performance appraisal methods they used for health professionals including nurses (Hamilton et al., 2007). From the survey responses the researchers identified seven approaches to performance appraisal:

1. appraisal/performance review,
2. reflection,
3. process review,
4. multisource feedback,
5. observation,
6. supervision, and
7. standards. (pp. 773–791).

Appraisal/performance review is a commonly used and traditional approach to performance appraisal. This approach consists of the manager evaluating the employee's performance and identifying areas for improvement. This approach may be combined with self-appraisal, where the employee also evaluates his or her performance. Reflection is an approach that is related to self-appraisal and may be used in combination with other approaches, such as clinical supervision and professional portfolios. Process review involves discussion of critical incidents, and is a technique that Hamilton et al. state may be less appropriate for assessing individual nurses. Multisource feedback (also referred to as MSF or 360-degree feedback) involves obtaining feedback from different sources, including peers, patients, and colleagues. Observation is an approach that is not used frequently. It is a time-consuming approach that can be criticized for focusing in on a brief period of performance when the employee knows he or she is being observed. Supervision, like observation, is a time-consuming approach that also can be criticized for focusing on brief encounters. The use of standards is an approach where performance is evaluated against predetermined standards of clinical practice.

Hamilton et al. (2007) reviewed the limited literature available regarding the accuracy of the above seven approaches to performance appraisal. They noted that no one method is inherently better, but how the method is implemented, including the education provided to the manager and employees about the process, may be an issue and that research on performance appraisals need to include this and not just the accuracy of the methods.

We believe that performance appraisals can be very time consuming for the manager, particular since today's nurse managers may have numerous nurses and other health care workers reporting directly to them. Given this, managers need to consider if there is evidence that performance appraisals improve motivation and performance, along with any other positive or negative outcomes to employees or to the organization. We also encourage nurse managers to consider using an approach other than the traditional appraisal/performance review. Many professional associations require nurses to use reflection and to document their learning goals, as part of their continuing competency program (see the Interview on page 224). This is an approach that may be more suitable for nurse managers to use than traditional performance appraisals because it recognizes that nurses are professionals. Similarly, considering the nature of clinical work and nurses' need for feedback about their nurse–client interactions to develop their practice, the use of observation and supervision merit attention. Finally, we believe there should be a focus away from evaluating individuals to evaluating teams and work processes. Nurses frequently work in teams and patient outcomes depend on teams who perform well. Chapter 11 on Quality Improvement discusses this issue in more depth.

Benefits of Performance Appraisals

Nickols (2007) identified a number of benefits of performance appraisals that he refers to as "supposed benefits." These benefits are: feedback, goal-setting, career management, objective assessment, and legal protection. With feedback, the hope is that employees improve the quality of their work. The feedback forms the basis for the employee and manager forming objectives. Ideally, these objectives are mutually accepted by the employee and manager and are directed at facilitating the goals of the organization. The feedback also helps with career management, because the employee's needs for development are identified. The performance appraisal process should provide an objective assessment, where employees are evaluated against fair performance expectations that are known to the employee, for example, through their job description. Performance appraisals can also useful to the organization in the event the decision is made to terminate an employee's employment.

In addition to the benefits of performance appraisals identified above, Schraeder, Becton, and Portis (2007) noted that performance appraisals facilitate communication between managers and employees. We agree that performance appraisals facilitate communication, and see them as creating a "forced" point of communication between the nurse manager and health care worker. Given that numerous employees may report to a nurse manager, it is easy for a nurse manager to communicate minimally with some of his or her employees. Due to the number of persons the nurse manager does talk to daily, the nurse manager may not even be aware that a long time has passed since he or she has spoken alone with a particular employee. There are always some vocal staff members who approach the manager regularly, sharing their concerns for the quality of health care and their own feelings and needs. However, there are also staff members who are less assertive in approaching a busy manager, and the performance appraisal meeting gives these persons the opportunity to discuss their individual concerns.

Additionally, we believe that performance appraisals provide the nurse manager with the opportunity to ask what to do, or stop doing, to facilitate each nurse's work. This provides the nurse manager with invaluable information to develop the manager's leadership skills. Thus, the performance appraisal meeting is a time that the nurse manager can use to obtain self feedback.

Cost of Performance Appraisals

Nickols (2007) believes the cost of performance appraisals outweighs the benefits. The list of costs is longer than the list of benefits, and includes both soft costs and hard costs. The soft costs are reductions in productivity, erosion of performance, creation of emotional anguish, damage to morale and motivation, emphasizing individual versus team and task versus process, fostering a short-term view, institutionalizing existing values and biases, fostering fear and lack of trust, and political gains. The hard costs are the direct and indirect financial expenses.

Soft Costs of Performance Appraisals (Nickols, 2007)

1. reductions in productivity
2. erosion of performance
3. creation of emotional anguish
4. damaging to morale and motivation,
5. emphasizing individual versus team and task versus process
6. fostering a short-term view, institutionalizing existing values and biases
7. fostering fear and lack of trust
8. political gains

Hard costs of performance appraisals (Nickols, 2007)

1. direct financial expenses
2. indirect financial expenses

Source: Nickols, F. (2007). Performance appraisal weighed and found wanting in the balance. The *Journal for Quality and Participation*, Spring, 11–16.

Reductions in productivity may occur following the performance appraisal. We are not clear why Nickols (2007) believes this is the case, but assume he is referring to persons who receive a good performance appraisal and then feel they can decrease their efforts for a while. We would add that other reasons for a reduction in productivity is the time taken for the performance appraisal meetings, the emotional anguish of anticipating the appraisal, and the negative effect caused by written negative feedback (which in our experience is perceived more negatively than verbal feedback).

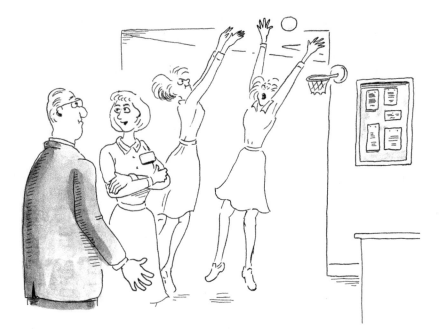

"Morale soared when we installed the Nurf basketball net."

Erosion of performance might occur if people set objectives that they can easily achieve. Perhaps if these objectives were not set, employees would be more visionary and work toward higher or more innovative objectives. Creation of emotional anguish occurs if employees dread the forthcoming performance appraisal. Performance appraisals may be damaging to morale and motivation, particularly if the employee views the feedback as unfair. In fact, if employees are provided negative feedback for their performance when there are environmental constraints on their performance, the feedback is likely to be damaging. For example, a nurse working in a busy department with inadequate staffing may have difficulty ensuring patients receive safe care for the treatments they are undergoing, yet be provided feedback that more time should be spent on family meetings or discharge planning. This can be particularly damaging as these are the activities the nurse probably wants to perform, yet he or she is consumed by dealing with or preventing crises.

Many nurses work on teams, and for quality patient care, the team needs to work well. Performance appraisal systems reward the individual and not the team. To make an analogy to a sports team, if rewards are given to players based on the points they score, players may focus on their own goals rather than assisting others to score a goal. This may result in a lower number of goals for the team. Emphasizing individuals rather than the team, and tasks performed by individuals rather than team processes, means that performance appraisals reward individual performance, a paradox since the organization really wants team performance.

Performance appraisals foster a short-term view by evaluating performance over the past year, while ignoring excellence in prior years or forthcoming contributions. Performance appraisals may institutionalize existing values and biases by rewarding the behaviours that management or the organization have identified as important, rather than new behaviours that may lead to different ways of doing things. Additionally, performance appraisals may foster fear and lack of trust in management, whereby employees learn to comply with what they think the employer wants.

Performance appraisals may be criticized as a process that is open to political games. While performance appraisal systems may strive to be fair by evaluating an employee through standards or seeking input from a variety of persons, ultimately the manager's perception of the employee affects the ratings. In cases where feedback is obtained from a number of persons, these persons may bring their biases or grudges to the table.

We would add to Nickols (2007) list of costs of performance appraisals the fact that managers need excellent communication skills and tact to provide an employee with negative feedback in a way that the employee is receptive to this feedback and uses it to grow and develop. Unfortunately, this is a skill that many managers, not only nurse managers, are still learning. Further, our experience is that written, negative feedback that becomes part of an employee's file may lead to anger and resistance. In contrast, asking an employee questions and helping him or her identify how to change may lead to growth.

Finally, do good performers improve their performance because of a good performance appraisal? Or are they motivated to provide quality care, regardless of any carrots or sticks thrown their way by managers? Think about yourself in a situation of providing patient care. In your relationship with the patient you identify what you can do to help the patient. Would your motivation to do the best you can for a patient change because of the performance appraisal you received? What type of feedback would you need to change your performance, and thereby the quality of your patient's care?

The hard costs of performance appraisals are the financial ones. First, there is the time spent on preparing and giving performance appraisals. There is also the cost of developing the appraisal system, training managers to use the system effectively, and dealing with appeals or grievances. Could this time be better spent on other projects? Has the development of complex, time-consuming performance appraisal systems by human resource departments improved the quality of patient care and/or served to justify the continued existence or expansion of human resource departments? We do believe that self-reflection about your nursing practice is essential. The challenge is to develop a system that encourages nurses' self-reflection and helps them develop their nursing practice, without the disadvantages that have been identified with some systems of performance appraisals.

Research Evidence

There is a dearth of research on performance appraisals in the nursing or health care literature. In management literature, research on performance appraisals has focused on the reliability and validity of different performance appraisal tools as well as comparing one type of performance appraisal to another type. For example, one study found appraisals were viewed more positively when employees felt the purpose of the appraisal was to identify employee development needs, and that upward appraisals were viewed more positively than peer appraisals (Bettenhausen & Fedor, 1997). A study that did look at the use of performance appraisals with nurses examined their acceptance of performance appraisals (Bettenhausen & Fedor, 1991). This study found the nurses accepted performance appraisals more when they thought the purpose was for identifying their developmental needs rather than for administrative use. Therefore, we believe nursing performance appraisals that focus on nurses' self-reflections and development of learning objectives may be more useful than traditional approaches to performance appraisal. Self-reflection and development of learning objectives is performed by nursing students during their studies and is required on an ongoing basis by professional associations.

SUMMARY ON PERFORMANCE APPRAISALS

Perhaps performance appraisals facilitate health care workers' motivation and performance, but perhaps there are other initiatives that would be more effective and efficient in improving the quality of patient care. Given that performance appraisals take much time of managers, health care workers and human resource employees, we need research that demonstrates their relationship with nurse performance. We also need research that demonstrates the relationship between performance appraisals and patient outcomes.

Despite the lack of evidence that performance appraisals improve motivation and performance, organizational operations are slow to change. Further, given that Accreditation Canada has a standard that says the performance of health care workers should be evaluated regularly and that this should be documented (Accreditation Canada, 2010), we can anticipate health care organizations will continue to implement performance appraisals. Therefore, unless you are working in a setting that does not seek accreditation, in all likelihood your organization will have a system of performance appraisals. Given this, we suggest you try to optimize the benefits of performance appraisals. For example, make use of the feedback opportunity to identify how you can improve your performance and seek development opportunities, provide your manager with information that can help support your needs and desires, use the feedback to help set objectives to help your career, and consider the feedback as an opportunity for you to learn more how others perceive you.

DISCIPLINARY PROCEDURES

When a nurse's performance falls below acceptable standards and nurse managers or educators are unable to improve the nurse's work performance through feedback or education, nurse managers or the professional association may be required to use a disciplinary process. Disciplinary action can be taken when a nurse does not follow the health care organization's policies or procedures, has attitudes or behaviours that are not congruent with providing good nurse care or being a team member, or is unable to provide nursing care that meets professional standards (Anderson & Pulich, 2001). A nurse may not follow ethical standards; develop a non-therapeutic relationship with a patient; or demonstrate incompetence due to a lack of education, nursing skills, or proper decision-making ability. It is not enough to be a skilled nurse, and the context within which nursing takes place requires the nurse to form therapeutic relationships with patients, clients, and residents and to work well with other team members. Taking disciplinary action is a difficult decision and process for all involved, but as professionals we have an obligation to the public to ensure safe patient care.

Traditionally, disciplinary action was seen as punitive, but current approaches try to emphasize constructive approaches that help the employee take responsibility to change their performance. This is done in part by treating employees fairly and with respect and engaging them to help meet the needs of the health care organization (Anderson & Pulich, 2001).

Progressive discipline is a constructive approach to discipline that is based on the belief that employees should receive several warnings regarding their performance or behaviour, in order that they have time to change. The warnings are accompanied by different repercussions for the employee (Anderson & Pulich, 2001; Princeton University Human Resources, 2010). For example, in a typical four-stage progressive discipline procedure, the nurse would first receive an oral warning. The emphasis is on helping the nurse learn how his or her performance or behaviour differs from what is expected. At this stage the manager offers assistance to help the nurse change. An organization's progressive discipline procedure may involve several such oral warnings before a letter is written. The oral warnings are not placed on the nurse's file, but the manager may document the meeting and ask the nurse to sign and add any comments. In the event the oral warnings do not lead to the desired change, the next meeting with the nurse may include a written letter of warning. Subsequent meetings may include suspension with or without pay, and ultimately termination when the manager believes the employee will not be able to change his or her performance or behaviour.

Stages of Progressive Discipline

1. Oral warning

2. Oral warning with written letter of warning

3. Suspension with or without pay

4. Termination

Progressive discipline is considered a positive approach to discipline in that it is based on managers' belief that employees can learn, develop, and change. Managers may have to help the nurse to be aware of the changes to his or her work performance and behaviour that are needed for the organization's success. While it may seem paradoxical, this process can result in improved communication and a better relationship between the nurse and manager (Anderson & Pulich, 2001).

In cases where the nurse's action are extreme, such as stealing narcotics or purposefully causing harm to a patient, the nurse may be terminated without use of progressive discipline. In these cases, the nurse may be put on paid leave until an investigation is completed. In such cases, the organization may be legally required to report the incident to the professional association and the professional association then review the complaint and decide if a disciplinary hearing is required.

Giving Effective Feedback in Organizations

We have outlined disciplinary procedures that have been described in the literature and that are in use in many health care organizations. However, organizations have human resources policies and/or collective agreement considerations that managers must use in dealing with performance issues.

The disciplinary process should not be used for nurses making an honest mistake (Johnstone & Kanitsaki, 2005), as was unfortunately done by both health care organizations and professional associations in the past. Honest mistakes are made even by expert clinicians (Reason, 2000), and using a disciplinary procedure to deal with these may reduce the reporting of errors, as well as demotivate the nurse and cause all nurses who are aware of the nurse's treatment to experience anger. Honest mistakes should be reviewed to look for root causes and analyze work processes to see how they can be improved to reduce errors (see Chapter 11, Quality Improvement).

While current approaches to discipline try to emphasize that they are helping the nurse to change, the use of the word "discipline" cannot but evoke negative feelings and reactions. This has implications not only for the nurse being disciplined but also for other

Interview

Beverley McIsaac

Beverley McIsaac is the Nursing Consultant Regulatory Services/Advanced Practice at the Association of Registered Nurses of Newfoundland & Labrador (ARNNL). She is responsible for implementing and evaluating the ARNNL's program to ensure nurses maintain their competency.

Q: When nurses in Newfoundland and Labrador renew their license, they complete a continuing competency program. Can you describe this program and its purpose?

A: A main component of this program is that each nurse reflects on his or her practice or service area, whether this practice is in direct care, administration, education, or research, and completes a self assessment of his or her learning needs. Another component is that each nurse takes one of his or her learning needs and develops a goal that is related to one of ARNNL's standards for practice. Next, the nurse develops a learning plan for this goal and this plan is for learning over the next year. At the end of the year, the nurse evaluates how the learning has made a difference in the care or

service he or she provides. An additional piece is that the program includes 14 hours of mandatory education a year, of which 7 have to be formal hours, such as inservice or conference hours, while 7 hours can be informal such as reading nursing journals, articles, etc.

The purpose of continuing competency programs is protection of the public. The public expects nurses to maintain their competence, and the regulatory body has the legal responsibility to ensure that all nurses are competent. Therefore, nurses as well as other professional groups have continuing competency programs.

Q: What do you see as the benefits of this continuing competency program?

A: The ARNNL initiated their continuing competency program in 2010, and since that time we have heard from many nurses that this program should have been implemented years ago. I met with nurses throughout the province to introduce the program, and the majority were already assessing their learning needs and attending education programs, and took great pride in how they continued to be active learners. Surprisingly, there is a small minority that is not participating in lifelong learning, and this was sometimes identified by other nurses who attended sessions. They would note that a particular nurse(s) who was not at the session really should be there, and go on and say things such as a nurse(s) had not even renewed CPR certification or a nurse(s) even took pride in the fact that he or she had not attended an educational session or read journal articles since graduation.

Fourteen hours is not a lot and most nurses were doing more even before implementation of the continuing competency program. However, this program ensures that the small minority who had not engaged in learning since graduating as a nurse would have at least 14 hours. This is important for the nursing profession, because as nurses we want all nurses to maintain and enhance competency. It is also important because as nurses we need to assure the public that nurses are competent. In fact, the regulatory body has an obligation to ensure all registered nurses maintain and enhance their competency, and one way to ensure competence is having a continuing competency program.

Q: How is the continuing competency program in Newfoundland and Labrador similar or different to continuing competency programs in other Canadian provinces?

A: All of the regulatory bodies in Canadian provinces have a continuing competency program, although they may give it a different name, and this program is similar to programs across Canada. However, Newfoundland and Labrador is the only province where nurses have a mandatory education hour requirement. Seven of these hours are structured learning, and for these hours the registered nurse is required provide evidence of this education such as a certificate of learning.

Newfoundland and Labrador has registered nurses who work in rural and remote areas. Therefore, our program has to be flexible for nurses, because all nurses need to be able to achieve what the program requests. Not all nurses live where there may be educational programs, and some may even work in areas with unreliable Internet access. That is why 7 of the 14 hours of mandatory education can be informal learning.

Our program includes auditing 5 to 10% of all registered nurses, while not all provinces audit nurses. However, to assure the public that nurses are maintaining their competence, we need to measure the degree to which nurses are participating in the continuing competency program.

Q: Have you heard feedback from nurses that participating in the continuing competency program has helped improve their performance or motivation at work?

A: We did a survey in 2012 and found the nurses' attitudes toward the program were positive. One item on the survey was to rate the statement "Registered Nurses must be accountable for their own learning" and 85% agreed with this statement. This represents a shift in nurses' opinions about who should be accountable for learning. When I met with nurses to introduce the program, many felt that employers should be responsible for nurses' learning, not the nurse. Now when I meet with nurses, I find that most see this as their own responsibility. In fact, many nurses speak with pride about how they assume responsibility for their own learning.

Q: Who has access to the learning plan developed by a nurse?

A: The only occasion a nurse needs to show someone his or her learning plan is if they are audited by the ARNNL. When we began our program, many nurses were concerned that if they wrote they needed to improve an area of practice, their manager would have access to this information and could use this against them. However, this is not the case because the learning plan belongs to each individual nurse.

Source: Interview with Beverley McIsaac. Reprinted by permission.

nurses who are aware of the process, generally through the disciplined nurse because managers will keep the process confidential. This awareness can be challenging for the nurse manager, as nurses are free to interpret their view of the situation while the nurse manager needs to keep the nurse's situation confidential. The nurse's colleagues may be relieved when a difficult employee is effectively managed, and it may improve everyone's motivation. At other times nurses may choose to side with the disciplined nurse, even if they had previously complained about this nurse. This polarization can have a negative impact on the climate of both the nursing department and the health care organization.

How nurse managers interact with nurses during disciplinary meetings is also important, as the way managers work with nurses can model how nurses work with patients, clients, and residents. A health care organization's philosophy of nursing and/or the theory(s) of nursing they use to guide nursing care typically describe working with clients in collaboration and in a relationship that demonstrates respect and caring and supports trust. Nursing leaders need to work with nurses in a way that is congruent with the organization's philosophy and theories of care.

SUMMARY

This chapter has outlined some of the key theories of work motivation, and suggested how these theories might relate to nurses' motivation and performance. In addition, this chapter has summarized research that examined nurses' sources of motivation, the outcomes of their motivation, and the level of their motivation. Issues considered were generational difference in motivators, how managers may have an impact on motivation and performance, and the role nurses may take in managing their own and their colleagues' motivation and performance.

Managers have a role in modelling the leadership behaviours and providing the environmental supports that nurses need to be motivated and perform well. Nurses are motivated in part by a need to make a difference in the lives of others and provide care, and managers can work toward creating workplaces where nurses have time to provide the type of care that led them to select nursing as a career. Managers can provide structures such as career ladders to help motivate nurses and keep them in direct care positions (see the Leading Health Care Example in this chapter). They can also help nurses who are not performing well by mentoring them and giving them feedback, and ultimately using progressive discipline when required.

Nevertheless, nurses have a huge role to play in their own motivation and performance. We believe that nurses want to be motivated and to perform well, because feeling motivated and knowing you have done a good job makes you feel good. In the event nurses are in a workplace where they do not feel motivated, they can consider the sources of motivation included in this chapter, as well as strategies such as developing a professional purpose statement. Ultimately, a nurse who is not motivated will not feel good about his or her performance. In the event a nurse is unable to identify factors in the work environment or relationships with colleagues or managers that he or she can change, it may be in this nurse's best interests to identify another type of nursing or working environment where he or she will feel motivated, and patients will receive the type of care they deserve.

Glossary of Terms

Baby boomers   Baby boomers were born from approximately 1946 to 1964.

Career ladders   A structure for promoting direct care nurses to a different level of clinical practice, based on their expertise, whereby nurses at different steps of the ladder have different responsibilities, and may have a different salary scale and job title.

Generation X   were born from approximately 1965 to 1981. They are more informal and place more importance on their non-work life than baby boomers.

Nexters   Nexters are also referred to as generation Y, the millennial generation, millennials, generation next, the net generation, or the echo boomers. Nexters were born approximately from 1982 to 2000 and are the generation who are currently entering the workforce. They are comfortable with computer technology and want a voice in decision making as new employees, and like generation X they place more emphasis on their non-work life than baby boomers.

Peer appraisals   Feedback for the purposes of a performance appraisal is obtained from the employee's peers or coworkers.

Progressive discipline   A constructive approach to discipline that is based on the belief that employees should receive several warnings regarding their performance or behaviour to have time to change.

Self-efficacy   Self-efficacy is a person's belief in his or her capacity to successfully perform a specific task.

360-degree feedback   Feedback for the purposes of a performance appraisal is obtained from a variety of other employees that the person interacts with on the job, as opposed to just from the manager.

Upward appraisals   Feedback for the purposes of a performance appraisal is obtained from the subordinates of the employee who is being evaluated.

Work engagement   Is the opposite of burnout and refers to positive feelings of enthusiasm, absorption, fulfillment, and dedication toward your work.

Work motivation   Is the intensity and persistence of an employee's work-related behaviour. It is "the extent to which persistent effort is directed towards a goal" (Johns & Saks, 2011).

CASE

Tonya had been working as a direct care nurse on a general medical unit since she graduated with a bachelor's degree in nursing a year ago. When she first started on the unit, she was nervous about whether she would be able to manage the workload and provide safe care. In her university nursing courses, her class had discussed the importance of taking breaks to avoid burnout. Tonya now felt good that she was assertive in telling other nurses what care her patients required while she was off the unit. She also felt she prioritized care, and set realistic objectives for her nursing care that prioritized safe patient care.

This morning, Tonya was scheduled to meet with her nurse manager for her first performance appraisal since starting to work. Tonya believed her nurse manager would give her a very positive appraisal. She was shocked when the meeting started with her nurse manager saying she had a number of concerns about Tonya's performance. The nurse manager then said that instead of focusing on tasks, Tonya needed to become concerned with the broader picture of what was happening on the entire unit as well as the broader picture about her patients' and their families' lives. She said most of the nurses on the unit felt Tonya "dumped" work on them and had tunnel vision when it came to helping them.

Tonya felt hurt and angry, and betrayed by the nurses who had complained about her. She stood up and went to the door while yelling, "If you were ever on the unit, maybe you would know what I did!" She slammed the door as she left the room.

Questions

1. What could the nurse manager have done differently, prior to the meeting?
2. What could the nurse manager have done differently, during the meeting? Suggest how the nurse manager could have worded the feedback.
3. Within the nurse manager's feedback, can you identify how this could be presented in terms of an opportunity for Tonya to become a more expert clinician?
4. What could Tonya have done differently to learn about the nurse manager's perception of her performance, during the past year?
5. Suggest how Tonya could have responded to the feedback.
6. Tonya wants to keep her position on the medical unit. Should she initiate a meeting with the nurse manager, and if so, what should be her plan for this meeting?

Critical Thinking Questions and Activities

1. Interview a nurse who works for an organization that uses a performance appraisal process.
   a. Describe the type of performance appraisal used.
   b. How does the nurse feel about the performance appraisal process?
   c. Compare your findings with the findings of other students in your class.

2. Divide into groups of six students. Debate the question "Should health care organizations continue to use performance appraisals?" Two students should present arguments pro, two students against, one student serves as moderator, and the remaining student identifies and rates the strengths of points made by both sides.

3. Interview a nurse you know who you believe demonstrates motivation for his or her nursing practice. Ask, "What motivates you about your nursing practice?" Following the interview, see if you can relate what the nurse says to any of the theories of motivation and work motivation discussed in this chapter.

4. What do you think is the role of the nurse in promoting his or her own motivation to nurse? What things can each nurse do to increase or maintain their motivation to nurse?

5. What can a nurse do to help his or her colleagues increase or maintain their motivation in the workplace?

6. Germain and Cummings (2009) identify five categories of nurses' perceptions of how their motivation and performance is affected. They note that nurses can have an impact on their own motivation by considering these factors, and two of their suggestions are provided in this text (build a trusting relationship with nursing colleagues and nurse managers, and inform managers of the resources nurses need to do their work). What other examples can you think of where nurses can affect these five categories to improve their own motivation and performance?

Self-Quiz

1. Factors in Herzberg's motivation-hygiene theory that lead to work motivation include:
   a. Salary
   b. Goal-setting
   c. Work-life balance
   d. Recognition

2. All of the following are discussed in Bandura's social cognitive theory *except:*
   a. Self-efficacy
   b. Self-esteem
   c. Self-evaluative reactions
   d. Performance

3. Maslow's hierarchy of needs:
   a. is a useful heuristic for prioritizing client needs
   b. is currently the best explanation of work motivation
   c. has been developed to include transcendence, outcome expectancy, and cognitive needs
   d. is criticized for its focus on the needs of professsionals

4. Benefits of performance appraisals include:
   a. goal-setting
   b. legal protection
   c. opportunity for manager to seek feedback about manager's performance
   d. emphasis on individual outcomes

5. Career development programs
   a. are a form of progressive discipline
   b. may include clinical ladders
   c. are hindered by professional purpose statements
   d. refer to graduate degrees in nursing

6. Kylee learns that a coworker who was recruited to her rural community centre to fill a vacant position was enticed to move to her area with a salary that was much higher than Kylee's salary. After Kylee learned this, she started placing less effort into participating on committees or volunteering when her manager asked for assistance. Kylee's behaviour can be most easily explained by:
   a. Self-efficacy theory
   b. Social cognitive theory
   c. Equity theory
   d. Expectancy theory

Useful Websites

The following website describes the Donner-Wheeler Career Planning and Development Model developed by two Canadian nurses, Gail Donner and Mary Wheeler. www.donnerwheeler.com/programs and services/career development.html

The Registered Nurses' Association of Ontario website has some information about career development.
http://rnao.org/page.asp?PageID=861&SiteNode ID=199

References

Accreditation Canada. (2010). *Qmentum Program Standards. Effective Organization*. Ottawa: Accreditation Canada.

Anderson, M., & Lavoie-Tremblay, M. (2008). Evaluation of the Executive Training for Research Application (EXTRA) Program: Design and early findings. *Healthcare Policy*, 4(2), e136–e148.

Anderson, P., & Pulich, M. (2001). A positive look at progressive discipline. *Health Care Manager*, 20(1), 1–9.

Asselin, M. (2003). Motivating LPNs. *Nursing management*, 34(8), 40–45.

Bandura, A. (1986). *Social foundations of thought and action: A social cognitive theory*. Englewood Cliffs, NJ: Prentice-Hall.

Bandura, A. (1997). *Self-efficacy: The exercise of control*. New York, NY: W. H. Freeman and Company.

Benner, P. (1982). From novice to expert. *American Journal of Nursing, 81*, 402–407.

Benner, P. (1984). *From novice to expert*. Reading, MA: Addison-Wesley.

Bettenhausen, K. & Fedor, D. (1991). Constructing evaluation realities: How the dual roles of giving and receiving peer feedback affect acceptance of a peer evaluation system. In M. Peiperl (Chair). *Peer evaluation revisited*. Symposium conducted at the 51st annual meeting of the Academy of Management, Miami, Florida.

Bettenhausen, K. & Fedor, D. (1997). Peer and upward appraisals. A comparison of their benefits and problems. *Group and Organization Management, 22*(2), 236–263.

Blegan, M. (1993). Nurses' job satisfaction: A meta-analysis of related variables. *Nursing Research, 42*(1), 36–41.

Boughn, S. (2001). Why women and men choose nursing. *Nursing and Health Care Perspectives, 22*(1), 14–19.

Buchan, J. (1999). Evaluating the benefits of a clinical ladder for nursing staff: an international review. *International Journal of Nursing studies, 36*, 137–144.

Burket, T., Greider, P., & Rohrer, E. (2010). Clinical ladder program evolution: Journey from novice to expert to enhancing outcomes. *The Journal of Continuing Education in Nursing, 41*(8), 369–374.

Canadian Nurses Association. (2001). *Framework for the practice of registered nurses in Canada*. Retrieved June 11, 2011, from www.cna-aiic.ca/CNA/documents/pdf/publications/RN_Framework_Practice_2007_e.pdf

Cianci, R., & Gambrel, P. (2003). Maslow's hierarchy of needs: Does it apply in a collectivist culture. *Journal of Applied Management and Entrepreneurship, 8*(2), 143–161.

Cooper, H., & Cottrell, R. (2010). Charting your career path through clear professional values and purpose. *Health Promotion Practice, 11*(1), 13–15.

De Cooman, R., De Gieter, S., Pepermans, R., Du Bois, C., Capers, R., & Jegers, M. (2008). Freshmen in nursing: Job motives and work values of a new generation. *Journal of Nursing Management, 16*(1), 56–64.

De Loach, R., & Monroe, J. (2004). Job satisfaction among hospice workers. What managers need to know. *The Health Care Manager, 23*(3), 209–219.

Freeman, T., & O'Brien-Pallas, L. (1998). Factors influencing job satisfaction on specialty nursing units. *Canadian Journal of Nursing Administration, 11*(3), 25–51.

Germain, P., & Cummings, G. (2010). The influence of nursing leadership on nurse performance: A systematic literature review. *Journal of Nursing Management, 18*, 425–439.

Hamilton, K., Coates, V., Kelly, B., Boore, J., Cundell, J., Gracey, J., McFetridge, B., McGonigal, M., & Sinclair, M. (2007). Performance assessment in health care providers: A critical review of evidence and current practice. *Journal of Nursing Management, 15*, 773–791.

Hertzberg, F., Mausner, B., & Snyderman, B. (1967). *The motivation to work*. New York: John Wiley & Sons.

International Council of Nurses. (1995). Career development for nurses. Working Document. Geneva: ICN.

Johns, G., & Saks, A. (2011). *Organizational behaviour: Understanding and managing life at work*. Toronto, Pearson Canada.

Johnstone, M., & Kanitsaki, O. (2005). Processes for disciplining nurses for unprofessional conduct of a serious nature: A critique. *Journal of Advanced Nursing, 50*(4), 363–371.

Kerr, J., & Jeans, M.E. (2006). The EXTRA difference: Leadership development. *ACEN Update, 19*(3), 24–27.

Kubicek, M. (2004). Turning appraisals around. *Training Magazine*, September, 20–22.

Laschinger, H., Wong, C., Ritchie, J., Danielle D'Amour, D., Vincent, L., et al. (2008). A profile of the structure and impact of nursing management in Canadian hospitals. *Healthcare Quarterly, 11*(2), 85–94.

Maslow, A. (1943). A theory of human motivation. *Psychological Review, 50*(4), 370–96.

McCabe, R., Nowak, M., & Mullen, S. (2005). Nursing careers: What motivated nurses to choose their profession? *Australian Bulletin of Labour, 31*(4), 384–406.

McClelland, D. (1955). *Studies in motivation*. New York: Appleton-Century-Crofts.

McClelland, D. (1975). *Power: The inner experience*. New York: Irvington.

MacPhee, M., & Bouthillette, F. (2008). Developing leadership in nurse managers: The British Columbia Nursing Leadership Institute. *Nursing Research, 21*(3), 64–75.

Martin, D., & Bartol, K. Performance appraisal: Maintaining system effectiveness. *Public Personnel Management, 27*(2), 223–230.

Meadus, R., & Twomey, C. (2007). Men in nursing: Making the right choice. *Canadian Nurse, 103*(2), 13–16.

Milliman, J., Zawacki, R., Norman, C., Powell, L. & Kirksey, J. (1994). Companies evaluate employees from all perspectives. *Personnel Journal, 73*(11), 99–103.

Mrayyan, M., & Al-Faouri, I. (2008). Nurses' career commitment and job performance: Differences across hospitals. *Nursing Research, 21*(2), e101–e117.

Newton, J., Kelly, C., Kremser, A., Jolly, B., & Billett, S. (2009). The motivation to nurse: An exploration of factors amongst undergraduate students, registered nurses and nurse managers. *Journal of Nursing Management, 17*, 392–400.

Nickols, F. (2007). Performance appraisal weighed and found wanting in the balance. *The Journal for Quality and Participation*, Spring, 11–16.

O'Brien-Pallas, L., Tomblin-Murphy, G., Birch, S., & Baumann, A. (2001). Framework for analyzing health human resources. In *Future development of information to support the management of nursing resources: Recommendations*. Ottawa: Canadian Institute of Health Information.

Princeton University Human Resources. (2010). *Disciplinary procedure*. Retrieved June 15, 2011, from www.princeton.edu/hr/policies/conditions/5.1/5.1.4/

Reason, J. (2000). Human error: Models and management. *British Medical Journal, 320*, 768–770.

Salyer, J. (1995). Environmental turbulence: Impact on nurse performance. *Journal of Nursing Administration, 25*(4), 12–20.

Schaufeli, W., Salanova, M., González-Romá, V., & Bakker, A. (2002). The measurement of engagement and burnout: A confirmative analytic approach. *Journal of Happiness Studies, 3*, 71–92.

Schraeder, M., Becton, J., & Portis, R. (2007). A critical examination of performance appraisals. *The Journal for Quality and Participation*, Spring, 20–25.

Stacey-Adams, J. (1963). Towards an understanding of inequity. *Journal of Abnormal and Social Psychology, 67*, 422–436.

Toode, K., Routasalo, P., and Suominen, T. (2011). Work motivation of nurses: A literature review. *International Journal of Nursing Studies, 48*, 246–257.

Vroom, V. (1964). *Work and motivation*. London: John Wiley.

Wahba, M., & Lawrence, G. B. (1974). Maslow reconsidered: A review of research on the need hierarchy theory. *Organizational*

Behavior and Human Performance, 15(2): 212–240.

Yildiz, Z., Ayhan, S., Erdoğmus, S. (2009). The impact of nurses' motivation to work, job satisfaction, and sociodemographic characteristics on intention to quit their current job: An empirical study in Turkey. *Applied Nursing Research, 22,* 113–118.

Zimmer, M. (1972). Rationale for a ladder for clinical advance. *Journal of Nursing Administration, 11*(6), 18–24.

Chapter 8
Nursing Roles and Nurse Staffing

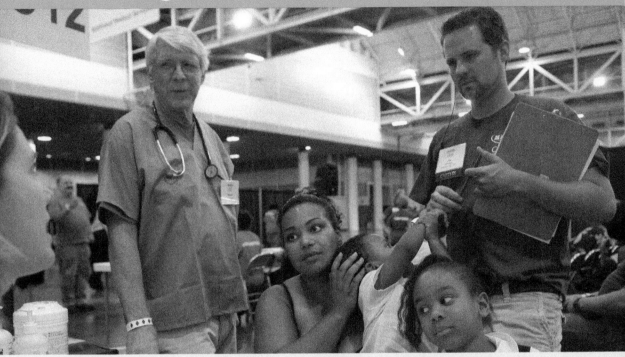

ROD LAMKEY JR/AFP/Getty Images/Newscom

Learning Objectives

After reading, studying, and reflecting on this chapter's content, you will be able to:

1. Describe regulated and unregulated nursing categories in Canadian health care organizations
2. Identify direct care nursing roles and categories of personnel involved in nursing care in Canadian health care
3. Discuss a variety of approaches to nurse staffing and the factors to be considered in establishing a staffing plan
4. Discuss the relationship between nurse staffing and outcomes for patients/clients, nurses, and the organization
5. Identify the range of staffing and scheduling policies that might be required in a health care organization and discuss the factors that must be considered in establishing such policies
6. Discuss the benefits, challenges, and considerations in establishing a system of self-scheduling

INTRODUCTION

In Chapter 2 we discussed the wide variety of health care occupations within the Canadian health care system and made reference to the numbers and kinds of regulated nursing and unregulated personnel who participate in nursing care in such organizations as hospitals and long-term care facilities. In the first part of this chapter, we discuss direct care roles and management roles involved in nurse staffing in health care organizations as well as the concepts of **skill mix/staff mix** and **scope of practice** and **scope of employment**. Understanding these roles and the concept of scope of practice/employment is important when planning staffing and staffing policies within a health care organization.

In the next section of this chapter we focus on a topic that will be of interest to you as a new graduate or a nurse entering a new workplace, that of staffing and staffing policies. During your career you might experience different staffing levels as you move from one work setting to another, if you encounter generalized nursing shortages, or if your work setting reduces staffing due to budgetary constraints. Staffing became a major focus of attention due to cost-cutting by Canadian hospitals during the 1990s. The job losses and reduced opportunities for nursing graduates in Canada led to increased migration of nurses, mostly to the United States, and decreased the enrollment of students in nursing schools. Shortages of nurses followed as the demand for nurses increased in the following decade along with the retirement of increasing numbers of older nurses. Nursing shortages were a problem in many countries of the world, including the United States, and led to questions about the numbers and categories of personnel who could most efficiently provide safe and quality nursing care. We will focus on what we have learned from experience and research in Canada and elsewhere about staff mix, staffing methods or approaches, and staffing policies. In particular, we will focus on how staffing influences patient/client, nurse, and organizational outcomes. In this section, we also discuss challenges in staffing and scheduling and some of the approaches used to address these problems. We highlight the importance that staffing has for patient care quality, work life quality, and outcomes for health care organizations.

DIRECT CARE ROLES IN NURSING

Direct care roles in nursing care delivery include those provided by members of regulated groups, who are in some settings, assisted by **unregulated health care workers**. When we refer to direct care roles, most of the time we are thinking about roles requiring direct physical contact with clients, such as in the role of the "bedside nurse" in a hospital or a staff nurse in a public health unit. However, there are some roles that would be considered direct care even without physical contact, as in the case of telenurses who engage in assessment activities and provide advice over the telephone, or roles involving the use of the internet or teleconference systems.

Regulated Nursing Groups

As discussed in Chapter 2, there are four groups of nursing personnel that are regulated:

- Registered Nurses
- Nurse Practitioners (who are also Registered Nurses)

- Registered Psychiatric Nurses (in Alberta, British Columbia, Manitoba, Saskatchewan, and Yukon)
- Registered Practical Nurses in Ontario, infirmières et infirmiers auxiliaires or nursing auxilliaries in Quebec, and Licensed Practical Nurses in the rest of Canada).

Health care organizations employ members of some or all of the groups mentioned above (depending on the province or territory) to meet the nursing care needs of clients/patients. As members of a regulated group, they are accountable for the standards of practice set by their registering/licensing body. Nurses in each of these groups are educated to work within their scope and to recognize the limits of their scope of practice within health care. As a registered nurse, you might move from one regulatory jurisdiction to another and encounter regulated groups that are new to you. It is important that you understand your scope of practice when you become licensed in a new jurisdiction as well as the scope of practice of members of regulated categories with whom you have not worked before. So, for example, if you are new to working in a Western province, you might work with registered psychiatric nurses for the first time in your nursing career.

It is also very important that employers of nurses have a clear understanding of the scope of practice of regulated groups and design positions in an organization that maximize that scope for the benefit of patients, the satisfaction of their nursing staff, and the most cost-effective use of nursing resources for the organization and the overall health care system.

For the purposes of this chapter, we will focus on some of the direct care roles of registered nurses, the largest group of regulated professionals, as they are the ones frequently encountered in health care. These include:

- **Staff nurses**. You are likely most familiar with this role in hospitals, but they exist in other settings as well, such as public health units, clinics, and long-term care facilities. They are often referred to as front-line nurses and bedside nurses, depending on the context.
- **Nurse Practitioners** (NP). This is a subset of Registered Nurses and they work in an **Advanced Nurse Practice** role. They constitute a regulated group and their title cannot be used by any nurse who has not been educated to this level and who is not licensed in this category. Depending on the province, they may be registered or licensed in different fields, for example, primary health care, adult acute care, pediatric acute care, and so on. These nurses work within their legislated scope of practice and carry direct care responsibilities, but aspects of their role involve education, consultation, leadership, and research. An acute care nurse practitioner may function in a role that requires specific expertise, for example, pain management for clients who receive inpatient and outpatient services from a hospital's Pain Management Service.
- **Clinical Nurse Specialist** (CNS). A CNS is a registered nurse in an advanced nursing practice role, but unlike NPs, they may not be part of a specific regulated group. They have graduate education in nursing that leads them to develop greater breadth and depth of knowledge and skill in a specialized area of nursing. They hold positions in hospitals and other settings where they provide direct care services to patients, but

also they engage in support, education, and monitoring of nursing staff; provide consultation throughout the hospital; and promote the conduct and uptake of nursing research to improve nursing care. There has been some concern about the sustainability of the role of the CNS in health care, unless, as a group, CNSs can establish a vision for their role and a national voice (Bryant-Lukosius et al., 2010).

Of the various kinds of direct care nursing roles, the most confusing and least understood are advanced practice nursing roles (Bryant-Lukosius, DiCenso, Browne, & Pinelli, 2004) and greater attention to their role is needed at a time when acute care NPs are being incorporated into hospitals in increasing numbers (Cummings, Fraser, & Tarlier, 2003).

In addition to these direct care roles, other kinds of nurses may provide support to nurses within health care organizations. For example, nurse educators are frequently employed by hospitals to provide educational support to nursing staff and other health care staff in the organization.

Unregulated Health Workers

In Chapter 2 there was a brief discussion of the category of unregulated health worker. This kind of worker may have some duties related to the direct care of patients or clients, working under the direction of a regulated health professional. Their job titles might reflect their role in direct care, such as personal support worker, health care assistant, or health care aide. A confusing array of titles for these workers is not limited to Canada, as Crossan and Ferguson (2005) note there is the same problem in the United Kingdom's National Health Service (NHS), with a frequent lack of clarity about what these individuals actually do. In Canada, individuals in these roles may have had a formal period of education, generally lasting weeks to a few months, or they may have received on-the-job training.

In Chapter 5, there was some discussion of the category of unregulated health workers in relation to delegation and assignment. You might want to review this section and that on decision-making about delegation to unregulated health care providers, as you may encounter these workers in your career. In times of nursing shortages and/or cost-cutting in health care, the numbers and kinds of unregulated personnel may increase. If the staffing plan in your health care organization includes unregulated workers in direct care activities, it is important that you know what activities and tasks can be safely assigned to them. In working with unregulated health workers, you will be in a leadership position with respect to assessing and assigning activities. In order to do so, you need to understand the scope of employment of the worker, which should be reflected in a position description.

NURSING SKILL MIX/STAFF MIX

The terms "skill mix" or "staff mix" as applied to nurse staffing refer to the numbers and types (regulated and unregulated) of personnel used to provide care to a group of patients or clients in a setting (CNA, June 2003). Both direct and indirect care activities are included in consideration of staffing requirements. Direct care refers to nursing activities with the client, while indirect activities are those away from the client, but necessary to direct care, such as charting, care planning, and obtaining supplies. Although some **staffing plans** in the past merely specified a ratio of nursing personnel to patients or clients, increasingly, health care organizations are seeking to refine their plans to identify the optimal mix of different types of personnel to obtain the most cost-effective outcomes. Staffing plans do not include nursing students. When you engage in clinical practice as a nursing student, you are not counted as part of the nurse staffing complement, because you are present for educational purposes, rather than for the purposes of providing service.

Skill mix has become a topic of concern in Canada, particularly in acute care settings. In *Staffing for Safety: A Synthesis of the Evidence on Nurse Staffing and Patient Safety*, it was noted that there was reason to be concerned about the declining quality of health care due to poor staffing (Ellis, Priest, MacPhee & McCutcheon, 2006). The authors noted the following:

- evidence of rising patient acuity and need for specialized care
- decreased staffing over the previous decade through replacement of registered nurses with non-registered nurses and unregulated personnel
- early retirement of experienced, senior nurses
- younger nurses leaving the profession

In the past several decades, greater research attention has been given to the appropriate mix of personnel in staffing plans and what difference the mix makes in terms of patient, nurse, and health system outcomes.

MANAGEMENT ROLES IN NURSE STAFFING

Staffing is a process that involves decision making at various levels. Three levels are described in the Registered Nurses Association of Ontario's (RNAO) document entitled *Healthy Work Environments Best Practice Guidelines: Developing and Sustaining Effective Staffing and Workload Practices* (2007):

- Strategic nursing decision making is the level that includes decisions that guide the approach to nursing care delivery in an organization. Included in strategic decisions are what the skill mix (RN, RPN, unregulated) will be, staff status mix (full-time, part-time, and casual), staffing levels, and model of care/philosophy and organization of care delivery). Decisions about the numbers and kinds of clients who are to be cared for by a team/unit are a part of strategic nursing decision making.
- Logistical nursing decision making generates directions on staffing for a team or unit within an organization. Decisions relate to normal staffing levels, replacement staffing method (such as float pool, agency staffing), and scheduling approaches and methods.
- Tactical nursing decision making refers to decisions that are made on a short-term basis (day-to-day or shift-to-shift) to adjust to changing client needs or changes in staff availability.

As you can see from the range of decisions, many nurses are involved in staffing decisions, a great deal of communication and feedback is required, and judgments are constantly required to ensure a match between patient needs and nurse supply.

In most health care organizations of considerable size, there are at least two kinds of nurse managers involved in or playing a leadership role in these decisions: a nurse executive(s) and nurse managers (who may be positioned at more than one level within the organizational structure). Nurse executives are key in strategic decision making about staffing, nurse managers of units are usually key in logistical processes, and tactical decision making is made by nursing staff teams/clinical leader on each unit as adjustments are required.

METHODS OR APPROACHES TO STAFFING

There are at least five approaches to staffing that are described in the nursing literature (Flynn & McKeown, 2009; McGillis Hall et al., 2006). These are:

1. Reliance on professional judgment and expertise to identify staffing requirements
2. Patient classification systems and workload measurement systems
3. Decision frameworks used to formulate staff mix and staffing plans
4. Use of standardized ratios—nurse-to-patient/client ratios
5. Dynamic and shared decision making

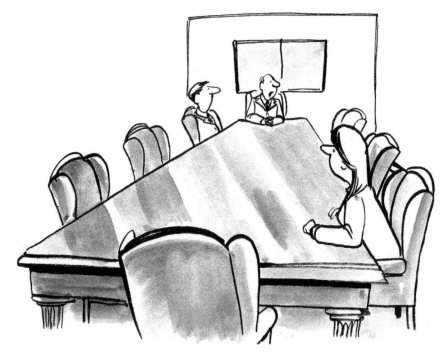

"How could anyone think that this department is under staffed?"

Cartoonresource/Shutterstock

Professional Judgment

Professional judgment, "gut" feeling, and intuition are the historical and traditional approaches that are still used to determine the appropriate numbers and mix of caregivers in a particular setting. Nurses and managers in a setting recognize when workload becomes too great, and identify the need for more staff when there are temporary changes or upward trends in **patient acuity** that call for readjustment of the traditional plan. Some nurses interviewed by McGillis Hall et al. (2006) thought professional judgment was used more often than more formal systems of staffing and that financial constraints were an influence as well.

Patient Classification/Workload Measurement Systems (WMS)

Patient classification systems refer to the grouping of patients based on the amount of direct nursing care they require and using such a classification scheme to predict the demand for nursing care. Patients may be classified into groups based on such characteristics as acuity of illness, or on the basis of critical elements of care required. **Workload measurement systems** (WMS) may use a patient classification and then established hours of care for the types of patients in the setting to calculate staffing requirements. Others may rely on tasks required and standard times required for these tasks to establish staffing requirements (RNAO, 2005). In this way, staffing is based on patient requirements, and a range of workload systems have been developed over the years to assist in making staffing decisions, mostly in acute care hospitals. Typically, patient classification data or a WMS may be used to justify budget requests or budgets for a nursing unit. Using estimates of average hours of care required by the typical range of patient categories on the unit, an average unit workload can be computed. In this way, these systems assist in establishing longer-range staffing for a unit, rather than determining day-by-day staffing requirements. In Table 8.1 you will see some of the strengths and limitations of such systems of workload measurement.

According to McGillis Hall et al. (2006, p. 264), "these [WMS] systems fell into disuse as a staffing tool because they often called for greater staffing than organizations were able to provide." The experience has been that when these tools indicate the need for more staff, it is rarely forthcoming and when the systems identify surplus staff based on the system, nurses are sent to work on other units (McGillis Hall; Berry & Curry, 2012). Many do not consider them consistent, useful, or reliable and while they may show trends in acuity or changes in patient acuity, they do not affect workload. You might continue to see these systems in your place of employment. In many settings, nurses continue to complete the forms required to track and report on workload, but they do not seem to drive staffing decisions in the way in which they were initially intended.

Table 8.1 Strengths and Limitations Related to Workload Measurement Systems

Strengths	Limitations
▪ It can be used by administrators to make resource allocation decisions between patient care settings and make strategic decisions based on cost per case and funding incentives.	▪ Some WLM systems have been integrated into patient documentation systems but the success of this has been inconsistent.
	▪ Not all WLM tools have been validated and may not accurately capture the work of nursing.
▪ Some WLM tools can now be integrated with computerized documentation systems to link workload to patient characteristics, clinical outcomes, and standards with financial data to determine costs.	▪ Not all nurses have a strong grasp of the potential of WLM or have unrealistic expectations regarding application of the tools.
	▪ Comparisons between similar health facilities are difficult because of the different methodologies and systems used in the hospital sector and the validity and reliability of data collected.
▪ Has the potential to contribute to quality of care and nursing's contribution to patient care by providing support for appropriate resource allocation.	▪ Reliability and validity can vary within the hospital sector as well—in part due to inadequate human resources and because the necessary supporting infrastructure is not provided to adequately support the system
	▪ WLM tools may be inappropriately used for purposes other than that for which they were created such as controlling costs; this can contribute to the lack of endorsement from staff to participate.
	▪ Some WLM tools do not capture the complexity of nursing knowledge and skill.

Source: Reprinted with permission from the *Best Practice Guidelines*, published by the Registered Nurses' Association of Ontario. All rights reserved.

Decision Frameworks for Staffing

Decision frameworks represent one approach to making staffing decisions and these frameworks can use principles (ANA, 1999) or a group of elements/factors to consider when making broad decisions about staffing (CNA, et al., 2005, 2012). Currently, a framework developed by the Canadian Nurses Association, the Canadian Council for Practical Nurse Regulators, and the Registered Psychiatric Nurses of Canada is designed as a resource for staff mix decision making in any health care setting. You will recognize the complexity of making these kinds of decisions by considering Figure 8.1. The framework identifies factors related to clients, staff, and the organization; five guiding principles; and client, staff, and organizational outcomes that are to be considered by staffing decision makers.

Staff Mix Decision-making Framework

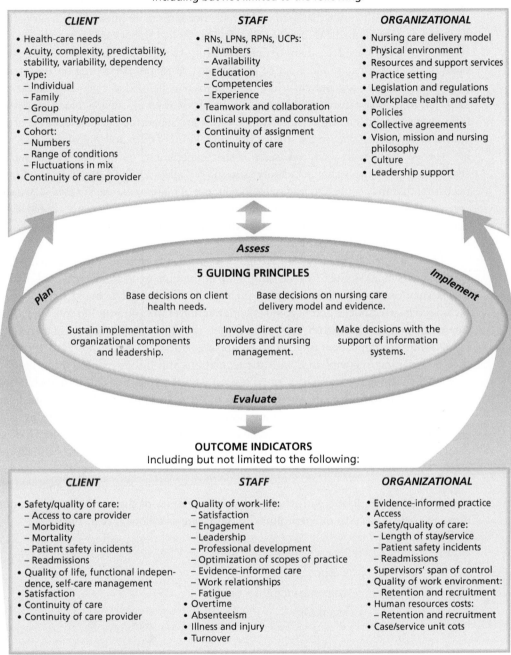

FACTORS TO CONSIDER
Including but not limited to the following:

CLIENT
- Health-care needs
- Acuity, complexity, predictability, stability, variability, dependency
- Type:
  - Individual
  - Family
  - Group
  - Community/population
- Cohort:
  - Numbers
  - Range of conditions
  - Fluctuations in mix
- Continuity of care provider

STAFF
- RNs, LPNs, RPNs, UCPs:
  - Numbers
  - Availability
  - Education
  - Competencies
  - Experience
- Teamwork and collaboration
- Clinical support and consultation
- Continuity of assignment
- Continuity of care

ORGANIZATIONAL
- Nursing care delivery model
- Physical environment
- Resources and support services
- Practice setting
- Legislation and regulations
- Workplace health and safety
- Policies
- Collective agreements
- Vision, mission and nursing philosophy
- Culture
- Leadership support

Assess

Plan

5 GUIDING PRINCIPLES

Base decisions on client health needs.

Base decisions on nursing care delivery model and evidence.

Implement

Sustain implementation with organizational components and leadership.

Involve direct care providers and nursing management.

Make decisions with the support of information systems.

Evaluate

OUTCOME INDICATORS
Including but not limited to the following:

CLIENT
- Safety/quality of care:
  - Access to care provider
  - Morbidity
  - Mortality
  - Patient safety incidents
  - Readmissions
- Quality of life, functional independence, self-care management
- Satisfaction
- Continuity of care
- Continuity of care provider

STAFF
- Quality of work-life:
  - Satisfaction
  - Engagement
  - Leadership
  - Professional development
  - Optimization of scopes of practice
  - Evidence-informed care
  - Work relationships
  - Fatigue
- Overtime
- Absenteeism
- Illness and injury
- Turnover

ORGANIZATIONAL
- Evidence-informed practice
- Access
- Safety/quality of care:
  - Length of stay/service
  - Patient safety incidents
  - Readmissions
- Supervisors' span of control
- Quality of work environment:
  - Retention and recruitment
- Human resources costs:
  - Retention and recruitment
- Case/service unit cots

Figure 8.1 Staff Mix Decision-making Framework

Source: *Staff Mix Decision-making framework for quality nursing care*. Ottawa. CNA, p. 8.,(c) Canadian Nurses' Association. Reprinted with permission.

Standardized Ratios

Standardized ratios or staffing norms for particular kinds of units and settings have frequently been used as a basis for staffing plans. Acute care hospitals have a variety of different kinds of specialty units that predictably have needs for more nursing hours per patient day than do general medical-surgical units. For example, critical care units in acute care hospitals typically have 1:1 patient to nurse ratios due to high patient acuity, while general medical-surgical units are more apt to range from 1:8 to 1:4, depending on the patient population and type of hospital. While these ratios may be used as a general guideline in facilities, so far mandatory ratios have not been established in Canada. Nurse-to-patient ratio approaches to staffing or standardized ratios are supported by some because of the consistency they can offer in the staffing of similar kinds of units and appeal to nurses who are worried about high workload, such as that experienced during widespread nursing shortages. Many believe that mandatory ratios do not allow for flexibility in responding to needs and that they could also lead to inefficient use of human resources at times. Another concern is that legislation that sets minimum levels of staffing may become viewed as the maximum level, so that even when more than the minimum set by law is required, an employer may not staff to that level.

The State of California introduced mandatory nurse-to-patient ratios in general acute care hospitals in 2004, the first (and only) state in the U.S. to do so (Serratt, et al., 2011). The regulations specify the maximum number of patients per licensed nurse (which includes registered nurses and licensed vocational nurses in California) in specific patient care units. Serratt, Harrington, Spetz, and Blegen (2011) studied the effects of mandatory ratios following implementation of the state regulations to see if hospitals increased their RN staffing in compliance with the regulations and if they reduced other kinds of personnel (non-regulated, support, or professional staff) in order to reduce the additional costs. The study took place during the early years of policy implementation and used data from 2000 to 2006. They found that most hospitals did increase their RN staffing by using employees as well as **agency nurses** to meet the mandated ratios and that they did not decrease the use of non-nurse staff. They concluded that the legislation had the desired result, which was to increase the number of licensed nurses caring for patients in general acute care hospitals. Approximately 9 percent of hospitals included in the study did not seem to be in compliance with the legislation. Examples of these mandated minimum nurse-to-patient ratios in different units by 2008 were as follows (see p. 134):

Critical care	1:2
Pediatric	1:4
Postpartum (mothers only)	1:6
Step down	1:3
Medical/surgical	1:5
Psychiatric	1:6

Despite improvements, the researchers noted that additional studies are required to determine if these improved nurse-to-patient ratios have improved patient outcomes. Cook,

Gaynor, Stephens, and Taylor (2012) did examine outcomes, but did not find relative improvements in the patient safety measures they included in their study. They did agree that the legislation had achieved the intended effect of decreasing patient-nurse ratios.

Similar legislation to that in California exists in Australia, where disputes between unions and state governments led to the Australian Industrial Relations Commission arbitration decision in Victoria state (Gerdtz & Nelson, 2007). The decision led to implementation of nurse-to-patient ratios, initially set at 1 to 4 on two shifts of medical-surgical units, but later changed to a more flexible system of 5 nurses to 20 patients on a unit as minimum staffing. This flexibility meant that a nurse could be assigned a variable number of patients, depending on patient needs, within the number minimally required on a 20-bed unit. In Western Australia, a similar decision brought about another staffing method, that of nursing-hours per patient-day (NHPPD). This approach mandated specified nursing hours depending on the classification of wards (units) with differing levels of patient acuity, turnover, patient complexity, and so on (Twigg, et al., 2011). McGillis Hall et al. (2006) found differing views on mandated ratios among the 20 participants who were interviewed about staffing methods in Canada. Many expressed fears the mandated ratios would be inflexible and inefficient and remove decision-making power from nurses (Buchan, 2005; Buerhaus, 2009; McGillis Hall et al., 2006). Despite concerns among nurses they interviewed, McGillis Hall et al. found that many nurses reported that ratios actually exist on an informal basis anyway. McGillis Hall et al. supported the idea of a pilot study on use of this method, as proposed by the Canadian Federation of Nurses Unions in 2005. Currently, persistent concerns about inadequate staffing have led to renewed calls to set legislated minimum nurse-patient ratios in Canada, or as an alternative, to implement **dynamic and shared decision-making staffing models** (Berry & Curry, 2012).

Dynamic and Shared Decision-Making Models

Dynamic and shared decision-making models refer to those approaches to staffing that involve front-line nurses working in collaboration with nurse managers to make day-to-day staffing decisions based on characteristics of patients and nurse competencies or characteristics. It is dynamic in the sense that decisions are made based on changes in the group of clients/patients and the nurses available. For example, the synergy model, described by Curley (1998), seeks to match the characteristics of patients (important to nurses) with the competencies of nurses (important to patients) in a "mutually enhancing" and synergistic way that improves outcomes. These characteristics and competencies are summarized in Table 8.2.

The ideas inherent in the synergy model have evolved and formed a model of care that has been used in workplaces in various ways, including as a way to determine appropriate staffing ratios (Kaplow & Reed, 2008). In Canada, a Saskatchewan staffing project (Rozdilsky & Alecxe, 2012) and a British Columbia nursing workload project (MacPhee, et al., 2010) used the synergy model as the basis for approaches to staffing that involved shared decision making. The British Columbia project is described in the Related Research box.

Table 8.2 Synergy Model: Patient Characteristics and Nurse Competencies

Patient Characteristics	Nurse Competencies
Stability	Clinical judgment
Complexity	Advocacy and moral agency
Predictability	Caring practices
Vulnerability	Facilitation of learning
Participation in decision making and care	Collaboration
Resource availability—personal, psychologcial, social, technical, financial	Systems thinking
	Response to diversity
	Clinical inquiry

Source: Curly, A., Patient-nurse synergy: Optimizing patients' outcomes. *American Journal of Critical Care* 7(1), 64-72. Reprinted with permission of the American Association of Critical Care Nurses.

As a consequence of ongoing complaints by nurses about heavy workloads and burnout, front-line nursing staff have expressed a desire to be involved in staffing decisions (Laschinger, et al., 2003). Increasingly, new approaches and technology tools are being tested in health care settings to address the calls for dynamic models that drive staffing decisions based on design input and monitoring by nursing staff and clinical managers (Fram & Morgan, 2012).

STAFFING PLANS AND POLICIES

From the earlier sections of this chapter, you will have a sense of how complex the function of staffing is in a health care organization, especially where staffing is needed on a 24/7 basis. Health care organizations vary in the degree to which staffing is centralized or decentralized, but typically, one of the functions of first-line nurse managers in a larger organization, such as a hospital, is staffing and scheduling. While the responsibility for planning and establishing the broad parameters guiding staffing may be centralized at the executive level (see organizational factors in Figure 8.1), nurse managers must work within those parameters to plan staffing and scheduling for one or more units or patient populations, making what RNAO (2007) refers to as logistical decisions. Staffing is an important management function and accountability for nurse managers—the challenge is to work within the staff policies and financial resources to match patient requirements with skilled nursing care providers.

A nurse manager is required to establish a staffing budget based on a staffing plan. The budget for the unit is established in terms of **full-time equivalents**, commonly referred to as FTEs. The unit's staffing budget is expressed in terms of FTEs paid for the standard work week, for example 35 hours per week. The unit may use a budgeted FTE by hiring two half-time employees (0.5 FTE each), to provide greater flexibility in staffing over 24-hour periods where staffing levels may vary by shifts. If a unit has 20 FTEs, the plan would indicate what percentage should be RNs and what percentage should be

RPN/LPN staff, as well as building in sufficient consideration for statutory holiday, vacation, and illness coverage using casual or agency nurses. Staffing plans must consider more
than the establishment of minimum numbers of various categories of nursing personnel
for a unit or workplace. A whole range of parameters affects the requirements for staffing
on a daily basis. Some of these are:

- Kinds of shifts (8-hour, 10-hour, 12-hour, split shifts) and rotation of shifts
- Full-time to part-time ratios, casual staff, and float pools
- Orientation policies
- Overtime guidelines and rules
- Flextime, temporary exchange of shifts, or work times
- Scheduling, self-scheduling
- Job-sharing policies
- Understaffing, replacement of absent staff, use of casual or agency personnel
- Length of a staffing cycle and length of time ahead it is known by everyone
- Policies on tardiness, absenteeism, emergencies
- Vacation time requests, requests for days off, resolving conflicts
- Overstaffing and reassignment to other units, crosstraining for other units
- Experience profile of staff, seniority rules

Settings will vary in terms of how these topics are addressed. In some workplaces, the
policy on a number of topics relevant to staffing may be part of a collective agreement between
an employer and a union. In larger organizations, human resources departments are responsible for designing and establishing proposals for topics such as absenteeism and broad orientation policies. In a small workplace, such as a primary health care clinic, these topics may be
included in an individual employment contract or not addressed at all, unless a question arises.

Scheduling

Among policies that affect job satisfaction and balancing the work and personal life of a
nurse are those related to scheduling. Scheduling can be a major issue, particularly for
hospital nurses, most of whom in Canada work rotating shifts. While there are some
scientific, mathematical, and technical skills involved in creating schedules that meet the
needs of a group of clients/patients, there is a creative aspect, or an art, to developing
schedules that work well for patients, nurses, and managers. It is absolutely key that scheduling be done in a fair and open manner, balancing needs for care with the flexibility that
enhances work–life balance for staff. The challenge for nurse managers is to achieve both
predictability and flexibility in staffing (Bailyn, Collins, & Song, 2007).

Some of the options in scheduling that have been tried include use of different shift
lengths, permanent staffing for less popular shifts for nurses who prefer them for personal
life reasons, finding a scheduling pattern that is desirable for the nursing staff on a unit
because of the time-on, time-off days, and self-scheduling approaches (Bailyn, Collins, &
Song, 2007; RNAO, 2007). The development of a schedule that is acceptable to a group

of nurses with different needs however, is a collective challenge and requires collaborative effort. See Box 8.1 for reasons to rework a schedule on a hospital unit(s).

Self-scheduling

There is a long history to self-scheduling. Some of the benefits that have been identified include empowering nurses to control and balance their personal and work lives, improving both the predictability and flexibility of schedules for a group of nurses, reducing the time managers require to spend on staffing, and improving cooperation in the workplace (Bailyn, Collins & Song, 2007). Approaches to self-scheduling may involve sign-up sheets for shifts for a pre-determined scheduling cycle, or software that enables nurses to enter shift requests on a computer. Self-scheduling systems require guidelines and parameters for making requests so that the system is fair to all involved, and it may not fully satisfy all requests. Therefore, not all self-scheduling efforts have been successful and problems in implementation can result from peer pressure, favouritism, and failure of nurses to adhere to the agreed-upon rules (Bailyn, Collins & Song, 2007; Teahan, 1998). Box 8.2 displays some of the parameters that must be considered in self-scheduling approaches.

WHY ARE STAFFING PLANS AND SYSTEMS IMPORTANT?

A great deal of attention has been given to staffing in the past few decades because of the experience of nurses during health care budget cutbacks in the 1990s and the subsequent nursing shortages. These shortages were not limited to Canada; research from around the world focused on a number of major concerns about staffing:

1. The impact on patient safety and quality of care of reductions in the qualifications and/or numbers of nursing personnel.

2. Lack of full-time positions and the difficulty of new graduates to obtain early experience in a stable position. Many new nurses had to either work outside of Canada or hold two to three part-time positions.

3. Excessive use of casual employees, making demands on the fewer full-time employees higher.

4. Pressure on regular staff to work overtime, leading to burnout and absenteeism.

5. Substitution of RNs with less expensive categories of personnel, including RPNs/LPNs and unregulated care providers/UHWs.

Patient/Client Outcomes

A growing body of evidence in the research literature notes that the level and mix of nurse staffing has an effect on client outcomes. Most of this research has been conducted in acute care hospital settings, although more is now being done in home-care and long-term care settings (Harris & McGillis Hall, 2012). Some examples of key findings regarding the effect on patients are:

- In a study of 19 teaching hospitals in Ontario, data were obtained from questionnaires, interviews, focus groups, and selected databases. Nursing staff mix was a significant predictor of the following patient outcomes: functional independence, pain, social functioning, and satisfaction with obstetrical care. Higher proportions of registered nurses and registered practical nurses were associated with better outcomes at the time of discharge. In terms of secondary patient outcomes, there were a higher number of medications and wound infections on units with lower proportion of RNs to RPNs. On units with less experienced nurses, wound infection rates were higher (McGillis Hall et al., 2001).

- In a study of hospital nursing characteristics and 30-day mortality at 49 acute care hospitals in Alberta, hospital nursing variables that were found to be associated with lower patient mortality were higher nurse education levels, a higher RN to non-RN skill mix, better nurse-physician relationships, and less use of casual and temporary employees (Estabrooks, et al., 2005).

- In a study that linked data from a survey of 3,886 registered nurse and registered practical nurse respondents to hospital outcome data for patients with specific diagnoses, researchers found that 30-day mortality rates were lower in hospitals with higher proportions of registered nurses, higher proportions of baccalaureate-prepared nurses, lower amount of nursing staff, and higher proportions of nurse-reported adequacy of staffing and other resources. No significant results were found for relationships to unplanned readmissions to hospital (Tourangeau et al., 2006). The researchers note that 30-day mortality rates are only partially explained in their study and that further research is required. However, they conclude that "… medical unit staffing should maximize the proportion of registered nurses in their nursing staff mix … (p. iv). This study suggests that staff mix, not just absolute staff numbers are key decisions in safe staffing.

- In a systematic review and meta-analysis of registered nurse staffing and patient outcomes, Kane, et al. (2007) found that a higher proportion of RNs had a positive effect on patient outcomes for intensive care and surgical units, including lower hospital mortality, **failure to rescue**, cardiac arrest, hospital-acquired pneumonia, and a reduction of other adverse events.

- In a retrospective observational study of nurse staffing in 43 units of an academic tertiary hospital for more than 175,000 shifts in the U.S., researchers found an association between RN staffing below planned/targeted hours and increased mortality (Needleman et al., 2011).

- In a study of patient outcomes of 665 hospitals in four U.S. states, researchers examined the impact of nurse staffing and level of nurse education in good, average, and poor work environments. Researchers found that there was a beneficial effect of increasing the percentage of nursing staff with baccalaureate in nursing degrees in all of the hospitals, decreasing the odds of 30-day inpatient mortality and failure to rescue by about 4%. They also found a decrease in the odds of deaths and failures of about 4% in the hospitals with average work environments, and by about 9% for deaths and 10% for failures in the best hospital work environments when nursing workload was decreased by about one patient per nurse. In poor hospital work environments, the decrease of workload had almost no effect in reducing these odds (Aiken, 2011).

- A multinational team examined nurse staffing, workload, work environment, and patient outcomes using five years of fiscal data (2001 to 2006) from the public hospital system in New South Wales, Australia. The longitudinal data indicated increased investments in nurse staffing over the years, but these were primarily in specialized nursing units. There was also increased use of casual staff (part-time hour rates higher) and "downward substitution" with conversion of nursing positions to assistive personnel positions. The researchers found more RN staff was associated with lower levels of adverse events (Duffield et al., 2011).

Nurse Outcomes

A wide range of nurse outcomes related to staffing and workload have been studied, particularly following the increased workloads that resulted from cutbacks in the 1990s and nursing shortages in the following decade. These outcomes include burnout, moral and psychological distress, fatigue and exhaustion, absenteeism, turnover, intent to leave one's position and/or nursing, and job satisfaction (Berry & Curry, 2012). A few examples of research findings are:

- In the McGillis Hall et al. (2001) study of 19 Ontario teaching hospitals, the majority of units had a staff mix of regulated and unregulated staff, usually RNs and unregulated workers. The higher the nurses perceived the quality of care to be on their unit, the greater the job satisfaction level. The lower that perception, the higher their level of job pressure, job threat, and role tension. Nurse leadership had an influence on all of the nurse outcomes; that is, the more positive perception of nurse leadership by nurses, the higher the job satisfaction and the lower pressure, threat, and tension.

- In a study of the impact and determinants of nurse turnover in Canadian hospitals, researchers found an average turnover rate of 19.9 percent. Higher turnover rates were associated with higher levels of role ambiguity and role conflict and lower job satisfaction. The researchers concluded that stable nurse staffing and support from managers was needed to promote job satisfaction (O'Brien-Palls, et al., 2010).

- In a study of fatigue among registered nurses, the CNA and RNAO (2010) conducted a study that included a national survey of more than 7,000 RNs across Canada in all health care sectors. More than 55% reported feeling fatigued at work "almost always," with 80% reporting fatigue following work. Nurses in the study identified "relentless and excessive workloads, ongoing staffing issues and sicker patients as the key reasons for their fatigue" (CNA, n.d., p. 4).

Organizational/Health System Outcomes

Policy makers in health care organizations and health care systems are interested in nurse staffing and its relationship to quality of care (patient outcomes), costs (to an institution and to the health system), and cost-effectiveness (is this staffing pattern the most effective use of resources?). Nurse staffing research related to costs or other impacts on an organization or the health system has been growing in the past 20 years or so. Here are some of the findings:

- In a systematic review of research examining the impact of nurse staffing on hospital costs and length of stay (LOS) of patients, Thungjaroenkul, Cummings, & Embleton (2007) identified 17 articles that met the inclusion criteria of the review and quality assessment. Thirteen were U.S. studies while the remainder were from Australia, Austria, Canada, and Taiwan. Results were mixed in the 12 studies that examined nurse staffing and costs, in that some studies reported that higher registered nurse-to-patient ratios reduced hospital costs while other studies found no significant relationship between skill mix and costs. Ten studies showed a relationship between registered nurse staffing and decreased length of stay. The authors concluded that both costs and LOS are affected by RN staffing levels and that consistency in measures is needed in future studies.

- In a scoping review of economic evaluation studies that examined the relationship between nurse staffing, skill mix within the nursing team, and between nurses and

RELATED RESEARCH

British Columbia's Nursing Workload Project

A Provincial Nursing Workload Project was conducted between 2006 and 2010 in British Columbia that involved union and employer associations as well as Ministry of Health Services funding. The overall project involved eight project sites, two each from acute care, long-term care, community health, and community mental health sites. An overall provincial committee steered the project, which was aimed at empowering nurses to make a positive change in the work environment, thus improving quality and safety of care, job satisfaction of nurses, and retention of nurses in the workplace. Site committees were made up of staff volunteers with a clinical nurse leader or educator, all of whom had guaranteed release time to work on the project. The project followed a participatory action research (PAR) approach, so that nurses defined problems, planned approaches to address

them, and reflected on changes, making adjustments as required.

In phase one, project teams learned about factors that promote high quality working environments and identified aspects of their own practice environment that had a negative effect on workload. Nurses developed action plans to address these issues. In phase two, they analyzed patient characteristics to develop staffing plans that provided a "fit" between patients and nurses. Phase three involved focus groups with all involved to consider the results of the project, develop toolkits of helpful resources, and plan how to sustain desired outcomes.

The synergy model was used by the site team in an acute care setting during phase two to look at patient characteristics on a unit. Many workload measurement systems used for staffing focus on tasks that must be completed rather other medical staff, 17 articles were selected that addressed these issues and met the standard when assessed for methodological quality. The authors found a positive relationship between more intensive nurse staffing and patient outcomes. However, care was more expensive, and therefore it was difficult to assess cost-effectiveness. The authors concluded that more rigorous economic evaluations are needed that looked at the effect of variations and levels of nurse staffing (Goryakin, Griffiths, & Maben, 2011).

In summary, studies of nurse staffing have demonstrated that level and mix of funding has an effect on patient/client outcomes and on nurse well-being and satisfaction with their job. Studies on the relationship between staff mix and costs have shown mixed results and although there have been increased costs associated with higher nurse staffing, cost-effectiveness has not been well assessed. In acute care hospitals in Canada, there has been a move to greater use of Registered/Licensed Practical Nurses, but few studies have been done to evaluate the outcomes of these recent changes in staff mix.

than patient characteristics. However, using eight patient characteristics in the model (see Table 8.2), nurses collected data over a number of 12-hour day/night shifts on the patient population, using a 1 to 5 scale, with 1 being the highest acuity. Although the synergy model also uses scores for nurse characteristics, they are only designed for RNs, and therefore nurse characteristics were not scored for this project. Instead, staffing decision rules were developed based on patient synergy scores, nurse scope of practice (categories of caregiver), years of experience, and experience on the particular unit. For example, rules such as assigning only an experienced RN with knowledge of the unit to patients with a synergy score of 1 to 2 were developed. When consensus was reached on staffing rules, they used these to try out staffing assignments for several shifts. In a future phase three, qualita-tive data would be collected from nursing staff to assess the extent that this experience and tools could be used to improve the staffing, staffing requests, and work environment. This innovative and dynamic approach to staffing generated synergy model tools for use by other sites and illustrated an approach to staffing that involves front-line nurses and leaders in shared decision making.

Discussion Questions

1. How could this approach be applicable to the current setting in which you work? What factors would be similar?

2. What challenges would your current setting face?

Source: MacPhee, M., Jewell, K., Wardrop, A., Ahmed, A., & Mildon, B. (2010). British Columbia's provincial nursing workload project: Evidence to empowerment. *Nursing Leadership, 2010, 23*(1), 54–63.

Registered Nurses and Licensed Practical Nurses in a long-term care facility in Newfoundland and Labrador were part of a project designed to enhance the attractiveness of working in long-term care by adopting a new staffing model on a pilot basis. The model enables nurses involved to spend 20 percent of their paid time in professional development activity. Originally, the 80/20 model RN staffing model was developed by the University Health Network (UHN) in Toronto and subsequently implemented in other settings, but this project was the first use of the model in a long-term care setting.

The intent of the project was to assist RNs to develop leadership and clinical skills and enhance the environment for residents in the facility. The organization wished to increase RN retention as well as increase the capacity of RNs for leadership. A steering committee included representatives from the government, union, regional authority, and project personnel. Nurse educators were involved as resource persons. An assessment of the needs of participating nurses was completed, educational resources were obtained/developed, and a comparison site was identified for evaluation of the results. Coverage of the hours of nurses involved in the project was provided by hiring part-time nurses for additional hours.

During the two-year time frame for the pilot project, six RNs and one LPN engaged in a variety of activities including distance-based university courses; completion of a post-basic gerontology diploma program and a diabetes educator diploma; and attendance at gerontology-related conferences, workshops, and seminars. Some participants worked on a falls-prevention program and palliative care policy for the organization.

The outcomes of the project in this setting were very positive in several respects, two of which are a high level of satisfaction by participants with the staffing model and sustained interest in engaging in professional development. For example, two participants registered for the post-basic program in gerontology at the end of the project, and three planned to write the Canadian Nurses Association certification exam in gerontology. Although there were no formal measures of outcomes in terms of resident care, some of the following observations were: decrease in resident falls, positive feedback from families on palliative care, and integration of the falls-prevention program into a regional program. Nurse participants also reported greater job satisfaction and intention to stay at the facility.

Despite the positive reports on this project, there was concern that the 80/20 model could not be maintained due to both costs and availability of human resources. The planning group discussed what other models might be feasible and plans were made to continue with an 85/15 model for a smaller number of participants for each semester for a period of time and to evaluate the results. This example illustrates that in order to achieve desirable work–life conditions for nurses that support and enhance their continuous learning, organizations must use staffing models that reflect such goals and commitment. Professional development of nurses is just one factor, although an important one, that must be built into an organization's staffing plans and policies.

Source: Stuckless, T., & Power, M. (2012). 80/20 Staffing model pilot in a long-term care facility. Newfoundland and Labrador, (45–50). In Canadian Federation of Nurses Unions (CFNU) and partner organizations. The research to action project. Applied workplace solutions for nurses. *Canadian Journal of Nursing Leadership*. Report available at www.longwoods.com/publications/nursing-leadership/special-issue

SUMMARY

A variety of approaches to staffing have been used in the last several decades and most of the published experience with and research on nurse staffing has focused on acute care settings. A great variety of factors must be considered in making decisions about staffing for nursing care and these are reflected in guides for decisions about staffing, for example in identification of principles and frameworks for staffing. These guidelines help in establishing the kinds of decisions that must be made and the parameters (some might say constraints) for decision making, for example legislation or collective agreements.

Decisions about staffing in health care have clearly been shown to have an effect on the quality of patient care, as evident in patient outcome research (ranging from a reduction in adverse events to higher mortality rates). Such decisions also have an impact on nurses (ranging from job satisfaction to burnout and leaving an organization and the profession) and affect outcomes for organization and health system (ranging from shorter lengths of stay to increased absenteeism costs). Despite the attention given to issues of workload and staffing in government and other reports on nursing and despite increased levels of research on the topic, there is still considerable dissatisfaction in practice settings and impatience with respect to staffing issues, although it varies from one setting to another. The following quote from a recent report summarizes this concern and the current call for new approaches:

> Principle-based staffing frameworks and workload measurement systems have failed to truly impact the system. Frontline nurses still lack the authority and autonomy to operationalize the staffing indicated by such measurement systems in timely ways, and there is little nursing input at the system level. These problems persist despite the overwhelming evidence that points to the need for adequate staffing to provide safe, high-quality care. What action can be taken at the front line to address their concerns, and ultimately improve the quality of care? The answer lies in staffing approaches that are transparent, responsive, and implementable at the unit level and that result in the right staffing for safe, quality patient care. Two major approaches to staffing may provide these answers: mandated standardized nurse-patient ratios, and staffing through dynamic, collaborative shared decision making. (Berry & Curry, 2012, p. 59)

Glossary of Terms

Advanced nurse practice or advanced nursing practice. Advanced nurse practitioner is used as an overall term to describe roles that involve in-depth nursing knowledge and skill in nursing and typically require a graduate degree in nursing. Nurse practitioners and clinical nurse specialists are engaged in advanced nurse practice.

Agency nurses refers to nurses who work for an organization that places them in health care organizations, usually on a per shift basis, to meet temporary staffing needs in that organization.

Clinical nurse specialist (CNS) an advanced nurse practice role, requiring graduate education in nursing, that was initially introduced to meet the growing specialization of care in hospitals and provide nursing expertise as well as support to staff nurses. The CNS has clinical expertise in specialized area, such as maternal-child health, critical care, gerontology, and so on, and provides an advanced level of nursing care. The CNS position incorporates roles of clinician, consultant, education researcher, and leader.

Dynamic and shared decision-making staffing models refers to models of staffing that involve direct care nurses and nurse managers adjusting day-to-day staffing requirements when there are changes in the number and characteristics (primarily acuity) of patients.

Failure to rescue is a concept used in research on nurse staffing and is an outcome measure that is a nurse-sensitive outcome (meaning a result that is considered to be sensitive to nursing care or reflective of nursing care). The outcome refers to death among patients following a treatable complication, now more frequently defined as hospital-acquired complications.

Full-time equivalent (FTE) refers to a full-time worker, as expressed in the staffing budget. For example, a nurse manager may establish an annual budget for 10 FTEs, but these may be made up from a mixture of full-time and part-time employees.

Nurse practitioner (NP) refers to a registered nurse "with additional education in health assessment, diagnosis and management of illnesses and injuries, including ordering tests and prescribing drugs" (CNA, 2003) and who is licensed/registered in a province or territory.

Patient classification systems refer to systems for determining patient requirements for nursing care. Patients may be classified into groups based on descriptions of their characteristics or based on critical indicators of care required.

Patient/client acuity refers to the degree of severity of illness/condition. High patient acuity means that staffing requirements are higher in terms of level of provider and/or number of providers.

Scope of employment refers to the roles and responsibilities of unregulated personnel in health care organizations that are specified by the employer and are limited by their education for those roles (CNA, 2012).

Scope of practice refers to activities that a care provider is educated and authorized by legislation to perform in the jurisdiction in which he or she practices. Legislation is supplemented by the authorizing/licensing body's development of standards, statements, and guidelines (CNA, 2012).

Skill mix/staff mix refers to the numbers and kinds of health care personnel that provide care to clients, for example on a unit of a hospital or in a primary health care setting.

Staffing plan refers to an organization or a unit's plan for staffing numbers and categories of staff to meet the predictable needs of that unit. The plan is needed to prepare the budget for the organization/unit, normally annually, and would include needs for full-time, part-time, and casual workers.

Standardized ratio also referred to as staffing norms or nurse-to-patient/client ratios, establishes a fixed relationship between the number of nurses to the number of patient/client(s). The ratio can be established for nursing personnel, for RNs, or other categories of care providers.

Unregulated health care worker refers to care providers or assistant personnel who provide some form of health service and who are not licensed or regulated by a professional or regulatory body. Those who assist with nursing care may have job titles like nursing aide, health care aide, personal support worker.

Workload measurement systems refer to ways of calculating workload that predict the amount of nursing required for a group of patients/clients, usually for the next shift. Different systems use different methodologies, including patient classification, to determine needs for care.

CASE

You are working on a busy surgical unit of a community hospital. The nurses complete the forms of a workload measurement system on a daily basis, but because of budgetary limitations, the unit rarely gets increased staffing when the measurement system indicates a need for more nurses. The nurse manager has asked you to join a committee to look at a new staffing plan for the unit because a budget is being prepared for the next year. You know that several of the experienced RNs on the unit will be retiring, and your colleagues are concerned that there will be a reduction in RNs or a decrease in the experience level of staff as part of a change in the staff mix.

Questions

1. What information do you think the committee will need to begin their work on a staffing plan?

2. What internal and external resources would be helpful to the committee in doing its work?

3. What principles do you think the committee members should agree to as they begin their task?

4. What kinds of evidence do you think the committee would need to formulate recommendations on a staffing plan? Where could they find this evidence?

5. What factors would the committee need to take into consideration in formulating a staffing plan?

6. How would you recommend that the committee justify its recommendations in a written report?

Critical Thinking Questions and Activities

1. Identify the kinds of nursing personnel that form the staff where you have had or currently have a clinical placement. What are the roles and responsibilities of the different categories of staff that a) provide direct nursing care, b) support direct care nurses in some way, or c) manage nursing care? Compare the staff mix and roles

with a different kind of health care organization where you have provided care.

2. How are decisions made in your workplace about the number of nursing personnel required each day or shift? How are decisions made (and by whom) to increase or decrease the number of direct care nursing staff on a daily or shift basis? How are requests made for additional staff?

3. Ask one or more nurses in the workplace if they have had variations in the workload that occurs in the workplace and what seems to account for the changes. Discuss with them: a) what happens when workload increases or decreases, b) what their experience has been when they are short of staff due to a nurse who is ill or is on vacation.

4. Using the current staff mix in your current workplace or a former workplace experience, review the Canadian Nurses Association (2005) Evaluation Framework to Determine the Impact of Nursing Staff Mix Decisions. Reflect on how you would answer questions related to structure, process, and outcome.

5. In pairs, work with a partner to role play a situation in which you have completed a shift in which you were concerned that staffing was insufficient on your unit. Ask your partner to adopt the role of nurse manager and you play the role of the staff nurse at a meeting to discuss your concerns about staffing. Reverse the roles.

Self-Quiz

1. Which of the following methods of making staffing decisions is **not** used in acute care in Canada?
   a. Mandated staffing ratios
   b. Workload measurement systems
   c. Professional judgement
   d. Best practice frameworks

2. Staff mix refers to which of the following?
   a. Requirements for regulated and unregulated practitioners
   b. Combinations of regulated and unregulated providers
   c. Varieties of nursing models used in practice setting
   d. Range of generalist and specialist nurses on a unit

3. Dynamic approaches to staffing refer to:
   a. methods that enable self-scheduling
   b. systems that use computerized tools
   c. principle-based staffing methods
   d. methods that enable daily and shift adjustments

4. You are working on a hospital unit that uses a patient classification approach to determine staffing requirements on a daily basis. You would expect greater staffing requirements for which of the following unit conditions?
   a. More elderly patients
   b. Fewer support services
   c. Increased acuity levels
   d. Higher surgical activity

Useful Websites

Canadian Federation of Nurses
Unions
www.nursesunions.ca

Canadian Health Services Research
Foundation
www.chsrf.ca

Canadian Nurses Association
www.cna-aiic.ca

NP Canada
http://npcanada.ca/portal/

Registered Psychiatric Nurses of
Canada
www.rpnc.ca

References

Aiken, L., Cimiotti, J. P., Sloane, D. M., Smith, H. L., Flynn, L., & Neff, D. (2011). Effects of nurse staffing and nurse education on patient deaths in hospitals with different work environments. *Medical Care, 49*(12), 1047–53.

American Nurses Association (ANA). (1999). *Principles for nurse staffing.* Washington, DC: ANA.

Bailyn, L., Collins, R., & Song, Y. (2007). Self-scheduling for hospital nurses: an attempt and its difficulties. *Journal of Nursing Management, 15,* 72–77).

Baumann, A., O'Brien Pallas, L., Armstrong-Stassen, M., Blythe, J., Bourbonnais, R., Cameron, S., Doran, D., Kerr, M., McGillis Hall, L., Vézina, M., Butt, M., & Ryan, L. (2001). *Commitment and Care: The Benefits of a Healthy Workplace for Nurses, their Patients and the System.* Ottawa: CHSRF. Available at www.chsrf.ca

Berry, L., & Curry, P. (2012). *Nursing workload and patient care. Understanding the value of nurses, the effects of excessive workload, and how nurse-patient ratios and dynamic staffing models can help.* Ottawa: CFNU.

Bryant-Lukosius, D., Carter, N., Kilpatrick, K., Martin-Misener, R., Donald, F., Kaasalainen, S., Harbman, P., Bourgeault, I., & DiCenso, A. (2010). The clinical nurse specialist role in Canada. *Nursing Leadership, 23*(Special Issue), 140–144.

Bryant-Lukosius, D., DiCenso, A., Browne, G., & Pinelli, J. (2004). Advanced practice nursing roles : development, implementation and evaluation. *Journal of Advanced Nursing, 48*(5), 519–529.

Buchan, J. (2005). A certain ratio? The policy implications of minimum staffing ratios in nursing. *Journal of Health Services Research & Policy, 10*(4), 239–244.

Buerhaus, P. I. (2009). Avoiding mandatory hospital nurse staffing rations: An economic commentary. *Nursing Outlook, 57,* 107–112.

Canadian Nurses Association. (June, 1998). *Ethical issues related to appropriate staff mixes. Ethics in Practice.* Ottawa: CNA.

Canadian Nurses Association. (2003). *The Nurse Practitioner.* Ottawa: CNA.

Canadian Nurses Association. (June, 2003). *Staffing decisions for the delivery of safe nursing care. Position statement.* Ottawa: CNA.

Canadian Nurses Association. (n.d.). *Taking action on nurse fatigue. Position statement.* Ottawa: CNA.

Canadian Nurses Association, Canadian Practical Nurses Association, Canadian Council for Practical Nurse Regulators & Registered Psychiatric Nurses of Canada. (2005). *Evaluation framework to determine the impact of nursing staff mix decisions.* Ottawa. CNA.

Canadian Nurses Association, Canadian Council for Practical Nurse Regulators, & Registered Psychiatric Nurses of Canada. (2012). *Staff mix. Decision-making framework for quality nursing care.* Ottawa. CNA.

Canadian Nurses Association and Registered Nurses Association of Ontario. (2010). *Nurse Fatigue and Patient Safety: Research Report*. Ottawa, ON, Canada.

Cook, A., Gaynor, M., Stevens, M. Jr., & Taylor, L. (2012). *The effect of a hospital nurse staffing mandate on patient health outcomes: Evidence from California's minimum staffing regulation*. Carnegie Mellon University, CMPO University of Bristol and NBER. Available from www.bristol.ac.uk/cmpo/publications/papers/2012/wp283.pdf

Crossan, F., & Ferguson, D. (2005). Exploring nursing skill mix: a review. *Journal of Nursing Management, 13*, 356–362.

Cummings, G. G., Fraser, K., & Tarlier, D. S. (2003). Implementing advanced nurse practitioner roles in acute care. An evaluation of organizational change. *Journal of Nursing Administration, 33*(3), 139–145.

Curley, M. A. Q. (1998). Patient-nurse synergy: Optimizing patients' outcomes. *American Journal of Critical Care 7*(1), 64–72.

Duffield, C., Diers, D., O'Brien-Pallas, L., Aisbett, C., Roche, M., Kings, M., & Aisbett, K. (2011). Nursing staffing, nursing workload, the work environment and patient outcomes. *Applied Nursing Research, 24*, 244–255.

Ellis, J., Priest, A., MacPhee, M., & Sanchez McCutcheon, A. (March, 2006). *Staffing for safety : A synthesis of the evidence on nurse staffing and patient safety*. Ottawa: Canadian Health Services Research Foundation. Document available at www.chsrf.ca

Estabrooks, C. A., Midodzi, W. K., Cummings, G. G., Ricker, K. L., & Ginovannetti, P. (2005). The impact of hospital nursing characteristics on 30-day mortality. *Nursing Research, 54*(2), 74–84.

Flynn, M., & McKeown, M. (2009). Nurse staffing levels revisited: a consideration of key issues in nurse staffing levels and skill mix research. *Journal of Nursing Management, 17*, 759–766.

Fram, N., & Morgan, B. (2012). Linking nursing outcomes, workload and staffing decisions in the workplace: the dashboard project. In Canadian Federation of Nurses Unions (CFNU) and partner organizations. The research to action project. Applied workplace solutions for nurses. *Canadian Journal of Nursing Leadership*. Report available at www.longwoods.com/publications/nursing-leadership/special-issue

Gerdtz, M., & Nelson, S. (2007). 5-20: A model of minimum nurse-to-patient ratios in Victoria, Australia. *Journal of Nursing Management, 15*, 64–71.

Goryakin, Y., Griffiths, P., & Maben, J. (2011). Economic evaluation of nurse staffing and nurse substitution in health care: A scoping review. *International Journal of Nursing Studies, 48*, 501–512.

Harris, A., & McGillis Hall, L. (2012). *Evidence to inform staff mix decision-making: A focused literature review*. Ottawa: CNA.

Kane, R., Shamliyan, T., Mueller, C., Duval, S., & Wilt, T. (2007). The association of registered nurse staffing levels and patient outcomes. *Medical Care, 45*(12), 1195–1204.

Kaplow, R., & Reed, K. (2008). The AACN model for patient care: A nursing model as a force of magnetism. *Nursing Economic$, 26*(1), 17–25.

Laschinger, H. K. S., Finegan, J., Shamian, J., & Wilk, P. (2003). Workplace empowerment as a predictor of nurse burnout in restructured healthcare settings. *Healthcare Quarterly, 1*(3), 2–11.

Lavoie-Tremblay, M., O'Brien-Pallas, L., C., G., Desforges, N., & Marchionni, C. (2008). Addressing the turnover issue among new nurses from a generational viewpoint. *Journal of Nursing Management, 16*(6), 724–733.

MacPhee, M., Jewell, K., Wardrop, A., Ahmed, A., & Mildon, B. (2010). British Columbia's provincial nursing workload project: Evidence to empowerment. *Nursing Leadership, 2010, 23*(1), 54–63.

McGillis Hall, L., Doran, D. I., Baker, G. R., Pink, G., Sidani, S., O'Brien-Pallas, L., & Donner, G. J. (2001). *A study of the impact of nursing staff mix models and organizational change strategies on patient, system and nurse outcomes*. A summary report of the nursing staff mix outcomes study, September 28, 2001, Faculty of Nursing, University of Toronto.

McGillis Hall, L., Pink, L., Lalonde, M., Tomblin Murphy, G., O'Brien-Pallas, L., Spence Laschinger, H. K., Tourangeau, A., Besner, J., White, D., Tregunno, D., Thomson, D., Peterson, J., Seto, L., & Akeroyd, J. (2006). Decision making for nurse staffing: Canadian perspectives. *Policy, Politics, & Nursing Practice, 7*(4), 261–269.

Needleman, J., Buerhaus, P., Pankratz, S., Leibson, C., & Stevens, S. (2011). Nurse staffing and inpatient hospital mortality. *New England Journal of Medicine, 364*, 1037–45.

O'Brien-Pallas, L., Tomblin Murphy, G., Shamian, J., Li, X., & Hayes, L. (2010). Impact and determinants of nurse turnover, a pan-Canadian study. *Journal of Nursing Management, 18*(6),1073–1086.

Registered Nurses Association of Ontario. (2005). *Reporting on…nursing workload measurement systems—A discussion of the issues*. Toronto: RNAO.

Registered Nurses Association of Ontario. (2007). *Healthy work environments best practice guidelines: Developing and sustaining effective staffing and workload practices*. Toronto: RNAO. Available from www.rnao.org

Rozdilsky, J., & Alecxe, A. (2012). Improving patient, nursing and organizational outcomes utilizing formal nurse-patient ratios. (103–113). In Canadian Federation of Nurses Unions (CFNU) and partner organizations. The research to action project. Applied workplace solutions for nurses. *Canadian Journal of Nursing Leadership*. Report available at: www.longwoods.com/publications/nursing-leadership/special-issue

Serratt, T., Harrington, C., Spetz, J., & Blegen, M. (2011). Staffing changes before and after mandated nurse-to-patient ratios in California's hospitals. *Policy, Politics, & Nursing Practice, 12*(3), 133–140).

Stuckless, T., & Power, M. (2012). 80/20 Staffing model pilot in a long-term care facility. Newfoundland and Labrador, (45–50). In Canadian Federation of Nurses Unions (CFNU) and partner organizations. The research to action project. Applied workplace solutions for nurses. *Canadian Journal of Nursing Leadership*. Report available at: www.longwoods.com/publications/nursing-leadership/special-issue

Teahan, B. (1998). Implementation of a self-scheduling system: a solution to more than just schedules! *Journal of Nursing Management, 6*(6), 361–368.

Thungjaroenkul, P., Cummings, G. G., & Embleton, A. (2007). The impact of nurse staffing on hospital costs and patient length of stay: A systematic review. *Nursing Economic$, 25*(5), 255–265.

Tourangeau, A., Doran, D., Pringle, D., O'Brien-Pallas, L., McGillis Hall, L., Tu, J. V., & Verma, A. (2006). *Nurse staffing and work environments: Relationships with hospital-level outcomes*. Ottawa: Canadian Health Services Research Foundation. Document available at www.chrsf.ca

Twigg, D., Duffield, C., Bremner, A., Rapley, P., & Finn, J. (2011). The impact of nursing hours per patient day (NHPPD) staffing method on patient outcomes: A retrospective analysis of patient and staffing data. *International Journal of Nursing Studies, 48*, 540–548.

Chapter 9
Quality of Work-Life Issues

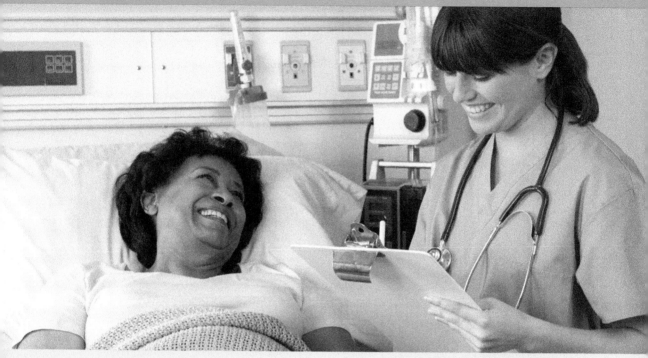

Monkey Business Images/Shutterstock

Learning Objectives

After reading, studying, and reflecting on this chapter's content, you will be able to:

1. Describe the characteristics of magnet hospitals
2. Describe theoretical models of work stress and burnout
3. Discuss the relationship of empowerment to outcomes for nurses and patient safety
4. Identify how the values and needs of nexters and nurses nearing retirement may differ from those of other nurses
5. Relate issues related to quality of work life to your practice setting(s)
6. Suggest ways nurses can work together to improve the quality of work life

INTRODUCTION

Terms such as "quality of work life," "professional practice environments," and "healthy work environments" are relatively new in the nursing literature. These terms reflect the growing realization that the quality of nurses' work life has important implications for patient care as well as nurses' own health.

In this chapter we will look at three areas of research that have helped nurses, health care administrators, and policy makers recognize the importance of the quality of nurses' work life. First, research about magnet hospitals (hospitals that attracted nurses to work in them even when hospitals in nearby areas had shortages of nurses) began to describe work environments that attracted nurses. Second, research about work-induced stress identified negative outcomes for nurses, such as burnout and high turnover of nurses from their job or even leaving the profession. This area of research later examined patient safety as an additional outcome of nurses' stress. Third, research findings that nurses felt disempowered, dissatisfied, and unsupported increased as researchers examined the impact on nurses of cuts to Canadian health care budgets in the 1990s. The budget cuts also resulted in fewer jobs for new graduates, who were therefore leaving nursing or the country. This led to Canadian researchers measuring nurses' empowerment, satisfaction, turnover intent, and related constructs and their outcomes for nurses and patients. Ultimately, health administrators and policy makers predicted that a national shortage of nurses was inevitable unless more students could be recruited into nursing and nurses could be retained in the profession.

In this chapter will also discuss research that indicates new graduates may have different needs and expectations from their workplace and work than previous generations. Therefore, health care administrators and policy makers may need to make adjustments to the workplace and work in order that different cohorts of nurses feel satisfied.

The recognition of a potential shortage of nurses and the varying needs of different cohorts of nurses, along with the research findings from research stemming from magnet hospitals, work stress, and the impact of budget cuts have led to many initiatives to improve **professional practice environments**. We will summarize one such initiative, a quality professional practice environments (QPPE) project, as an example of how nurses working together can become empowered and resolve issues they identified as hindering their ability to provide patient care.

The issue of workplace violence, including bullying and incivility in the workplace, is another important issue that has an impact on quality of work life, and is discussed in Chapter 10, Team Building and Managing Conflict.

MAGNET HOSPITALS

In the United States, during the 1970s and 1980s there was a shortage of nurses. Despite this shortage, McClure and colleagues (1983) discovered that some hospitals did not have such a shortage even when neighbouring hospitals within the same city did. They used the term "magnet hospitals" to describe hospitals that attracted and retained nurses despite the shortage of nurses in nearby hospitals (Kramer, 1990). Nurses were aware that these hospitals were good employers, and they actively sought work at these hospitals.

Although this research was done in the United States, it has implications for any country, because when there are more nursing positions than nurses, nurses will seek out good employers.

Researchers (for example, Scott et al., 1999, Upenicks, 2002) examined the characteristics of magnet hospitals in an attempt to learn how other hospitals could attract and keep nurses. They found that magnet hospitals had a number of characteristics, including:

- Fewer hierarchical levels: Magnet hospitals had fewer layers of management. This may facilitate the concerns of clinical nurses reaching the senior administrative nurse.

- More autonomy for nurses: Nurses had increased discretion in making decisions about the care they provided patients. Primary care nursing was often the care delivery model.

- More control in decision making: Nurses had input into decisions affecting how care was provided in their department. In some cases, shared governance was in place.

- Support from supervisors and coworkers: For example, direct care nurses were encouraged to continue their formal education. Supervisors and coworkers supported their attendance at in-services or committee meetings by adjusting their schedule and/or patient assignment and by assisting with their patient care when they were away from the unit. Nurses were engaged in more collaboration with physicians than in non-magnet hospitals.

- Effective leadership: Nurses felt trusted and valued. The chief nurse executive was included on the senior executive team. Systems of nurse scheduling were flexible.

- Manageable workload: Workload was not overly stressful and enabled nurses to provide quality patient care.

In short, these magnet hospitals provided nurses with the opportunity to have a high level of involvement in decisions around the care they gave, in decisions related to their nursing units, and in decisions involving nursing at the hospital.

Researchers examining the unique characteristics of magnet hospitals also looked at outcomes, such as nurses' job satisfaction, turnover, and absenteeism. These studies showed that nurses in magnet hospitals had higher levels of job satisfaction (for example, Aiken, Havens, & Sloan, 2000) and less burnout (for example, Aiken, Havens, & Sloan; Friese, 2005) than nurses in non-magnet hospitals, and that nurses at magnet hospitals had lower rates of turnover than their colleagues at other hospitals (Kramer & Schmalenger, 2003).

A team of Canadian researchers examined the impact of magnet characteristics in a survey of nursing homes. Responses to surveys sent to the directors of nursing at Canadian nursing homes found that nursing homes with strong magnet characteristics had higher levels of nurse and resident satisfaction, a work culture of participatory decision making, more resources spent on staff education, and a lower rate of vacant nursing positions (Rondeau & Wagar, 2005).

There is growing evidence that magnet characteristics lead to improved patient outcomes, although a recent systematic review found that more evidence is required before we can conclude that patients in magnet hospitals have better outcomes. For example, one study in this area that found that characteristics of magnet hospitals, specifically autonomy, control, and collaboration, reduced nurses' feelings of burnout and increased nurses' trust in management (also called organizational trust), which in turn affected job satisfaction and the quality of patient care as assessed by the nurses themselves (see Figures 9.1 and 9.2) (Laschinger, Shamian, & Thomson, 2001). Other studies have found lower patient mortality in magnet hospitals than in matched hospitals (Aiken, Smith, & Lake, 1994; Aiken, Sloane, & Lake, 1997). A number of studies have found that the rate of patient mortality is associated with various characteristics of magnet hospitals (Kazanjian et al., 2005).

Since 1993, American hospitals can apply to the American Nurses Credentialing Center for magnet designation to recognize their nursing quality, and more recently this has been extended to other countries and health care organizations. While a few hospitals outside of the United States have obtained official magnet designation from

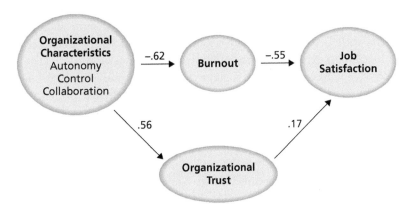

Figure 9.1 Final Job Satisfaction Model

Source: Stuckless, T. & Power, M. (2012). 80/20 Staffing model pilot in a long-term care facility. Newfoundland and Labrador, (45–50). In Canadian Federation of Nurses Unions (CFNU) and partner organizations. The research to action project. Applied workplace solutions for nurses. *Canadian Journal of Nursing Leadership*. Report available at www.longwoods.com/publications/nursing-leadership/special-issue.

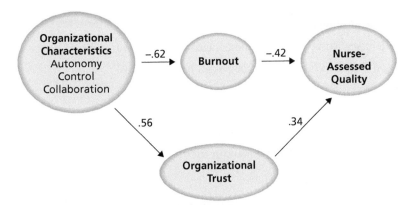

Figure 9.2 Final Nurse Assessed Quality Model

Source: Stuckless, T. & Power, M. (2012). 80/20 Staffing model pilot in a long-term care facility. Newfoundland and Labrador, (45–50). In Canadian Federation of Nurses Unions (CFNU) and partner organizations. The research to action project. Applied workplace solutions for nurses. *Canadian Journal of Nursing Leadership*. Report available at www.longwoods.com/publications/nursing-leadership/special-issue.

this American centre, to date there are no Canadian health care organizations with this official designation. Health care organizations are sometimes described as having official magnet designation, being in the application process for magnet designation, or having the characteristics or the reputation of a magnet health care organization.

The Joanna Briggs Institute published a systematic review of studies that examined the impact on nursing and patient outcomes of hospitals having official designation as magnet organizations, planning to apply for magnet status (Magnet-Aspiring), having the reputation of magnet organizations (Reputational Magnet), or not having magnet status (non-Magnet) (Salmond et al., 2009). The authors of this systematic review summarized the results of 17 research studies of hospitals with different magnet designations to determine what we can conclude about the relationship of magnet designation and outcomes for nurses, patients, and the organization. The review included both qualitative and quantitative studies. Of interest is that outcomes for nurses were more positive in magnet hospitals. For example, nurses in magnet hospitals felt they had more autonomy, worked in conditions with better staffing and resources, and had better managers. Nurses in magnet hospitals also experienced less burnout and felt more satisfied.

In contrast, the research did not support the idea that physician–nurse relationships were better in magnet hospitals. In addition, there was insufficient evidence that nurses in magnet hospitals felt a stronger nursing focus with clear standards of patient centred care, had fewer occupational health outcomes, or better patient outcomes. This does not mean that the nursing focus is not stronger in magnet hospitals or that there are not fewer occupational health outcomes or that the patient outcomes are not better—it only means that additional research is required before we could have confidence in stating magnet hospitals are different in these areas.

To summarize the key findings about magnet hospitals:

- A stronger professional practice environment for nursing
- No difference in the quality of nurse–physician relationships

To summarize the key findings related to nurses in magnet hospitals, the nurses:

- Felt more autonomous
- Believed they worked in departments with better staffing and resources
- Believed they had nursing managers with higher ability
- Experienced higher satisfaction
- Experienced less burnout
- Believed quality of patient care was higher
- Felt more likely to intend to remain in their nursing position for the next year

More research is needed to determine:

- If nurses in magnet hospitals believe their workplace has a stronger nursing focus and clear standards of patient care
- If there is a difference in health outcomes for nurses in magnet hospitals
- If there are better patient outcomes in magnet hospitals

Implications of Magnet Hospitals for Nurse Leaders

Nurse leaders and other key stakeholders are interested in learning about practices at magnet hospitals in order to implement similar practices at non-magnet hospitals with the goal of attracting and retaining nurses. Nurse leaders who attempt to use the practices of magnet hospitals in an effort to create a work environment where nurses feel involved and satisfied with their workplace may need to change the way they work with nurses. Such changes in management practices can be difficult to implement and some require a lot of training. For example, nurse managers may feel that they support their nurses and that they do involve them in decisions, but in reality, the nurses do not feel supported. In these cases, managers need to learn the specifics of what behaviours they should change. Nurse managers may wish to empower clinical nurses, but they may not know what they need to do for nurses to become empowered. Similarly, some clinical nurses who want to be involved in decision making may benefit from staff development programs that help them develop skills such as team work, collaboration, consultation, and negotiation.

In the spirit of trying to become a magnet hospital, a number of nursing departments in Canada and throughout the world have adapted practices to increase nurses' involvement. **Shared governance** has frequently been implemented with the goal of flattening the organizational hierarchy and involving nurses in unit decisions. Shared governance refers to an organizational structure where decision making is shared with staff. Porter-O'Grady (1992) applied shared governance to nursing, involving nurses within an organization in decision making related to their professional practice. See the Leading Health Care Example in this chapter for another example. Depending on the organization, there may be several councils, such as one each for clinical practice, nursing education, nursing leadership, and nursing research with an overall executive council that the other councils report to.

Self-scheduling is another workplace initiative that some believe will decrease nurses' dissatisfaction with their schedule. With self-scheduling, nurses within a department work together to develop their own work schedules rather than the nurse manager developing the schedule. A number of organizations are also implementing quality of work-life initiatives, whereby nursing staff on a unit identify their concerns and work to improve them. For example, Lavoie-Tremblay (2004) describes working with staff and managers of a long-term care unit in the province of Quebec. Through team meetings, staff and managers identified their work concerns and developed action plans to address these concerns. The goal was for managers to develop a participatory way of working with staff, thereby building a stronger team and increasing trust among staff.

WORK STRESS, BURNOUT, AND TURNOVER
Work Stress and Burnout

Nurses frequently say they feel "stressed" and "burned out"; however, their use of these terms may not be consistent with the definitions of these terms in the research literature. For example, it has been suggested that nurses say they are stressed instead of saying they are dissatisfied with their work because stress is a concept they find more acceptable than dissatisfaction with nursing (Barley & Knight, 1992). When nurses say they are stressed, they mean they have too much work, and this is something they are happy to let others know about in the hope of improving working conditions. However, to say they do not like their job is to say they do not like nursing, and nursing is seen as caring for others. As nurses value caring for others, they may not wish to be seen as not finding this type of work satisfying (Barley & Knight, 1992). In contrast, physicians generally say they do not like their job but do not say they are stressed, because they value being able to deal with any patient situation and they equate stress with incompetence (Barley & Knight, 1992).

The term burnout is also often used incorrectly, for example when nurses who are feeling temporarily exhausted say that they feel "burned out." However, burnout involves not only exhaustion but also other outcomes. Further, the type of exhaustion that is experienced in burnout is a state of emotional, mental, and physical exhaustion resulting from too high levels of stress for too long.

Definition of Work Stress

Work stress is the psychological and physical response to the strain that results from work stressors, or job demands. Work stress occurs when an employee is unable to meet job demands. Typically, the work stressors or job demands occur on a regular basis, and therefore chronic stress is experienced. Work stressors lead to strain that in turn leads to work stress. Work stress has a negative effect on productivity, psychological well-being, and health. An aspect of the work environment may be a work stressor for some nurses, while other nurses may not find this aspect to be a work stressor. For example, taking care of certain types of patients may be a work stressor for some nurses while other nurses enjoy working with these patients. Some nurses may find ambiguous situations stimulating, while others may find these stressful.

Definition of Burnout

Burnout, as defined by Maslach and Leiter (1997), is a state that includes three outcomes: 1) emotional exhaustion, 2) feelings of cynicism and detachment from work, and 3) feelings of being ineffective at work. Burnout is the outcome of a high level of stress experienced over time. Professionals who work with people, such as health care workers and teachers, often experience burnout. A person who is experiencing burnout feels exhausted and has impaired functioning, including feeling unable to provide support for other persons.

Maslach's measure of burnout includes three scales: emotional exhaustion, personal accomplishment, and depersonalization (Maslach, Jackson, & Leiter, 1996). A person who is experiencing burnout is high on emotional exhaustion and depersonalization, and low on personal accomplishment.

Theoretical Framework of Work Stress

A frequently used model to explain work stress is the person-environment fit model. The lack of fit between the employee's values and needs and the work environment leads to stress (Caplan et al., 1980; Edwards & Van Harrison, 1993; French, Caplan, & Harrison, 1982). The stress in turn may lead to turnover, absence, and burnout.

Another model of work stress is Karasek's job strain model (Karasek & Theorell, 1990). According to this model, high psychological demands combined with low autonomy to make decisions leads to job strain. The job strain leads to physical and psychological health problems, which are reduced by social support.

Lazarus and Folkman (1984) believe that people use different coping strategies when faced with stressors. Their cognitive appraisal of work stressors, along with the use of these coping strategies, explains differing levels of strain when individuals face the same stressor(s).

Negative Impact of Work Stress

Low to moderate levels of stress can be stimulating and have positive effects on nurses, such as challenging them to work better. However, high levels of work stress can have detrimental effects. Work stress has been shown to have a negative effect on job satisfaction, organizational commitment, absence, turnover, burnout, and health (Jacobson et al., 1996; Ganster & Shaubroeck, 1991) including cardiovascular disease (Kasl, 1996). Prolonged work stress has also been shown to have a negative effect on personal relationships (Baumann et al, 2001).

One study of Ontario nurses found a strong correlation between overtime and sick leave (O'Brien-Pallas et al., 2001). It is likely the overtime was a work stressor, which in turn led to increased absence. Further, a cross-sectional study of 8,044 Ontario nurses found that nurses' claims to the Ontario Workplace Safety and Insurance Board due to musculoskeletal injuries were higher in hospitals where nurse-physician collaboration was lower (O'Brien-Pallas, et al., 2004).

Work Stressors: The Predictors of Work Stress

Work stressors are aspects of the work environment that lead to strain, which in turn leads to the experience of work stress. A number of work stressors, including role ambiguity, role conflict, role overload, and work pressure, have been shown to predict all three dimensions of burnout (Lee & Ashforth, 1996; Jamal & Baba, 2000). Many other work stressors have been examined for nurses' stress including shift work (Skipper, Jung & Coffey, 1990), patient acuity (McLauglin & Erdman, 1992), unit type (Foxall et al., 1990), and ethical conflicts (Gaudine & Thorne, 2012).

A cross-sectional survey examined the stress of hospital nurses working in Alberta during health care restructuring in the mid-1990s (Maurier & Northcott, 2000). The work stressors in this case included the threat of being placed on recall, having a coworker bumped or laid off, and perceived job security and were associated with poor physical health. Poor physical health was particularly experienced by those who viewed these work situations as threatening. The researchers also identified coping strategies that decreased or increased the effect on physical health and depression.

Other Work Stressors: Patient Safety and Abuse of Nurses

Recent studies on patient safety have increased nurses' awareness of the frequency of errors in patient care. While aware that errors in care occur all too often, nurses may be asked to work overtime, staffing may be less than optimal, the pace of work too fast, and the workload heavy. Consequently, in addition to those work stressors, nurses may experience the stressor of fear of causing harm to a patient (Hughes & Clancy, 2009). More research is needed to examine the prevalence of this work stressor and its outcomes.

Recently, the issue of abuse of nurses in the workplace has gained much attention. There is evidence that nurses feel such abuse is part of their work, that the abuse may have been caused by their incompetent behaviour, and that they are expected to cope with it (Deans, 2004). This abuse may take the form of physical or verbal aggression or sexual harassment, and is clearly a work stressor (Hughes & Clancy, 2009).

RELATED RESEARCH

Workplace Intervention to Reduce Work Stress

Peterson, Bergström, Samuelsson, Åsberg & Nygren (2008) conducted a randomized control trial studied the effectiveness of peer-support groups (see Figure 9.3 Flowchart of Respondents). The study began with 3,719 health care workers (including physicians, nurses, nursing assistants, social workers, allied therapists, and so on) in Sweden completing a burnout measure. Those who were above the 75th percentile for emotional exhaustion (N = 660) were invited to participate in the study and 131 agreed to participate. Health care workers in the intervention group received a peer-support intervention. They met with a group leader for ten, two-hour sessions as well as a follow-up session four weeks later. The first session involved getting to know each other and discussing issues related to the group such as confidentiality. In the second session, discussion occurred around the question "What do you believe causes stress and burnout? In the remaining sessions, the health care workers discussed possible solutions and ways to prevent stress and burnout. All sessions began with 10 minutes of guided relaxation.

Participants in both the intervention and control groups completed questionnaires following the 10-week sessions, and at 7 and 12 months. The intervention group showed statistically different effects for general health, perceived quantitative demands at work, participation and development opportunities at work, and support at work. In addition, the evaluation of the peer-support intervention included a qualitative component. At 7 and 10 months, participants in the intervention group were asked to describe changes in their working conditions over the past 6 months. Seven categories were identified from this qualitative data: talking to others in a similar situation, knowledge, sense of belonging, self-confidence, structure, relief of symptoms, and behavioural change.

This study demonstrates that a relatively low cost peer-support intervention may help to reduce stress in health care workers. Study limitations include only 22.9 percent of the potential participants agreed to participate, the majority of participants were female, and outcome measures relied on self-reported data. While it does not state in the article whether the control group was offered the intervention at the end of the study, this can be done following clinical trials, particularly when the intervention is found useful.

Source: Peterson, U., Bergström, G., Samuelsson, M., Åsberg, M., & Nygren, Å. (2008). Reflecting peer-support groups in the prevention of stress and burnout: Randomized controlled trial. *Journal of Advanced Nursing, 63*, 506–516.

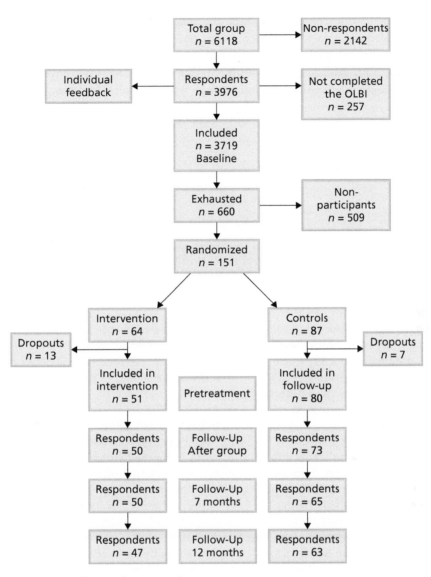

Figure 9.3 Flowchart of Respondents

Source: Peterson, U., Bergström, G., Samuelsson, M., Åsberg, M., & Nygren, Å. (2008). Reflecting peer-support groups in the prevention of stress and burnout: Randomized controlled trial. *Journal of Advanced Nursing, 63*, 506–516. Reprinted with permission of John Wiley and Sons.

Implications for Nurse Managers

Reducing work stressors helps prevent burnout and detrimental health outcomes. Sometimes people experience stress because their particular job is not a good fit for their needs and values. In these cases, it might help to find a different unit or nursing specialty. Offering social support and aiding nurses to develop coping strategies to help them with their work stressors can lessen the effects of stress. Ultimately, if the work environment has many stressors, such as fast pace of work, work overload, and role conflict, the job itself needs to be reviewed. Workload may need to be reduced through adding more staff, changing the staffing mix, or eliminating any unnecessary work processes. Effective leadership can help reduce work stressors. For example, a leader who clarifies employee roles might reduce role ambiguity, and a leader who helps team members to communicate effectively with each other can reduce work conflict. Incidents of nurse abuse should be followed up to prevent further abuse and to support the nurse.

RELATED RESEARCH

Nurses' Work Environment and Patient Safety

Research on nursing work environments has started to look at the impact of the work environment on patient safety outcomes. In a study by Lashinger and Leiter (2006), a survey with 8,597 nurse participants working in hospitals in two Canadian provinces, Ontario and Alberta, measured the work environment, burnout, and patient safety outcomes.

The aspects of the work environment measured were strong leadership, nurse–physician collaboration, involvement in policy development, staffing adequacy, and use of a nursing model of care (as opposed to a medical model). Burnout was measured by the Maslach Burnout Inventory – Human Service Scale (MBI–HSS) that includes three subscales for emotional exhaustion, depersonalization, and personal accomplishment. Patient safety outcomes were measured by nurses' ratings of the frequency of four adverse patient events in the past year: falls, nosocomial infections, medication errors, and patient complaints. The survey's hypothesis was that burnout is a mediator between aspects of nurses' work environment and patient safety outcomes. The term "mediator" is used in research to describe a variable that is the outcome of

one variable and the precursor of another variable. For example, in the following diagram, B is a mediator in the relationship between A and C, and there are two paths in this model (one path is between A and B and the second path is between B and C).

A → B → C

In the diagram below (an abbreviated form of the model tested in this study), burnout is the mediator between aspects of nurses' work environment and patient safety outcomes.

Aspects of nurses' work environment → Burnout → Patient safety outcomes

All paths in the study's model were supported (with the exception of the path from emotional exhaustion to adverse events). Thus, patient safety is affected by nurses' working environments, including leadership, either directly or through the effect of these variables on aspects of burnout (emotional exhaustion, depersonalization, and personal accomplishment).

Source: Laschinger, H.K.S., & Leiter, M.P. (2006). The impact of nursing work environments on patient safety outcomes: The mediating role of burnout/engagement. *The Journal of Nursing Administration, 36*, 259–267.

Turnover of Nurses

Turnover refers to when employees leave the organization either for voluntary reasons, such as for a new job, or for involuntary reasons, such as when asked to leave or the employee contracts a long-term illness or suffers a disability. Turnover can result from stress and burnout. Turnover is always expensive for an organization because of the cost of recruiting and orienting new employees. The time spent to orient nurses to specialty units such as operating rooms, ICUs, and labour and delivery makes turnover particularly expensive for these departments. Even when nurses stay in the same organization, when they transfer to a new department they may require specific orientation, and the nurses who replace them also require orientation.

Health care administrators are particularly concerned about the financial cost of turnover. However, turnover has important implications for other groups because it has a negative impact on nurses, nursing departments, health care organizations, and patient care.

Negative Impact of Turnover on Nurses

High turnover on a nursing unit has a detrimental effect on nurses as it increases the workload of the remaining nurses (O'Brien-Pallas et al., 2001). When a nurse resigns, the position may be temporarily vacant or the nurse replaced with a casual nurse or newly hired nurse who is assigned fewer or less complex patients. The remaining nurses may not only be assigned to the more complex patients on the unit, but will also have to orientate or oversee the work of the casual or newly hired nurse. This means the nurses' remaining time will largely be spent on ensuring patients on their unit receive safe medical care. The need to focus on the medical aspects of care may leave less time for providing the type of care that nurse find satisfying: the type of care that is based on a nursing model and is associated with magnet hospitals. As the remaining nurses become frustrated with not being able to provide care based on a nursing model and tired of continually orientating new nurses, the new nurses may not be emotionally supported or treated with the level of respect that they deserve. Similarly, nursing students doing clinical placements on the unit may not feel welcome, further exacerbating the vacancy rate when they decide not to apply for a job on the unit.

A high rate of turnover can also lower the morale of the remaining nurses (Cavanaugh & Coffin, 1992). The remaining nurses may come to feel they are being left behind in their careers. The nurses who leave are seen as heading to "greener pastures" where working conditions are better—to a unit with better shifts or a lower workload, or to a position such as a nurse educator or manager.

Negative Impact of Turnover on Nursing Departments

Nursing departments with high turnover can develop a poor reputation among nurses, making it difficult to fill vacant positions. The unit's reputation may be affected by the turnover on the team. As members of the team are constantly changing, staff may be less cohesive and experience more conflict (Mobley, 1982). The unit may also gain a poor reputation because of poor quality of nursing care. It can take a year or longer for a new nurse to be able to manage the same number and complexity of patients as an experienced nurse, depending on the nursing specialty. If a unit is staffed with the same number of nurses regardless of their level of experience, the unit will likely function less efficiently, and patients will suffer.

As work stresses increase from turnover, the remaining staff may decide to leave, causing a spiraling turnover in the department (Staw, 1980).

Negative Impact of Turnover on Health Care Organizations

Given the financial costs of turnover and the increasing shortage of nurses in Canada and elsewhere, turnover is an important issue for health care organizations. Turnover can be problematic when it leads to a budget deficit and an administrator feels the nursing department needs to reduce staff or have a different skill mix of staff to attain a balanced budget. Instead, spending on developing the characteristics of a magnet hospital can improve the unit's reputation, serve to attract nurses, and lead to cost savings through reducing turnover and absence.

Negative Impact of Turnover on Patient Care

Turnover affects staffing, and poor staffing has been linked to poor patient outcomes (for example, Sasichay-Akkadechanunt, Scalzi, & Jawad, 2003). For a more detailed discussion of staffing and patient outcomes, see Chapter 11, Quality Improvement.

Benefits of Turnover

Turnover can also have benefits (Abelson & Baysinger, 1984). New nurses can bring new ways of doing things and improvements in care in the unit. The enthusiasm of new graduates is infectious and might help all nurses feel motivated. Sometimes the nurses who leave a unit have been unhappy there and this can have a negative effect on the satisfaction of other nurses. Nurses may leave the unit to become full-time students, and later return to the unit with new ideas and enthusiasm.

Theoretical Framework for Turnover

While there are a number of theories to explain turnover (Hayes et al., 2006), one theoretical framework commonly referred to is "person-environment fit." This framework suggests that a misfit between the employee's values and needs and the work environment leads to stress (Caplan et al., 1980; Edwards & Van Harrison, 1993; French, Caplan, & Harrison, 1982). Stress in turn leads to decreased organizational commitment, increased absenteeism, and increased turnover (Jackson & Schuler, 1985). When employees feel less committed to the organization, they may withdraw through absence or turnover.

Predictors or Precursors of Turnover

Because of the costs of turnover to nurses, nursing units, health care organizations, and patients, much research has been done on the causes of turnover. Age, tenure, job satisfaction, organizational commitment, perceptions of other job opportunities, and supervisor relations are known to predict turnover (Tai et al., 1998). Other predictors of turnover that have been investigated in numerous studies include workload, stress, burnout, leadership style, workplace empowerment, opportunities for promotion, and scheduling (Hayes et al., 2006).

Burnout has been shown to be one predictor or precursor of turnover. A survey of 667 nurses in Atlantic Canada found work life predicted burnout, which in turn predicted nurses' intent to turnover (Leiter & Maslach, 2009). Another survey of 612 Canadian nurses found that two of the dimensions of burnout, emotional exhaustion and cynicism, along with supervisor incivility, predicted turnover intentions (Spence Laschinger, Leiter, Day & Gilin, 2009).

More recently, trust in the employer has been studied as a predictor of turnover and has been found to predict organizational commitment, job satisfaction, and intent to stay (Dirks & Ferrin, 2002; Gregory et al. 2007, Laschinger et al., 2001, Turnley & Feldman, 1998, 1999).

One survey of nurses in three teaching hospitals in Ontario examined how nurses' preference for a different employment status, the importance of income to them, and stress affected their intent to stay. Preference for a different employment status was measured by asking nurses if they were full-time, part-time or casual, and if this was the work they preferred. Importance of income was measured by asking how important their income was to their family's economic well-being. The analysis for all respondents (N = 1,396) showed that stress and preference for a different employment status positively predicted the intent to leave the hospital, while the importance of income to the family negatively predicted intent to leave the hospital. When the analysis was repeated for only full-time nurses, preference for a different employment status was no longer significant, and when the analysis was repeated for only part-time nurses, importance of income to the family was no longer a significant predictor.

Relationship Between Turnover and Absence

In one survey of hospital nurses living in Ontario (1,362 nurse respondents), full-time nurses were less likely than part-time nurses to respond that they intended to resign (Burke & Greenglass, 2000). Interestingly, full-time nurses were more likely to be absent from work than part-time nurses. In part this may be because part-time nurses are not paid for sick days and because part-time nurses have more time to recover from stressful workdays. While full-time and part-time nurses in this survey had similar job satisfaction, full-time nurses had higher emotional exhaustion. Another explanation for full-time nurses having higher absence but lower turnover than part-time nurses is that full-time nurses may need the income from full-time work and therefore feel unable to resign, but they are able to withdraw from work by using sick time.

Implications for Nurse Managers

Some of the predictors of turnover such as age and tenure cannot be modified. However, most of the predictors such as job satisfaction, organizational commitment, supervisor relations, workload, stress, burnout, leadership style, workplace empowerment, opportunities for promotion, scheduling of shifts, work status (full-time, part-time, or casual), and trust in employers can be modified.

RESEARCH FROM BUDGET CUTS IN THE 1990s

Budget Cuts and Work Process Innovations

In the 1990s provincial governments across Canada made significant cuts to their health care budgets. Administrators at hospitals and other health care organizations struggled to deal with these budget reductions as best they could. In some cases, they were able to provide services more efficiently by changing the way in which they provided care. For example, instead of admitting patients the day prior to surgery, patients were admitted on the day of surgery. Further, for certain surgical procedures patients were no longer admitted to hospital but were cared for in day care surgical departments. Emphasis was placed on discharging patients as soon as possible through coordinating care with community nurses and other health care providers in the community. These changes in the way care was provided are examples of **work process innovations**.

Budget Cuts and Nursing Work Life

Unfortunately for most organizations, such work process innovations provided only part of the needed budget reduction. Nursing personnel and supplies generally account for more than half of the overall budget for hospitals, and thus nurses had to deal with working with fewer colleagues. At the same time, departments providing **allied health professional services** and **support services** often dealt with their own cuts by reducing services that helped nurses with their workload. For example, the blood procurement department or the physiotherapy department may remove their workers from night or weekend shifts, leaving nurses to provide essential services in these areas. The housekeeping department might eliminate services on the night shift, leaving nursing to do jobs such as cleaning the case room between patients.

As a result, while hospital nurses had to deal with working with fewer nurses and/or with a skill mix of staff that had fewer nurses and more licensed practical nurses (LPNs) and/or unregulated nurses' aides, they also lost help from support services. Hospital nurses became stressed, their absent time increased, and some left nursing. Their vacant positions further increased the workload and stress of the remaining nurses. Direct care nurses were rarely consulted about budget cuts, nor were management nurses' concerns always listened to.

Canadian Research Initiatives in Quality of Nurses' Work Life

The worsening work environment for nurses along with the increased vacancy rate led to much research on the quality of work life of nurses. In particular, Heather Laschinger, PhD, RN, at the University of Western Ontario, undertook a series of studies that examined aspects of the work environment and outcomes such as job satisfaction. The Nursing Health Research Unit, a collaborative project of McMaster University and the University of Toronto Schools of Nursing, was started in 1990, funded by the Ontario Ministry of Health. The Canadian Health Services Research Foundation (CHSRF) was formed in 1997 and has been instrumental in bringing decision makers and researchers together. Further, nurses lobbied for and obtained a $25 million endowment in 1999 from the federal government and a 10-year agreement was created between the government and CHSRF, which administered the fund. This Nursing Research Fund was created to build nursing research capacity, nursing research output and use, and it should be noted that the program has contributed substantially to nursing work life research in Canada.

Early research into the quality of work life focused on nurse outcomes (for example, stress, burnout, nurses' health) and the cost implications for employers (for example, absenteeism, turnover) and was largely ignored by hospital administrators and policy makers. Then, researchers linked nurses' workload and other aspects of a poor work environment with patient outcomes (for example, morbidity, mortality, patient safety) (Aiken, Clarke, & Sloane, 2002) and the public and health care administrators began to take notice.

The next section discusses key research findings about nurses' work environment, focusing on Canadian studies, in particular, Laschinger's program of research. Implications for nurses and nurse managers and directions for future research are suggested.

Empowerment and Quality of Work Life

Heather Laschinger is a well-known Canadian nurse researcher who has conducted many studies over the past few decades with various colleagues. Her research has focused on aspects of quality of work environments and their outcomes for nurses and patients. Laschinger has conducted a number of studies to examine how nurses' empowerment has an impact on outcomes for nurses and patients. Much of Laschinger's research uses Kanter's (1977; 1993) theory of organizational empowerment and Spreitzer's (1995) concept of psychological empowerment as part of theoretical framework in her studies on nurses' empowerment. In addition, Laschinger's research has looked at aspects of quality work environments, including the characteristics of magnet hospitals.

Kanter's Theory of Organizational Empowerment

Kanter believes that employees respond to how the work environment is structured, or conditions in the work environment. When organizational structures enable employees to have information and the resources they need for their work, to receive support, and to have opportunities to learn, employees feel empowered. With these resources, they are able to accomplish their work. Kanter proposes that when employees feel empowered they feel more positive about work and strive to meet work challenges. **Psychological empowerment** is the psychological experience that employees have when they feel empowered (Spreitzer, 1995).

Laschinger's Research

In a survey of 404 Ontario nurse participants, it was found that **structural empowerment** led to psychological empowerment, which in turn led to job satisfaction (Laschinger et al., 2001).

The relationship between structural empowerment and magnet hospital character-istics was examined in a secondary analysis of data that had been gathered in Ontario for three surveys (Laschinger, Almost, & Tuer-Hodes, 2003). Two of these surveys were with hospital nurses and one with acute care nurse practitioners. The model tested in this secondary data analysis was that high structural empowerment was associated with magnet hospital characteristics, and high levels of empowerment and magnet hospital characteristics were associated with high job satisfaction. Structural empowerment was measured by an overall score from an empowerment measure (total empowerment) as well as by the four subscales that make up this measure (opportunity, information, support, resources). In addition, empowerment was calculated with scales to measure formal power, informal power, and a global empowerment measure. Magnet hospital characteristics were measured by an overall scale (Nursing Work Index or NWI-R) and three subscales from this scale: autonomy, control over practice, and collaboration. The correlations between the study variables for all three studies support the study's model. For example, total empowerment as measured in study one showed a strong correlation with magnet hospital characteristics as measured by the NWI-R (.605) and with job satisfaction (.625).

The relationship between empowerment and respect and affective organizational commitment to the organization was examined in a survey of 70 registered nurses and 75 registered practical nurses (LPNs elsewhere) working in Ontario nursing homes (DeCicco, Laschinger & Kerr, 2006). Respect was examined in part because clinical nurses were saying that they did not feel respected (Canadian Nursing Advisory Committee, 2002) and in part because of the finding that nurses' perceptions of respect are significantly correlated with their intent to resign (an outcome of particu-lar importance to organizations) and with structural empowerment (Laschinger, 2004). **Affective organizational commitment** was defined by Meyer and Allen (1991) as the employee's affective ties to the organization, such as their identification and involvement with the organization. Researchers and practitioners are interested in affective organizational commitment because it is correlated with turnover in an organization (Wagner, 2007). This study found support for the hypotheses that struc-tural and psychological empowerment were positively associated with perceptions of respect, and that nurses who perceived high levels of structural and psychological empowerment and felt respected had higher affective commitment to their place of work.

Another study was performed to test a model of nursing work life that includes empowerment, magnet hospital characteristics, job satisfaction, and perceptions of patient care quality (Laschinger, 2008). The purpose of this study was to test a more complete model of the nursing work-life environment by examining a number of variables in the same study. While a number of studies, including those outlined above, have exam-ined one or more of these variables, the goal of this study was to test a more complete model. Therefore, nurses working in tertiary care hospitals in Ontario were surveyed and 234 nurses responded. The analysis (structural equation modelling) found support for structural empowerment and magnet hospital characteristics affecting both job satisfac-tion and nurses' perceptions of quality of nursing care.

Limitations of the Studies

The studies on empowerment and quality of work life summarized above are limited in that survey data were collected at one time (cross-sectional design) and therefore it is difficult to say if a given variable caused another variable. Further, the studies relied on self-reported data or nurses' ratings of the variables. This is less than ideal, particularly for measuring the quality of patient care. Finally, the studies were limited to Canadian nurses living in specific regions of Canada, most studies included only acute care hospital nurses, and the survey response rates were not 100 percent (for example, the response rate was 59 percent in study five), making it difficult to generalize findings to nurses living in other countries and working in other settings.

These limitations are typical of survey research and of most of the research that has been done on nurses' work life. Despite these limitations, the fact that a number of the studies point to similar conclusions helps support the validity of the studies' findings.

Implications

Laschinger's program of research is important to nursing because it suggests aspects of the work environment that clinical nurses and nurse leaders can change, thereby improving outcomes for nurses and patients. Since structural empowerment is associated with psychological empowerment, changing structural factors in the work environment may improve psychological empowerment. Nurse leaders can examine structures in their workplace that facilitate nurses' autonomy and their collaboration with physicians. Traditionally, nurse managers felt they had to control care. For example, clinical nurses were asked to report on their patients to the charge nurse, who in turn reported this information to their administrator. This was time-consuming activity, and appears to be based on the assumption that the senior nurse in the hospital needs knowledge about patients in order for them to receive safe care. Instead of focusing on such activities, nurse managers could focus on how they can change structural factors, for example, by working with other departments so that supplies are received on the unit on time, by working to improve relations between other departments and their unit staff, by acknowledging when nurses may need help with providing care for their patients, and by holding staff meetings where nurses are involved in decisions about operating the unit.

Structural empowerment is also associated with the characteristics of magnet hospitals and nurses' job satisfaction. Therefore, changing structural factors in the work environment may enable nurse leaders and clinical nurses to foster the characteristics of magnet hospitals, which, together with structural empowerment factors, is associated with nurses' job satisfaction.

Structural and psychological empowerment are associated with feeling respected in the workplace and affective commitment to the hospital. In recent years, nurses have objected to the lack of respect they feel in the workplace (Canadian Nursing Advisory Committee, 2002). Interventions to help nurses feel more respected in the workplace are important for nurses' well being and ultimately for hospitals, because nurses who feel respected may not resign and they may strive to provide excellent care. Affective commitment is known to predict turnover, with persons with low affective commitment more apt to turnover. Thus, both feelings of respect and affective commitment are important outcomes for nurse leaders to foster, given the current shortage of nurses in Canada and elsewhere.

Quality of work life is also related to outcomes such as burnout and patient outcomes. Burnout can lead to increased numbers of absent days, including long-term sick leaves, as well as to leaving the organization and/or the profession. However, it is the link of aspects of the work environment to patient outcomes that may help administrators and policies understand the importance of improving work environments. The work of Laschinger and other researchers who have provided evidence of this link is important because nurse leaders can use it to support their request for the resources their department needs. Further, the public is becoming aware of the factors that are associated with patient safety in hospitals. Their awareness should be useful in supporting health care policy at the provincial and organizational levels that takes into account the research on nurses' work environments and patient outcomes.

Health care budget cuts in the 1990s also resulted in restructuring of hospitals, usually at the expense of the number of nurse managers and clinical nurse specialists. In some cases, nurse managers were replaced with non-nurse managers. Given the research evidence from Laschinger's work as well as studies on magnet hospitals, such cuts were short-sighted and may have contributed to nurses feeling less empowered. Effective nurse leaders work to provide nursing care from a nursing model, a characteristic of magnet hospitals. As shown in Laschinger's research, effective nurse leaders help create structural aspects of the work environment that facilitate psychological empowerment, decrease burnout and strain, and improve nurses' job satisfaction and patient outcomes.

Progress in Quality of Workplace Environments

As noted by Shamian and El-Jardali (2007), research on quality workplace environments has been slow to be translated into policy and changes in organizational practices. In light of the mounting evidence relating nurses' work life to patient safety, as well as the evidence relating nurses' work life to turnover at a time of an increasing shortage of nurses, it is time for research evidence to be transferred to provincial health policy and to the administrative practices of health care organizations.

Shamian and El-Jardali note that there have been improvements at a system level, such as funding for higher enrollment in nursing school and accreditation standards that include consideration of quality of nurses' work life. Other initiatives at some health care organizations include flexible staffing, more full-time permanent positions instead of part-time and/or temporary positions, and phased-in retirement.

An initiative that would help nurses with their high work demands and help them feel valued and respected is an 80–20 balance. This initiative involves nurses providing direct care 80% of the time and engaging in professional development 20% of the time. An 80–20 balance recognizes the needs and values of today's nurses for time to reflect on their care and and to continue to learn, as well as time to recuperate from stressful situations (Leiter, 2007). There are anecdotal reports that an 80–20 balance leads to reduced absenteeism costs, thereby recouping some of the costs of this initiative (Leiter, 2007).

Nurses' Fatigue

Given the ongoing shortage of nurses, to continue operating the health care system, managers have placed demands on nurses to work extra shifts and overtime, and to carry heavy workloads. It is one thing to have an occasional workday with a heavy workload or to occasionally do an extra shift or overtime. However, when nurses are required to do this continuously, these work stressors lead to fatigue.

A joint research report by The Canadian Nurses Association (CNA) and the Registered Nurses' Association of Ontario (RNAO) entitled *Nurse Fatigue and Patient Safety* presented the findings of a literature review, interviews, and focus groups, and a national survey on the topic of nurse fatigue and patient safety (CAN, 2010). Based on their literature review they defined nurse fatigue as:

> . . .a subjective feeling of tiredness (experienced by nurses) that is physically and mentally penetrative. It ranges from tiredness to exhaustion, creating an unrelenting overall condition that interferes with individuals' physical and cognitive ability to function to their normal capacity. It is multidimensional in both its causes and manifestations; it is influenced by many factors: physiological (e.g., circadian rhythms), psychological (e.g., stress, alertness, sleepiness), behavioural (e.g., pattern of work, sleep habits) and environmental (e.g., work demand). Its experience involves some combination of features: physical (e.g., sleepiness) and psychological (e.g., compassion fatigue, emotional exhaustion). It may significantly interfere with functioning and may persist despite periods of rest. (CNA, 2010, p. 12)

As noted in the above definition of nurse fatigue, the experience of nurse fatigue includes other outcomes to nurses, such as physiological and psychological outcomes, which include emotional exhaustion—a component of burnout. The report also notes the alarming association between nurse fatigue and patient safety.

The researchers make recommendations to policy makers, accreditation bodies, unions, administrators, nursing schools, and nurses about how to reduce nurse fatigue. For example, governments need to fund health care organizations and nursing schools so that they can employ adequate numbers of nurses and enroll adequate numbers of nursing students, respectively. Nursing schools can teach students how to recognize signs of fatigue and the need to care for themselves (Box 9.1). These recommendations for direct care

Box 9.1

1. Nurses learn to be aware of and recognize signs, symptoms, and responses to personal fatigue.

2. Nurses understand and work within the policies related to safe patient care within their organizations and within professional practice expectations.

3. Nurses take responsibility for mitigating and managing fatigue while at work, including using professional approaches to decline work assignments. When deciding to work extra shifts or when planning work or non-work related activities, nurses act on their ethical obligation to maintain fitness to practice.

4. Nurses work through their professional associations, nursing unions and regulatory bodies to advocate for safe patient care through safe scheduling practices in the work environment.

5. Nurses support policies, procedures, and health promotion initiatives that manage fatigue in the workplace.

Source: *Nurse Fatigue and Patient Safety Research Report.* Reprinted by permission of the Canadian Nurses' Association.

nurses are particularly relevant to you. Many provincial nursing associations have developed policies or information guides for nurses to help them prevent fatigue as well as how to manage it if they become fatigued.

ISSUES RELATED TO AGE COHORTS OF NURSES

The Ideal Work Environment for Nexters

Generation next, also known as generation Y and commonly referred to as nexters, refers to persons born around 1981 and after (Hicks & Hicks, 1999). Nexters grew up in an age of technology, with personal computers, the internet, cell phones, and ipods, and share much personal information using frequent text messaging and internet sites such as Facebook. Generation X was born between 1966 and 1980 and the baby boom generation between 1946 and 1966. Like baby boomers, nexters are motivated to work hard; however unlike baby boomers, they prefer collaborative approaches to work rather than competitive ones and will probably change their place of work much more frequently (Clausing, et al., 2003). Baby boomers and nexters may conflict with each other in the workplace if they don't understand their respective values.

Much of the research on nurses' work life has been done with the baby boom generation, and to a lesser extent, generation X. As nexters enter the workplace, they are being supervised by persons from other generations, who may use technology differently, communicate differently, and not understand their motivations. Nexters are entering the nursing force at a time when large numbers of baby boomers will be retiring, and therefore it is particularly important to understand what will engage this generation in the workplace. Statistics about how many new graduates leave their first position soon after graduating are alarming. For example, 38 percent of respondents to British Columbia's New Graduate Registered Nurse Study left their first position within their first year of employment due to the work environment, including poor staffing (Regan, 2003). While these nurses may move to another nursing position and not leave the profession, the costs of recruiting and orienting new nurses for the vacated positions and the continued emphasis on orientating new nurses draw upon scarce resources that could be used to support factors associated with magnet hospitals.

One correlational descriptive study with nexter nurses is a survey of nurses living in Quebec who were born after 1981 (Lavoie-Tremblay, Wright, et al., 2008). Some of the findings are that 53.4% of the 309 respondents had high psychological demand, 58.3% had low decision latitude, and 43.4% had high job strain. These findings are alarming given the need to retain new nurses in the workforce.

Traditionally, nurse educators have asked managers in practice for feedback about the performance of new graduates, with the goal of modifying the curriculum. Nurse educators work in close contact with students and through discussing their clinical experiences, they develop an understanding of what is important to their students. Nurse educators and managers could schedule time each year, to exchange ideas about engaging the new generation of nurses. Much has been written about how "nurses eat their young." Instead, we need to support new nurses, engage them in decision making, and not expect that they can assume the same workload as nurses with many years of experience.

The Ideal Work Environment for Older Nurses

With an increasing worldwide nursing shortage, there has been recent interest in looking at the needs of older nurses. Many nurses, particularly direct care nurses, choose to retire before they are 65 years of age, often because of the stresses of carrying a heavy workload and the physical nature of their work. Administrators have become interested in learning more about nurses who may take early retirement in order to learn if there are ways to keep them in the workplace.

One study interviewed 84 nurses who were over 50 years of age and working in England, Scotland, Wales, and Northern Ireland (Watson et al., 2003). The nurses mentioned the pace of work as well as their ability to meet the physical demands of their job as major issues. They suggested the following may help them delay retirement: flexible working hours, reduced hours, work settings such as outpatient departments or long-term care facilities, and returning to clinical work instead of working as a charge nurse. Further, nurses would be more apt to stay employed if they had pension plans that did not penalize them for working reduced hours, or for moving to less stressful jobs with lower remuneration.

In Canada, organizations may not be able to implement some of the above suggestions without negotiating these changes with nursing unions. Given the growing need to retain nurses in the workforce, and that retaining these nurses may reduce the stress of younger nurses, such contract changes may be warranted.

NURSES' QUALITY OF WORK LIFE AND PATIENT OUTCOMES

Earlier in this chapter we discussed research findings that support magnet hospitals being associated with better patient outcomes. Researchers have also studied the relationship between different aspects of nurses' working conditions and patient outcomes. A systematic literature review that included studies published from January 2000 to October 2009 (Bae, 2011) found eleven studies (nine American, one Canadian, and one Japanese). In all, 69 relationships between nurses' work life and patient outcomes were reviewed, including aspects of nursing work life such as autonomy, supervisor support, co-worker cohesion, nurse participation in hospital affairs, and staffing and resource adequacy; and aspects of patient outcomes such as medication errors, failure to rescue, patient falls, and catheter-associated urinary tract infections. Only 21 of these 69 relationships showed a positive impact on patient outcomes, 40 showed no statistical difference, and 8 showed a negative impact on patient outcomes.

The author of this systematic literature review concludes that we do not have sufficient research evidence to conclude a positive association between nurses' quality of work life and patient outcomes. Research in this area is complex because there are many factors that may be affecting the benefits to nurses from a particular aspect of work life. As well, there are many factors that have an impact on patient outcomes. Longitudinal studies that look at how nurses' work life and patient outcomes change over time, and intervention studies that look at how patient outcomes change as an aspect(s) of nurses' work life changes, are needed before we can conclude that the quality of nurses' work life has an impact on patient outcomes.

In contrast, a systematic review of the literature on the relationship between nursing workload and staffing, and a healthy work environment for nurses concluded there is a strong relationship (Pearson et al., 2006). This review located 171 research publications, some of which also looked at client outcomes, allowing the authors to also conclude there is a strong relationship between nursing workload and staffing and outcomes for clients. Workload and staffing may be key attributes of nurses' work environment with implications for patient outcomes.

Leading Health Care Example

Quality Professional Practice Environment (QPPE) Project in Newfoundland and Labrador

The Quality Professional Practice Environment (QPPE) Program, a joint initiative of the Association of Registered Nurses of Newfoundland and Labrador (ARNNL) and the College of Licensed Practical Nurses of Newfoundland and Labrador (CLPNNL), has been helping nurses in the province create and maintain workplaces that support professional practice and value personal well-being since 2005.

QPPE was initiated in response to feedback from nurses throughout the mid-1990s that they felt disempowered and dissatisfied, and were questioning their ability to meet their professional practice standards that would ensure the best quality patient care. Recent changes to the health system in the province had led to increased span of control for nurse managers that meant they were no longer readily available to support unit nurses, or obtain nurses' input into decisions that were affecting these nurses in their daily practice. Nurses reported they felt they were often working in "silos," not as collaborative partners with other service and health care providers. Put simply, nurses felt their time to deliver patient care was being compromised by inefficiencies in the system they had to deal with, such as obtaining laundry supplies on the weekend. Workplace stress and job dissatisfaction were seen as major contributors to many nurses leaving the province.

In a proactive response to these concerns, the ARNNL and CLPNNL took a leadership role with a diverse group of professionals, including nurses representative of all domains of nursing, to discuss what they could do to support nurses and enhance their workplace environment. The resulting QPPE Program was developed around six standards that provide the theoretical framework for the program. These standards are related to workload management, nursing leadership, control over practice and work life, professional development, organizational support, and communication and collaboration.

The goal of the QPPE Program is to empower nurses to a change in thinking from "They will fix it" to "How can I help to make it different?" In her role as QPPE Coordinator, JoAnna Bennett assists select groups of unit nurses to implement the formal QPPE Program over a period of 18 to 20 months. The start-up phase occurs over three months where all unit nurses go through an orientation to the program and complete an environmental questionnaire that rates their unit against the six cornerstone standards. This data then provide the basis for a representative working group (WG), consisting of six to eight nurses, to work with throughout the remainder of the program. This WG always includes the manager and clinical nurse responsible for the day-to-day operations of the unit as well as direct care nurses.

In preliminary discussions, site managers agree to provide relief for nurses to attend working group meetings. These orientation meetings focus on education about empowerment, leadership, and communication in addition to getting to know key individuals in the organization such as the professional practice coordinator, who meets with the group to discuss their specific roles.

The action research approach utilized in the program is part of the orientation as group members learn the process of experience, reflection, learning, and action planning that provides a safe and supportive environment for both challenging the status quo and experimenting with innovative practice. It incorporates a "learn by doing" model that supports empowered nurses to plan for and implement change while continuing to monitor and evaluate success and capture key learning.

In addition to these activities, the WG develops working guidelines that ensure any conflict or diverse opinions are effectively managed, all members can fully participate and each meeting ends with a set of action plan strategies for improvements. A communications strategy is developed to ensure the flow of information to and from unit nurses with the goal of engaging all nurses in the process. One part of this strategy is a "buddy" system that links each unit nurse with a member of the WG.

Following the start-up phase which includes two full-day sessions, the WG meets approximately every eight weeks

for either a half or full day. They work on selected priority issues identified in the questionnaire completed at the start of the program. All these meetings are facilitated by the QPPE Coordinator who also mentors members of the WG to develop their leadership skills with the goal of group ownership following completion of the QPPE program.

The formal program concludes with an evaluation that includes repeating the initial questionnaire to see how items have changed, including sub-scales that can identify changes in job satisfaction, morale, leadership, and participation. The evaluation also includes an analysis of action plans implemented by the working group and how they link with the six cornerstone standards. Discussions at this time also focus on how the initiative can be sustained. Sometimes this occurs in a formal manner with regularly scheduled meetings while other times it occurs more informally where nurses respond to issues arising in their workplace by getting together in a "QPPE huddle" and asking "If this was QPPE, what would we do to solve the issue?"

In her role as facilitator, JoAnna Bennett has been involved with a number of QPPE initiatives in different settings including acute care, urban and rural hospital units, long-term care, and a primary health care team. While nurses in all these initiatives have been creative, innovative, and committed in their strategies for changes to make their workplaces "better places to work" a similar theme emerged from discussions at three sites that led these nurses to challenge the status quo of how they delivered care. Using the QPPE process they responded to concerns related to scope of practice, role confusion, workload, and continuity of care and moved to a model of patient

(Continued)

care that promoted full scope of practice, more equitable workload distribution across the team, and increased accountability for quality patient care. Staff morale and job satisfaction increased while the team became more cohesive and productive.

Other initiatives include promoting preceptors and mentors for students and nurses new to the unit, improving physical and human resources, providing input into improved organizational orientation programs and policies, developing patient education pamphlets, supporting ongoing educational activities, and numerous initiatives to promote value and respect amongst peers and colleagues, just to mention a few.

The QPPE program has involved over 500 nurse participants in 15 sites since it began in 2005. The program and its achievements have been acknowledged at all levels of nursing across the regions as program participants report their successes. These nurses say the program has "been a wonderful opportunity to empower us as nurses," and "has really helped me understand how the unit is managed and how decisions are made." Nurses also feel they "have some control back in [their] work life," and are "excited that we are taking charge of our future."

Source: Personal communication with Joanna Bennett, Quality Professional Practice Environment Coordinator, Association of Registered Nurses of Newfoundland and Labrador.

SUMMARY

This chapter has discussed three streams of research that contributed to the recognition that quality of nurses' work life is an important topic. Research on magnet hospitals, nurses' stress, and nurses' disempowerment following budget cuts in the 1990s brought awareness to the topics of quality of work life and professional practice environments.

There has been much research in Canada on nursing work environments in the past couple of decades. We now have the evidence that poor work environments have detrimental effects on nurses and patients. While some of this evidence has been translated into changes in practice, most Canadian clinical nurses still work in challenging conditions. One example of a hospital where nursing has made much progress is the Ottawa Hospital, and this is described in the interview with Dr. Ginette Rodgers in Chapter 5.

Future research on nursing work environments is needed to build on the recent trend of testing interventions to improve work environments. Much of the research in quality work environments has focused on hospital settings, clinical nurses, and urban locations. We know less about community, long-term care, or rural settings, or about LPNs, NPs, or nurse managers. Given the need to attract people into the profession and to keep new graduates in nursing, we need to learn more about nexters and how to help them feel engaged and committed to health care organizations.

Glossary of Terms

Affective organizational commitment This term was coined by Meyer and Allen (1991) who defined affective commitment to the organization as the employee's emotional ties to the organization, such as their identification and involvement with the organization. Meyer and Allen's measure of organizational commitment includes scales for affective, normative (employee is committed to organization because he or she feels obligated to maintain connections), and continuance commitment (employee is committed to organization because he or she needs to continue ties, for example for financial reasons).

Allied health professionals Health professionals other than nurses and physicians, for example, speech therapists, physiotherapists.

Burnout Burnout was a state defined by Maslach and Leiter (1997) as including emotional exhaustion, feelings of cynicism and detachment from work, and feelings of being ineffective at work. Burnout is often the outcome of experiencing work stress for a long period of time. Maslach's measure of burnout includes three scales: emotional exhaustion, personal accomplishment, and depersonalization (Maslach, Jackson, & Leiter, 1996). A person who is experiencing burnout is high on emotional exhaustion and depersonalization, and low on personal accomplishment.

Magnet hospitals Hospitals that attract and retain nurses despite a shortage of nurses in nearby hospitals.

Professional practice environment Work environment that supports the professional practice of nursing.

Psychological empowerment Spreitzer defines psychological empowerment as the psychological feelings employees experience when they are empowered.

Self-scheduling In self-scheduling, nurses within a department work together to develop their work schedules rather than the nurse manager developing the schedule.

Shared governance Shared governance refers to an organizational structure where decision making is shared with staff. Porter-O'Grady (1992) applied shared governance to nursing, involving nurses within an organization in decision making related to their professional practice. Depending on the organization, there may be several councils, such as one each for clinical practice, for nursing education, for nursing leadership, and for nursing research with an overall executive council that the other councils report to.

Structural empowerment Kanter believes there are organizational structures that lead to employees feeling empowered, specifically access to information and to resources required to do your work, support, and learning opportunities.

Support services Services that provide assistance to accomplishing core services. For example, providing meals to hospital patients is necessary for patients who need to stay in hospital for health services.

Turnover refers to when employees leave the organization either for voluntary reasons such as for a new job or for involuntary reasons such as when asked to leave or contracting long-term illness or disability.

Work process innovations A new way of performing work that involves a number of steps.

Work stress Work stress is the psychological and physical response to the strain that results from work stressors, or job demands. Work stress occurs when an employee is unable to meet job demands.

Work stressors Aspects of the work environment that lead to strain, which in turn leads to the experience of work stress.

CASE

Jessica was the manager for two units of a large, long-term care centre that was part of a larger organization. She reported to Sara, the manager who had overall responsibility for the nursing care at the centre. Sara spent much of her time at meetings on other sites, and Jessica's contact with her was often limited to a monthly meeting of managers at the site, and a monthly, one-hour individual meeting. Jessica was responsible for the management of her two units, including the budget, staffing, hiring staff, performance appraisals, and quality improvement. She often spent several hours a day phoning staff at home to see if they would replace staff members who were absent. Jessica also felt pressured to produce quality improvement reports and monthly budget analyses.

The staff on Jessica's units included registered nurses, licensed practical nurses, and unregulated health workers, and they felt Jessica was generally not visible or available to them and questioned what she did all day. The registered nurses felt over-worked, and often felt they were working while the unregulated health workers took long coffee and lunch breaks. The unregulated health workers felt their opinions were not valued, and that the registered nurses and licensed practical nurses ordered them around. The licensed practical nurses felt they were not working to their full scope of practice because the nurses were afraid they would end up taking nurse positions.

Jessica noted the number of adult disposable diapers her units were using was steadily increasing, and was over the amount that had been budgeted for. This concerned her because the rehabilitation plan for a number of clients included continence retraining. However, what was really making her units go over budget was the increasing amount of absenteeism. She replaced some of the absent staff with casuals, some of whom she had to replace at an overtime rate, and sometimes she was unable to find a replacement.

Questions

1. What are the work stressors of Jessica? Of the registered nurses? The licensed practical nurses? The unregulated health workers?

2. How could all of the staff work together to improve the quality of continence retraining? How could this be done to help empower the nurses, the licensed practical nurses, and the unregulated health workers?

3. What suggestions do you have for how Jessica could work with the staff to decrease absence calls?

4. What could Jessica do to help her staff understand why she is not visible? Would it be possible for her to become more visible to her staff, and if so, how could she do this?

5. As a direct care nurse on the unit, if you identified the problem of nurse work overload, how could you work with other nurses and Jessica to improve this situation?

6. How do you suggest Jessica and her staff investigate the reasons for the increasing use of disposable diapers?

7. How do you suggest Jessica and her staff investigate the reasons for the increasing rate of absent calls?

Critical Thinking Questions and Activities

1. **a.** Interview a nurse who was employed as a clinical nurse in a hospital during the 1990s about his or her experience of working at a time of significant budget reductions.

   b. Interview a nurse who was employed as a nurse manager in a hospital during the 1990s about his or her experience of working at a time of significant budget reductions.

2. Identify characteristics of a local hospital that are similar to the characteristics of magnet hospitals.

3. **a.** What aspects of nurses' work environments need to be considered if nurses are to provide comprehensive care to patients?

   b. Have you seen accommodations made for nurses who are less experienced, have physical limitations resulting from years of practice, or have complex demands outside of their work?

   c. What actions of clinical instructors or other nurses help you to feel empowered for providing clinical care? Trusted? Respected?

4. **a.** Describe a work setting and an intervention that you believe would improve the psychological empowerment of nurses in this setting.

   b. What direct practice issue challenges you the most? Do you think this has an impact on your "psychological empowerment"?

5. Describe a work setting that you believe has the potential to retain nurses.

   a. If you were the nurse manager, what would you do to reduce the rate of turnover?

   b. As a clinical nurse on the unit, what could you do to decrease the rate of turnover?

6. **a.** Describe a work stressor you experienced in a clinical setting where you have practised.

   b. Did all of the nurses or nursing students in this clinical setting find this work stressor equally stressful? Why or why not?

7. In this chapter, the suggestion is made that "Workload may need to be reduced through adding more staff, changing the staffing mix, or eliminating any unnecessary work processes." Many nurses may feel it is no longer realistic to reduce workload through eliminating any unnecessary work processes.

   a. Can you identify any work processes that are inefficient? For example, how long is spent in change of shift report, and in reporting information to supervisors? Can any of this be eliminated and if so, what benefits may be lost?

   b. Would electronic charting at the bedside save time? What are the pros and cons of electronic bedside charting? Do you feel the cost is warranted?

Self-Quiz

1. The characteristics of magnet hospitals include:

   a. Fewer layers of managers
   b. Shared decision making such as shared governance
   c. Nursing models of care
   d. All of the above

2. High structural empowerment is:

   a. related to magnet hospital characteristics
   b. a precursor of turnover

    c. more important to baby boomers than nexters

    d. a concept that is similar to the concept of resilience

3. The predictors of turnover are of interest to nurse managers because:

    a. Turnover predicts organizational commitment

    b. Turnover allows the nurse manager to hire new nurses

    c. The manager may be able to influence some of the predictors

    d. The predictors of turnover are the same as the predictors of wellness

4. Which of the following is *not* a work stressor?

    a. Role ambiguity

    b. Burnout

    c. Role conflict

    d. Ethical conflict

Useful Websites

Canadian Nurses Association. (2010). Taking Action on Nurse Fatigue
www2.cna-aiic.ca/CNA/documents/pdf/publications/PS112_Nurse_Fatigue_2010_e.pdf

Canadian Nurses Association. (2010). Nurses Fatigue and Patient Safety Research Report
www2.cna-aiic.ca/CNA/practice/safety/full_report_e/files/fatigue_safety_2010_report_e.pdf

Nursing Health Services Research Unit (NHSRU)
www.nhsru.com/

Statistics Canada website – work stress among health professionals
www.statcan.gc.ca/daily-quotidien/071113/dq071113a-eng.htm

RNAO (Registered Nurses Association of Ontario) website – Healthy workplaces
www.rnaoknowledgedepot.ca/strengthening_nursing/phwe_what_is_a_hwe.asp

RNAO (Registered Nurses Association of Ontario) website – Healthy Work Environments (HWE) Best Practice Guidelines (BPG)
http://rnao.ca/sites/rnao-ca/files/Workplace_Health_Safety_and_Well-being_of_the_Nurse.pdf

RNAO (Registered Nurses Association of Ontario) website – Nursing shortage
www.rnaoknowledgedepot.ca/strengthening_nursing/rar_the_nursing_shortage.asp

References

Abelson, M.A., & Baysinger, B.D. (1984). Optimal and dysfunctional turnover: Toward an organizational model. *Academy of Management Review, 9,* 331–341.

Aiken, L.H., Clarke, S.P., & Sloane, D.M. (2002). Hospital staffing, organization, and quality of care: Cross-national findings. *Nursing Outlook, 50,* 187–194.

Aiken, L., Havens, D., & Sloan, D. (2000). The magnet nursing services recognition pro-gram: A comparison of two groups of magnet hospitals. *American Journal of Nursing, 100,* 26–35.

Aiken, L.H., Sloane, D.M., & Lake, E.T. (1997). Satisfaction with inpatient acquired immunodeficiency syndrome care: A national comparison of dedicated and scattered-bed units. *Medical Care, 35,* 948–962.

Aiken, L.H., Smith, H.L., & Lake, E.T. (1994). Lower medicine mortality among a set of hospitals known for good nursing care. *Medical Care, 32*, 771–787.

Bae, S. (2011). Assessing the relationships between nurse working conditions and patient outcomes: Systematic literature review. *Journal of Nursing Management, 19*, 700–713.

Barley, S., & Knight, D. (1992). Toward a cultural theory of stress complaints. In *Research in organizational behavior*, JAI Press.

Baumann, A., O'Brien-Pallas, L., Armstrong-Stassen, M., Blythe, J., Bourbonnais, R., Cameron, S., et al. (2001). *Commitment and care: The benefits of a healthy workplace for nurses, their patients and the system*. Ottawa, Ontario, Canada: Canadian Health Services Research Foundation.

Burke, R.J., & Greenglass, E.R. (2000). Effects of hospital restructuring on full time and part time nursing staff in Ontario. *International Journal of Nursing Studies, 37*, 163–171.

Canadian Nurses Association. (2010). Nurse Fatigue and Patient Safety Research Report www2.cna-aiic.ca/CNA/practice/safety/full_report_e/files/fatigue_safety_2010_report_e.pdf

Canadian Nursing Advisory Committee. (2002). *Our health, our future: Creating quality workplaces for Canadian nurses*. Retrieved February 20, 2004, from www.hc-sc.gc.ca/hcs-sss/pubs/care-soins/2002-cnac-cccsi-final/index_e.html

Caplan, R., Cobb, S., French, J., Harrison, R., & Pinneau, S. (1980). *Job demands and worker health: Main effects and occupational differences*. Ann Arbor, MI: Institute for Social Research.

Cavanaugh, S.J., & Coffin, D.A. (1992). Staff turnover among hospital nurses. *Journal of Advanced Nursing, 17*, 1369–1376.

Clausing, S., Kurtz, D., Prendeville, J., & Walt, J. (2003). Generational diversity: The nexters. *AORN Journal*. Retrieved on January 22, 2010 from http://findarticles.com/p/articles/mi_m0FSL/is_3_78/ai_109352507/pg_2/.

Deans, C. (2004). Who cares for nurses? The lived experience of workplace aggression. *Collegian, 11*, 32–36.

DeCicco, J., Laschinger, H., & Kerr, M. (2006). Perceptions of empowerment and respect. Effects on nurses' organizational commitment in nursing homes. *Journal of Gerontological Nursing, 32*, 49–56.

Dirks, K.T., & Ferrin, D.L. (2002). Trust in leadership: Meta-analytic findings and implications for research and practice. *Journal of Applied Psychology, 87*, 611–628.

Edwards, J.R., & Harrison, R.V. (1993). Job demands and worker health: A three dimensional reexamination of the relationship between P-E fit and strain. *Journal of Applied Psychology, 78*, 628–648.

Foxall, M.J., Simmerman, L., Standley, R., & Bene-Captain, B. (1990). A comparison of frequency and sources of nursing job stress perceived by intensive care, hospice, and medical-surgical nurses. *Journal of Advanced Nursing, 15*, 577–584.

French, J., Caplan, R., & Harrison, R. (1982). *The Mechanisms of Job Stress and Strain*. New York: Wiley.

Friese, C. (2005). Nurse practice environments and outcomes: implications for oncology nursing. *Oncology Nurse Forum Online, 32*, 765–72

Ganster, D.C., & Shaubroeck, J. (1991). Work stress and health. *Journal of Management, 17*, 235–271.

Gaudine, A., & Thorne, L. (2012). Nurses' ethical conflict with hospitals: A longitudinal study of outcomes. *Nursing Ethics*. doi: 10.1177/0969733011421626

Gregory, D.M., Way, C.Y., LeFort, S., Barrett, B.J., & Parfrey, P.S. (2007). Predictors of registered nurses' organizational commitment and intent to stay. *Health Care Management Review, 32*, 119–127.

Hayes, L.J., O'Brien-Pallas, L., Duffield, C., Shamian, J., Buchan, J., Hughes, F., et al. (2006). Nurse turnover: A literature review. *International Journal of Nursing Studies, 43*, 237–263.

Hicks, R., & Hicks, K. (1999). *Boomers, Xers, and other strangers: Understanding the generational differences that divide us*. Wheaton, IL: Tyndale House.

Hughes, R.G., & Clancy, C.M. (2009). Complexity, bullying, and stress. Analyzing and mitigating a challenging work environment for nurses. *Journal of Nursing Care Quality, 24,* 180–183.

Jackson, S., & Schuler, R. (1985). A meta-analysis and conceptual critique of research on role ambiguity and role conflict in work settings. *Organizational Behavior and Human Decision Processes, 36,* 16–78.

Jacobson, B.H., Aldana, S.G., Goetzel, R.Z., et al. (1996). The relationship between perceived stress and self-reported illness-related absenteeism. *American Journal of Health Promotion, 11,* 54–61.

Jamal, M., & Baba, V.V. (2000). Job stress and burnout among Canadian managers and nurses: An empirical examination. *Canadian Journal of Public Health, 91,* 454–458.

Kanter, R.M. (1977). *Men and Women of the Corporation.* New York: Basic Books.

Kanter, R.M. (1993). *Men and Women of the Corporation.* 2nd ed. New York: Basic Books.

Karasek, R., & Theorell, T. (1990). *Health work: Stress, productivity and the reconstruction of working life.* New York: Basic Books.

Kasl, S.V. (1996). The influence of the work environment on cardiovascular health: A historical, conceptual, and methodological perspective. *Journal of Occupational Health Psychology, 1,* 42–56.

Kazanjian, A., Green, C., Wong, J., & Reid, R. (2005). Effect of the hospital nursing environment on patient mortality: A systematic review. *Journal of Health Service Research Policy, 10,* 111–117.

Kramer, M. (1990). The Magnet hospitals: Excellence revisited. *Journal of Nursing Administration, 20,* 35–44.

Kramer, M., & Schmalenger, C.E. (2003). Magnet hospital nurses describe control over nursing practice. *Western Journal of Nursing Research, 25,* 434–452.

Laschinger, H.K. (2004). Hospital nurses' perceptions of respect and organizational justice. *Journal of Nursing Administration, 34,* 354–364.

Laschinger, H.K.S. (2008). Effect of empowerment on professional practice environments, work satisfaction, and patient care quality: Further testing the nursing worklife model. *Journal of Nursing Care Quality, 23,* 322–330.

Laschinger, H.K.S., Almost, J., & Tuer-Hodes, D. (2003). Workplace empowerment and magnet hospital characteristics: Making the link. *Journal of Nursing Administration, 33,* 410–422.

Laschinger, H.K.S., Finegan, J., & Shamian, J. (2001). The impact of workplace empowerment, organizational trust on staff nurses' work satisfaction and organizational commitment. *Healthcare Management Review, 26,* 7–23.

Laschinger, H.K.S., Finegan, J., Shamian, J., & Wilk, P. (2001). Impact of structural and psychological empowerment on job strain in nursing work settings. *Journal of Nursing Administration, 31,* 260–272.

Laschinger, H.K.S., & Leiter, M.P. (2006). The impact of nursing work environments on patient safety outcomes: The mediating role of burnout/engagement. *The Journal of Nursing Administration, 36,* 259–267.

Laschinger, H.K.S., Leiter, M., Day, A., & Gilin, D. (2009). Workplace empowerment, incivility, and burnout: the impact on staff nursing recruitment and retention outcomes. *Journal of Nursing Management, 17*(3), 302–311.

Laschinger, H.K.S., Shamian, J., & Thomson, D. (2001). Impact of magnet hospital characteristics on nurses' perceptions of trust, burnout, quality of care, and work satisfaction. *Nursing Economic$, 19,* 209–219.

Lavoie-Tremblay, M. (2004). Creating a healthy workplace: A participatory organizational intervention. *Journal of Nursing Administration, 34,* 469–474.

Lavoie-Tremblay, M., Wright, D., Desforges, N., Gélinas, C., Marchionni, C., & Drevniok, U. (2008). Creating a healthy workplace for new-generation nurses. *Journal of Nursing Scholarship, 40,* 290–297.

Lazarus, R.S., & Folkman, S. (1984). *Stress appraisal and coping.* New York: Springer.

Lee, R.T., & Ashforth, B.E. (1996). A meta-analytic examination of the correlates of the three dimensions of burnout. *Journal of Applied Psychology, 81,* 123–133.

Leiter, M.P. (2007). Deepening the impact of initiatives to promote teamwork and workplace health: A perspective from the NEKTA study. *Healthcare Papers, 7,* 79–84.

Leiter, M.P., & Maslach, C. (2009). Nurse turnover: the mediating role of burnout. *Journal of Nursing Management, 17*(3), 331–339.

Maslach, C., Jackson, S.E., & Leiter, M.P. (1996). *Maslach Burnout Inventory Manual.* 3rd ed. CA: Psychology Press.

Maslach, C., & Leiter, M.P. (1997). *The Truth About Burnout: How Organizations Cause Personal Stress and What To Do About It?* San Francisco: Jossey-Bass.

Maurier, W.L., & Northcott, H.C. (2000). Job uncertainty and health status for nurses during restructuring of health care in Alberta. *Western Journal of Nursing Research, 22,* 623–641.

McClure, M.M., Poulin, M., Wandelt, S.M., & Wandelt, M. (1983). *Magnet hospitals: Attraction and retention of professional nurses.* American Academy of Nursing Task Force on Nursing Practice in Hospitals. Kansas City, MO: American Nurses Association.

McLaughlin, A.M., & Erdman, J. (1992). Rehabilitation staff stress as it relates to patient acuity and diagnosis. *Brain Injury, 6,* 59–64.

Meyer, J.P., & Allen, N.J. (1991). A three-component conceptualization of organizational commitment. *Human Resource Management Review, 1,* 61–89.

Mobley, W.H. (1982). *Employee turnover, causes, consequences, and control.* Menlo Park, CA: Addison-Wesley.

O'Brien-Pallas, L., Shamian, J., Thomson, D., Alksnis, C., Koehoorn, M., Kerr, M., & Bruce, S. (2004). Work-related disability in Canadian nurses. *Journal of Nursing Scholarship, 36,* 352–357.

O'Brien-Pallas, L., Thomson, D., Alksnsis, C., & Bruce, S. (2001). The economic impact of nurse staffing decisions: Time to turn down another road? *Hospital Quarterly, 4,* 42–50.

Pearson, A., O'Brien Pallas, L., Thomson, D., Doucette, E., Tucker, D., Wiechula, R., Long, L., Porritt, K., & Jordan, Z. (2006). Systematic review of evidence on the impact of nursing workload and staffing on establishing healthy work environments. *International Journal of Evidence Based Healthcare, 4,* 337–384.

Peterson, U., Bergström, G., Sameuelsson, M., Åsberg, M., & Nygren, Å. (2008). Reflecting peer-support groups in the prevention of stress and burnout: Randomized controlled trial. *Journal of Advanced Nursing, 63,* 506–516.

Porter-O'Grady, T. (1992). *Implementing shared governance: Creating a professional organization.* St. Louis: Mosby.

Regan, S. (2003). Keeping new graduate registered nurses in B.C.: It's about quality practice environments! *Nursing, 35,* 23–24.

Rondeau, K., & Wagar, (2006). Nurse and resident satisfaction in magnet long-term care organizations: Do high involvement approaches matter? *Journal of Nursing Management, 14,* 244–250.

Salmond, S., Begley, R., Brennan, J., & Saimbert, M. (2009). A comprehensive systematic review of evidence on determining the impact of magnet designation on nursing and patient outcomes: Is the investment worth it? *JBI Library of Systematic Reviews, 7*(26), 1144–1203.

Sasichay-Akkadechanunt, T., Scalzi, C.C., & Jawad, A.F. (2003). The relationship between nurse staffing and patient outcomes. *Journal of Nursing Administration, 33,* 478–485.

Scott, J.G., Sochalski, J., & Aiken, L. (1999). Review of magnet hospital research: Findings and implications for professional nursing practice. *Journal of Nursing Administration, 29,* 9–19.

Shamian, J., & El-Jardali, F. (2007). Healthy workplaces for health workers in Canada: Knowledge transfer and uptake in policy and practice. *Healthcare Papers, 7,* 6–25.

Skipper, J.K., Jung, F.D., & Coffey, L.C. (1990). Nurses and shiftwork: Effects of physical health and mental depression. *Journal of Advanced Nursing, 15*, 835–842.

Spreitzer, G. (1995). Psychological empowerment in the workplace: Dimensions, measurement, and validation. *Academy of Management Journal, 38* (5), 1442–1462.

Staw, B.M. (1980). The consequences of turnover. *Journal of Occupational Behavior, 1*, 253–273.

Tai, T.W.C., Bame, S.I., & Robinson, C.D. (1998). Review of nursing turnover research, 1977–1996. *Social Science & Medicine, 47*, 1905–1924.

Turnley, W.H., & Feldman, D.C. (1998). Psychological contract violations during corporate restructuring. *Human Resource Management, 37*, 71–83.

Turnley, W.H., & Feldman, D.C. (1999). The impact of psychological contract violations on exit, voice, loyalty, and neglect. *Human Relations, 52*, 895–922.

Upenicks, V.V. (2002). Assessing differences in job satisfaction of nurses in magnet and nonmagnet hospitals. *Journal of Nursing Administration, 32*, 564–576.

Wagner, C.M. (2007). Organizational commitment as a predictor variable in nursing turnover research: Literature review. *Journal of Advanced Nursing, 60*, 235–247.

Watson, R. et al. (2003). Older nurses and employment decisions. *Nursing Standard, 18*, 35–40.

Chapter 10
Team Building and Managing Conflict

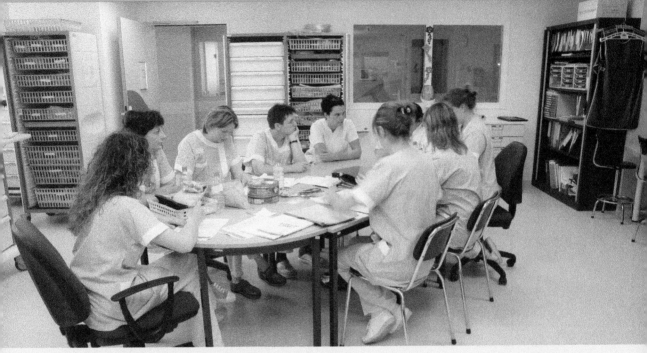

BSIP SA / Alamy

Learning Objectives

After reading, studying, and reflecting on this chapter's content, you will be able to:

1. Discuss how effective and ineffective teams develop
2. Suggest ways nurses can promote team building in their own work setting
3. Discuss strategies for effectively managing conflict in the workplace
4. Debate the pros and cons of conflict in the workplace
5. Suggest how health care organizations with and without unions can resolve disputes
6. Identify how nexters and nurses nearing retirement may be engaged in lateral violence (perhaps unknowingly) with their own and the other age cohorts
7. Discuss how the nurses' values related to decision making in organizations might lead to nurses' conflict with hospitals
8. Recommend a plan for how a conflict in the workplace that you have been involved in could be managed

INTRODUCTION

Most direct care nurses work on nursing teams as well as interdisciplinary teams. In addition, nurses may be part of other work teams, such as committees and research teams. When these teams function smoothly, nurses probably feel satisfied and patients may benefit. In contrast, when there is conflict among team members or between different teams, nurses may feel stressed, they may be absent from work more or resign, and patient care can suffer. Conflict on teams or between teams occurs for reasons such as differing views of what is best for a patient, how scare resources should be spent, or how nursing rotations or assignments are made. Unfortunately, conflict in the workplace can also occur when nursing colleagues abuse or bully each other (horizontal violence, also referred to as lateral violence), when managers abuse persons who report to them (vertical violence), or when nurses abuse their managers or nursing students abuse nursing instructors (upward violence).

Although conflict in nurses' work environment has negative outcomes, such as stress and a detrimental impact on patient care, can it also have positive outcomes? How can conflict be managed to reduce negative outcomes and/or improve positive outcomes? How can nurses work to create the type of team that everyone would like to work on? While you see yourself as a caring person, is it possible that your colleagues would see you as contributing to horizontal violence, or your nursing instructor or nurse manager believes you bullied them? This chapter discusses the characteristics of effective teams and suggests how nurses can help work with conflict effectively, build supportive and effective work teams, and reduce bullying in the workplace.

SUCCESSFUL WORK TEAMS

Teamwork in the workplace involves two or more employees working together to achieve a work-related goal that in many cases can only be achieved through teamwork or is achieved more effectively through teamwork. It has become a frequent saying among health care professionals that sports teams spend months training to learn to play as a team, while health care disciplines train their professionals separately, and upon graduation, expect them to work well on a team (Fry et al., 1974; Clark, 2009). Some nursing teams or interdisciplinary health teams may come together and function well, but other teams need to be "built" or need help in learning to function well together. The following sections discuss the characteristics of successful teams, the competencies needed by leaders and team members and leaders for effective teams, and team building. Knowledge about the characteristics of successful teams and the competencies of team leaders and members that are associated with successful teams can be used to help teams learn to function well (team building).

Characteristics of Successful Teams

While there are a number of characteristics of successful teams, Clark identified six that we agree contribute to well functioning nursing or interdisciplinary health care teams. These characteristics are:

- shared goals
- group norms

- roles
- horizontal leadership
- communication
- collocation (Clark, 2009).

Learning about the characteristics of successful teams is important because teams that are not functioning well may be able to assess how they operate compared with these characteristics. Nevertheless, it is important to note that much of the literature about the characteristics of successful teams is based on observations, descriptions, and theories rather than empirical studies, and this is particularly the case for successful health care teams.

Shared Goals

For a team to function well, team members must have shared and clear goals (Hall et al., 2005). A nursing team has a shared goal when, for example, all members of the team are aware that the team's goal is to provide family-centred care, and all agree with this goal and work to ensure it is attained.

Group Norms

Teams also have norms, which are the unwritten guidelines about how group members behave. Norms of effective groups are such things as communicating together to resolve conflicts, respecting members' ideas, and individual accountability (Parsons, 2006). An example of a norm for a nursing team is if nurses on a unit help their colleagues when one of their patients becomes very ill or they have a heavy assignment.

Roles

Different team members have different roles, which may be based on their expertise, job title, or consensus (Ducanis & Golin, 1979). **Role bending**, means members are flexible about assuming another member's role if required, and **role overlap**, occurs when roles are not exclusively held by one member (Clark, 2009; Molyneux, 2001). Role bending and role overlap are important features of effective teams in that members' ease with filling in for each other allows the team to operate smoothly (Clark, 2009; Molyneux, 2001). Role bending occurs when, for example, the physiotherapist is usually assisted by an aide to help a patient to ambulate but the aide is not on the unit, then another member of the team volunteers to assist the physiotherapist. Role overlap occurs for registered nurses and licensed practical nurses because they have significant overlap in their roles of providing client care.

Horizontal leadership

Horizontal leadership refers to a leadership style in which the leader does not dictate to other team members, but guides team members to discuss their ideas to reach consensus and to attain goals (Clark, 2009; Molyneux, 2001). This is in contrast to **vertical leadership**, where the leader directs team members. Leadership within a team with horizontal leadership may be carried out by different members at different times, as the type of leadership required can change over time. This is consistent with role bending, where in this case different members fill the role of leader (Clark, 2009). An example of horizontal leadership in a nursing department occurs when nurses work as a team to develop patient care guidelines for patients in their department. When the charge nurse is not available and an issue comes up, another nurse may fill in and respond to this issue, which is another example.

Communication

Communication is essential for a successful team, because good communication helps to prevent and resolve conflict and helps team members learn about and accept the strengths, weaknesses, and differences among group members (Clark, 2009). It is through communication that team members are able to work as a team and not as separate individuals. Good communication on a successful nursing team happens when nurses have differing opinions about how the care for a patient's wound, but they are able to discuss this and a consistent approach for all nurses on the unit is selected.

Collocation

Another characteristic of successful teams is **collocation**, or the situating of team members together in the same location, thereby facilitating their communication. Team members are able to sort out their differences when they share a physical location and interact frequently. Not all successful teams are located in the same physical space, but collocation does facilitate the networking that helps members work toward their shared goals. Placing the offices of all the nurses, physiotherapists, social workers, home care workers, and physicians responsible for home care services in the same section of a building is collocation.

Characteristics of Managers of Successful Teams

The characteristics and skills of managers or leaders who are successful in building and facilitating teams may differ from the characteristics that make someone a good vertical leader. Five key characteristics of managers or leaders of successful teams identified by Gilley, Gilley, McConnell, & Viliquette (2010) in their review of the literature include skills in:

1. coaching,
2. motivating,
3. communicating,
4. engaging team members in decision making, and
5. developing team members. (Gilley & Boughton, 1996; Gilley & Gilley, 2007; Gilley, Gilley, McConnell, & Veliquette, 2010)

The ability of a team manager to motivate team members will affect the team's success in obtaining their goals. Coaching is the way a team manager guides team members in their work, providing them with the knowledge, skills, and support to do their work. Managers of successful teams communicate effectively, conveying enthusiasm about the work of team members and the goals of the team. They give feedback about progress to goals, interacting in collaboration with employees to coach them to meet the team's goals. Managers of successful teams engage team members in decision making. This improves the quality of decisions because different perspectives are considered. Further, engaging team members in decision making improves the commitment of team members to the work and success of the team. Managers who foster the development of their team members help these members enjoy and feel committed to their work.

Researchers tested whether these characteristics of managers of successful teams were related to "a manager's ability to facilitate and build teams" (Gilley et al., 2010. p. 34). A survey was given to 689 masters and doctoral students at five universities in the United States. The graduate students were asked how often managers in their current or most recent place of work showed different behaviours as well as the extent to which managers facilitated teams and teamwork. Their analysis showed that the top five characteristics that predicted the respondents' view of managers' ability to facilitate and build teams were:

1. involving employees in decision making,
2. coaching employees,
3. appropriate communication with the employees,
4. motivating employees, and
5. facilitating employees' growth and development. (Gilley et al., 2010)

While this study provides some evidence for the type of leadership behaviours that are associated with successful teams, there is a need for additional research, including studies with nurses and other health professionals. For example, further research can examine the characteristics of team members and leaders of successful nursing and interdisciplinary teams in a variety of health care settings (multi-site large acute care hospitals, community hospitals, community services, residential care, and so on).

Competencies of Team Members for Successful Teams

In reviewing the literature on skills, knowledge and attitudes required by team members, Gilley, Morris et al. (2010) identified six areas where team members need to develop competencies:

1. conflict resolution
2. problem solving,
3. communication,
4. decision-making skills,
5. goal setting and performance management skills, and
6. planning and task coordination.

Conflict resolution competencies include skill at recognizing conflict that can lead to new ideas and positive changes, and distinguishing this useful type of conflict from undesirable conflict between members. Skill in conflict resolution, including the ability to collaborate and to identify win–win solutions (see the section on Responses to Conflict on page 300), is useful for resolving undesirable conflicts (Stevens & Campion, 1999). Competency in identifying problems and approaches to solving the problems and attaining the group's goals are important for the success of the team (Giley & Giley, 2007). Good communication among team members, including good presentation and writing skills (Klein et al., 2009), as well as respectful listening to the ideas of those in another competency, are required for the success of teams. The good decision-making skills involve the proper evaluation and consideration of all alternatives, and selection of the alternative that helps the team meet their goals. Team members also need to be able to select goals for the team, set these goals, and monitor their progress to attaining the goals (Steven & Campion, 1999). Finally, team members require skill in planning and task coordination in order to divide and coordinate work among members, and to balance the workload among members with different work task roles (Klein et al., 2009; Steven & Campion, 1999).

Team Building

In recent years, the term **team building** has increasingly been used to describe the efforts of team members, team leaders, and/or staff developers to improve the smooth functioning and effectiveness of work teams (Cummings & Worley, 2005; Gilley, Morris, Waite, Coates, & Veliquette, 2010). Team building refers to helping work teams develop their skills to work together, solve problems together, communicate well with each other, develop and recognize the strengths of individual members, increase members' commitment to working with other team members, and enhance horizontal leadership skills (Gilley, Morris et al., 2010; Pellerin, 2009). This team-development work helps teams to meet their work goals. In the health care sector, team building is seen as important for nursing and interdisciplinary health teams; there is nursing research evidence that group cohesion and job satisfaction affects the retention of nurses (Lucas, Atwood, & Hagaman, 1993; Parsons et al., 2006; Shader et al., 2001), and improved patient safety (Clark, 2009).

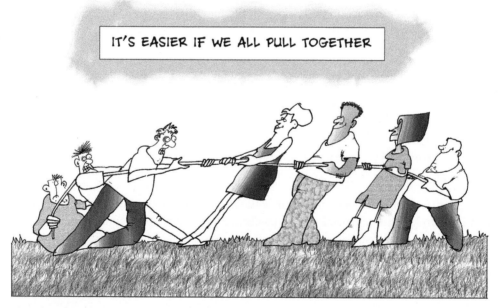

Fran/Cartoon Stock Ltd.

A study that examined the impact of a team-building intervention found improvements in group cohesion, nurse–nurse interactions, and job enjoyment, and a reduction in turnover (DiMeglio, Padula, Piatek, et al., 2005). What is noteworthy is that the team-building intervention consisted of three one-hour sessions. Therefore, this is a relatively low-cost intervention that does not consume much time, and therefore is not overly costly to implement.

A Canadian researcher in the province of Quebec, Dr. Lavoie-Tremblay, used a participatory process where direct care nurses identified their work constraints. Then the work groups met daily for six days to develop an action plan to improve the work constraint. During these meetings, staff developed their communication, collaboration, problem identification, and problem-solving skills. This team-building approach empowered the direct care nurses to take control over their work environment (Lavoie-Tremblay, 2004).

CONFLICT AT WORK

Conflict that is associated with disruptive clinician behaviour, discussed later in this chapter, is conflict that we should all work to prevent. However, much conflict in the workplace is a result of real individual differences in what different employees believe is the best decision or course of action, how objectives should be met, and so on. In this case, the conflict may actually be good as it can lead to innovative and creative decisions, and to positive changes (Rahim, 1986).

Groupthink—The Dangerous Outcome of Avoiding Conflict

In fact, when work group members want to avoid conflict and agree with everyone on the team even when they disagree, group members might continue on a problematic course of action. When group members decide they will not bring up their contrary views about a decision, the group proceeds without critically evaluating divergent opinions. The group is harmonious but their work may be faulty. When a group does not bring up and evaluate divergent opinions because they want to remain cohesive, this is known as "**groupthink**" (Janis, 1982). Groupthink is more likely to occur when members are similar to each other, the leader states his or her opinion early in the decision-making process and encourages others to agree with him or her, and the team's work process does not include procedures for evaluating the data they used for making the decision.

One strategy for avoiding groupthink is to allow all group members to brainstorm all possible options, during which time members do not discuss if they like or dislike the options. Other ways to avoid groupthink include:

1. generating a list of pros and cons for each option,
2. influential team leaders not supporting one course of action during discussions,
3. inviting outsiders to meet with the team to introduce differing points of view, and
4. critically examining the selected decision for everything that could go wrong.

Groups in which members are similar may be more harmonious and have fewer conflicts. However, groupthink is more apt to occur in these groups. Therefore, to avoid groupthink, dissimilar persons should be included in the group and team members should learn to manage conflict (Buckingham & Clifton, 2001).

Responses to Conflict

Individuals have different tolerances for conflict and respond differently to conflict. In the 1970s, researchers identified five types of responses to conflict (Thomas & Kilmann, 1978), and work in this area still supports these five categories of responses (Wilmot & Hocker, 2001; Sportsman & Hamilton, 2007). The five responses to dealing with conflict are:

1. competition,
2. collaboration,
3. compromise,
4. avoidance, and
5. accommodation.

These responses vary in their amount of assertiveness and cooperation. Competition occurs when both individuals focus on winning. Both parties are high in assertiveness and low in cooperation as they both focus on arguing for their desired outcome. Generally, competition results in the stronger party winning, and the type of solution from this type of approach is therefore referred to as a "win–lose" solution. Collaboration occurs when both individuals try to work together to find the best solution. To collaborate, both parties are high in assertiveness and cooperation. Collaboration involves looking at the needs of each person and searching for a solution that will meet the needs of both sides. Rather than each person advocating for what each initially wanted, they try and see if there is a new solution that both individuals will find favourable. Hence, solutions found through collaboration are sometimes referred to as "win–win" solutions. In contrast, when individuals who have a conflict engage in compromise, generally they find a solution that meets some of each of their needs but is not ideal for either person. When compromising, both parties are medium in assertion as well as medium in cooperativeness. Compromising results in "lose–lose" solutions, as neither party ends up a solution that he or she would consider ideal. Avoidance occurs when both individuals decide not to deal with the conflict. In this case, both individuals are low in assertiveness and cooperation. As the conflict is not dealt with, there is no solution, resulting in a "lose–lose" situation. The final type of response to conflict is accommodation. With accommodation, one individual decides to allow the other individual to have what the other person wants. In this case, the individuals are low on assertiveness but high in cooperation, and a "win–lose" solution occurs.

Individuals tend to favour one of the five approaches to dealing with conflict, and to use their favoured style when they experience conflict at home or at work. A number of research studies involving direct care nurses have found that these nurses tend to use avoidance when faced with conflict (for example, Baker, 1995; Eason & Brown, 1999).

> ## Approaches to Dealing with Conflict
>
> - Competition—a win–lose solution
> - Collaboration—a win–win solution
> - Compromise—a lose–lose solution
> - Avoidance—a lose–lose solution
> - Accommodation—a win–lose solution

One study found that both direct care nurses and nurse managers used avoidance as their main approach to conflict, followed by accommodation (Eason & Brown, 1999). There are a number of reasons why nurses might avoid conflict. First, nurses are busy persons, engaging in conflict takes time and energy, and they may have immediate patient care needs to meet (Vivar, 2006). Further, direct care nurses report to a nurse manager, and they may be concerned about how their manager will perceive the conflict (Vivar, 2006). A study that included 65 bachelor- and master-of-nursing students in Texas found that compromise was the primary approach to conflict, followed by avoidance (Sportsman & Hamilton, 2007).

Since collaboration results in a win-win solution that is high on assertiveness and high in cooperation, is it always the right style to use? Perhaps surprisingly, the answer is "no." The best style may depend on the situation. Collaboration can result in innovative solutions that had not yet been considered; hence collaboration is ideal when possible solutions may exist that have not yet been explored, and when there is time to do this exploration. An example of a conflict resolved through collaboration is a situation when a nurse refuses to preceptor a nurse who has just been hired, and the nurse manager insists that she should orient the new hire. Through discussion, the manager learns that the nurse does not want to orient someone because she has already agreed to be in charge, and there will be a group of eight nursing students also working on the unit, which means the nursing station and medication room will be rather crowded. Through collaboration, the nurse and her manager agree that another nurse who is working evenings can work days and be in charge, freeing this nurse to work evenings and orient the nurse when the unit is quieter. This is a win–win solution because the nurse attains her goal of not orientating someone while she is in charge when there are also nursing students on the unit, and the manager attains her goal of having the nurse whom she believes has the capability to provide an excellent orientation work with the new nurse.

Similarly, should avoidance be avoided because it is low in assertion and low in cooperation? Health care professionals are busy, and if they were to discuss every disagreement they had all day long, patient care would undoubtedly suffer! You undoubtedly have heard the expression "choose your battles." For the sake of good relations with others as well as time, it may be worthwhile to not take up every issue you disagree with. It may also be worthwhile to make a few concessions on issues that are less important to you, so that you are not always disagreeing with someone and can push your agenda forward for an issue that you find important.

The five approaches just discussed were identified in the literature in the 1970s and are still recognized as responses to conflict. In addition to these five approaches, other responses to conflict that are more extreme and dysfunctional are sabotage and violence.

Sabotage involves actions intended to thwart the goals or actions of another person or group. Sabotage can occur if a committee interviews several nurses and makes a selection. However this is someone who the team member who requested references does not agree should be selected. The person who calls for references can then neglect to email the referees and much later can tell the selection committee members that the references still haven't arrived. Violence, including different types of this disruptive clinician behaviour, is discussed later in this chapter in the section on disruptive clinician behaviour.

PREVENTING OR RESOLVING CONFLICTS BETWEEN NURSES AND MANAGERS

Communication Approaches for Assertive and Aggressive Responses

Conflicts between nurses and managers can be resolved using any of the five approaches to resolving conflict discussed in the previous section (competition, collaboration, compromise, avoidance, and accommodation). As well, there are certain communication approaches that can de-escalate or escalate a conflict, such as the use of "I" statements as opposed to "you" statements, the use of "you should" statements, and the use of "we" statements as opposed to "I" statements. These communication approaches are associated with assertive or aggressive communication.

Assertive behaviour is associated with being able to:

1. say no

2. ask for what you want

3. express negative and positive comments; and initiate, continue, and end an interaction (Arnold & Boggs, 2011)

When asking for what you want or expressing your own thoughts, you should use "I" statements (Arnold & Boggs, 2011). For example, "I believe I should be assigned to Mr. Smith today because I was his nurse two days ago." and "I do not agree with you putting in your resignation on December 10 for December 24 because the Christmas schedule is made and the other nurses have already made plans if they were scheduled off on December 25."

When someone uses an "I" statement to share feelings in response to a conflict with another individual, the other individual is less apt to take offence than when a "you" statement is made. For example, if a nurse is upset because she feels her patient assignment is too heavy, she could reply "I am feeling stressed and angry because I feel my assignment is heavier than the other nurses' assignments." "I" statements are useful because the other person learns the effect on you of his or her behaviour. The manager in this case may respond to the fact that the nurse is stressed, and rather than responding angrily, she may either explain her rationale for the assignment, suggest a solution such as providing some assistance to the nurse, or changing the assignment. Typically, "I" statements represent an assertive response to a conflict.

In contrast, the nurse who feels her assignment is too heavy could reply with a "you" statement: "You gave me an unfair assignment." In this case the nurse manger may feel she is being attacked, and therefore is more apt to respond emotionally and by defending herself rather than examining the nurse's assignment. If the nurse responds with a "you should" statement—"You should not have given me this assignment"—the nurse manager may become angry because not only is she being attacked, she is being told what she should have done, much as a parent tells a child what he or she "should" do. "You" statements are typically associated with aggressive responses (Arnold and Boggs, 2011), and "you should" statements, which direct another person, can be particularly irksome to the person you are communicating with.

There is also a passive way to respond to a heavy workload that is believed to be unfair: simply saying nothing and proceeding with the workload that one perceives is too heavy. In addition, there is a passive–aggressive approach, for example if the nurse says nothing to the nurse manager, but talks to numerous other nurses about how unfair the manager was to him or her.

"We" statements can be annoying, for a nurse manager or team member says "We believe that it doesn't look professional when nurses drink coffee at the nurses' station" and you haven't been consulted and are not sure if you agree with this. However, "we" statements can be inclusive when used to discuss the group's achievements, for example, "We have made a number of changes on the unit over the past year, and these have improved patient care." In this case, the use of "we" provides a sense of inclusiveness among team members. When team managers use the word "I" to discuss accomplishments, this can be particularly annoying to team members who are aware of their input into the accomplishment. In addition, using "we" statements when experiencing conflict can be useful in trying to move from what each party is advocating to focusing on common objectives (Northam, 2009).

Communication Strategies within Organizations

One way to prevent conflicts is to obtain different viewpoints prior to making a decision. Managers can email drafts of decisions, guidelines, or policies or place them on the intranet. Health care professionals are then given an opportunity to provide feedback about these drafts before these are finalized. This feedback can be given through email, the health care organization's intranet, meetings with union representatives, or staff meetings that are held as open forums for all employees or at the departmental level. It is particularly important to consult widely with all employees in a health care organization when the decision affects everyone or when a decision is one that is not desired by all parties. In this case, at least when the decision is announced the manager will be able to acknowledge that not all will think this is the best decision, that the opposing viewpoints were heard, and provide a rationale for the decision that includes acknowledging the different viewpoints.

The advantage of consulting widely with everyone involved is that all are given an opportunity to voice an opinion. However, such a consultation process consumes the time of all involved. If this process were used for all decisions, employees might become tired of being included in the consultation and may disengage from it. To provide safe patient care, there are times when changes in procedures need to be made immediately and quickly.

- consult widely
- email decisions
- meet with unions
- hold open forums
- meet with staff
- hold committee meetings

- acknowledge when a decision is not what all wanted
- acknowledge mistakes and revise decisions if necessary
- communicate in a style consistent with organization's stated values

It is difficult to communicate with everyone in a large organization, particularly when there are some who may choose to not read email or attend staff meetings. We know many managers who feel they spend much time communicating what is happening in the health care setting, and then feel frustrated when clinicians tell them they were unaware of impending changes. The importance of communication in a health care setting cannot be understated. The challenges in reaching everyone, every day, with every decision are huge.

One strategy to improve communication on a specific topic or issue is to have a representative from every department on a committee, and this person provides feedback at the unit level. One difficulty with this approach is that, depending on the number of departments, committees may end up with more members than are expedient for them to function smoothly. Another difficulty with this approach is that the representatives might miss a meeting or be negligent in passing on information.

Managers do make decisions that affect nurses, and these decisions can reflect errors in judgment. At times, this could be because a decision was needed quickly, and when more information is obtained, the manager may realize it was not the best decision. At other times, a manager may think he or she has all the information required for a decision, and fails to consult with all parties. Similarly, direct care nurses make decisions and may act or say things to nurse managers that reflect errors in judgment. In these cases, it is amazing how conflict or anger can be quickly resolved when the nurse manager or the nurse admits a mistake was made and apologizes. Further, reversing a decision shows others that you have heard them and that you are open to reconsidering your position.

A final communication strategy managers can use to reduce conflict with health care professionals is to ensure that their communication is congruent with the stated values of the organization. Leaders of health care organizations generally identify organizational values that they wish all employees to share, to display in their work with clients, and to become part of the organization's culture. These values are demonstrated by how members of the organization communicate and act. For example, respect, caring, and transparency are values that might be adopted by health care organizations. Nurses are taught that respect and caring are important for therapeutic communication. When these values have also been adopted as values for the health care setting, it implies all employees should act consistently with these values. While it is relatively easy to communicate in a respectful, caring, and transparent manner when you agree with another employee, at times of conflict it is challenging to remember these values, but doing so can help de-escalate the conflict.

DECISIONS IN HOSPITALS: THE CONFLICT BETWEEN NURSES' VALUES AND HOSPITAL ADMINISTRATORS' VALUES

There are several types of conflict that nurses may experience, for example, conflict about patient care decisions or conflict about how decisions should be made in the workplace. This section focuses on nurses' conflict with how they believe decisions *should* be made versus how they *are* made in their workplace. Underlying this conflict is a conflict between nurses' values as they relate to decision making and how decisions are made reflecting these or other values. We believe that nurses' conflict with how decisions are made in large health care organizations is a major source of discontentment for nurses, and that understanding the difficulties in changing practices in these organizations can help lessen this discontentment.

We have noticed that health care professionals are increasingly referring to the value "transparency." Professionals who work with clients in collaboration, an approach to working with clients where nurses and clients share information and agree to the plan of care, value transparency and collaboration. Within the workplace, transparency reflects the expectation of today's workers to know what decisions are made by managers as well as how these decisions are made.

Our observations lead us to believe that today's health care workers expect organizations to operate not only with transparency, but also as participative democracies (see Pateman, 1970, for a description of participation and democracies), wherein all clinicians participate in decisions made in the workplace. Participative democracy is consistent with the fact that clinicians, as professionals, are educated to make patient care decisions that are in a patient's best interest (Colvin, 1987). Yet hospitals are hierarchical and bureaucratic organizations, in which the chain of command is important and there are many policies (Colvin, 1987). As noted by Colvin (1987), professionals' expectation of how they decide to meet their patients' needs is at odds with this hierarchical, bureaucratic nature.

We believe that with the current emphasis on patient safety, the need for hospitals to develop policies on patient care and for administration to make quick decisions to improve patient care are evident. We also believe that the expectations of today's nurses for transparency and for participative democracy call for a new paradigm of decision making if nurses are to be happy with their workplace. We acknowledge that shared governance (Porter-O'Grady & Malloch, 2009) (see Chapter 5 for an overview of shared governance) is probably the best organizational structure to date that maintains the hospital's need to make quality decisions and enforce policies with professionals' need to participate. In shared governance, committees that include administrators and direct care nurses focus on decisions related to the standard of nursing practice, and this committee structure operates concurrently with the hierarchical hospital and nursing administration structures.

Unfortunately, the vast majority of nurses in most organizations that employ shared governance are unaware of and uninvolved in the work of the committees that are part of the shared governance model. This is particularly the case in very large, multi-site health care organizations. Further, the rapid time frame required for many decisions may mean many decisions are made by administration rather than through the committees. Therefore, hospitals with shared governance are still open to nurses feeling that decision making isn't transparent, and feeling at odds with the way administrators are making decisions.

The challenge for the next generation of nurse leaders is to identify how to structure large health care organizations where decisions can be transparent and nurses are part of a participative democracy. One possible way is to implement shared governance in a way that convinces all nurses in the hospital that they are involved in decision making and decision making is transparent, while at the same time ensuring that the development and implementation of policies can be quick, to ensure patient safety. Alternatively, the challenge for the next generation is to identify a new model of administration or decision making, a model that will reduce the conflict or tension between a nurse's expectations for practice and the hospital's need to ensure patient safety. Such a model would no doubt decrease nurses' conflict with hospital practices. Until large health care settings are transparent, engage all nurses, and become nimble at implementing policies and making changes to ensure safe care, nurses may find they are working in an organization structured to ensure safe care but not in their ideal work setting.

Dispute-Resolution Processes

Even when nurse managers and the nurses who report to them have excellent communication skills, differences in opinion may not be resolved. It is normal that persons may view a situation differently given individual differences in values, history, roles, and present circumstances. When nurses disagree with their nurse manager, they should first ask to meet with the manager to discuss the issue. If a meeting does not resolve the issue, the nurse might decide to submit a written complaint, which may take the form of a **grievance** in a unionized health care setting.

Unions are helpful for both their members and managers in dealing with differences of opinion. A good union representative will listen to the nurse and help the nurse to clarify the specific issue(s). This can also help to defuse negative emotions evoked by the dispute. Further, the union representative might tell the employee whether he or she has a legitimate complaint, given the employee's contract with the organization. In many cases, the union representative educates the nurse about his or her roles and responsibilities, and the nurse may gain an understanding of the manager's decision. This helps not only the nurse but also the manager, as the union explains the issues related to the complaint rather than the manager. In cases where the health care setting is not unionized, it falls on the manager to explain why a complaint is not valid. Given that the manager will be seen by the nurse to have a conflict of interest, the nurse may not accept the manager's position as valid.

A complaint procedure is valuable for a number of reasons. Managers do make mistakes and therefore a process for bringing these mistakes to their attention is needed (Forman & Merrick, 2003). Further, if employees do not have a legitimate route for addressing their complaints, it is possible that they would resort to insubordination, a work slowdown, a legal or illegal strike (Forman & Merrick, 2003), or acts of sabotage. (Note that a strike is illegal if notice is not given to management according to the union contract and/or provincial guidelines.) In addition, a contract may not cover all potential issues, or the wording of the contract may be unclear. In these cases, a grievance can help identify issues where the union contract requires revision (Forman & Merrick, 2003).

When a grievance is submitted in a unionized health care setting, the organization's management reviews the grievance through their internal process. In the event that management is unable to resolve the grievance, the complaint may go to **arbitration** (Forman & Merrick, 2003). In this case, both sides present their case before an arbitrator. The arbitration process is similar to a legal process in which two parties bring a dispute before a judge. The arbitrator makes a decision about how the grievance should be resolved. The union contract generally specifies that both management and the union will agree to follow the arbitrator's decision.

In health care organizations that are not unionized, the organization may have developed a policy for a dispute resolution. This may involve discussions at different levels within the organization. If the dispute is not resolved through early discussions, there may be a final review with a decision being made by a senior executive or a panel of employees from within the organization, or an outside party who is hired for this meeting (Forman & Merrick, 2003). In other nonunionized organizations, **mediation** may be employed (Ridley-Duff & Bennett, 2011). With mediation, the two disputing parties work to find a solution that they both agree on. They do this in the presence of a mediator who facilitates the process but does not identify the solution (Ridley-Duff & Bennett, 2011). For mediation to work, both parties have to want to resolve their conflict. Therefore, mediation may work best if used when conflicts are relatively recent, because when conflicts occur for a long time, both parties may become entrenched in their positions.

Although health care settings that are unionized generally use the grievance process, including arbitration when a grievance is not solved, we note that mediation could be used within unionized settings either before or after a grievance is submitted. We recognize that the union should be consulted when parties within a unionized setting agree to mediation, as they may see this as undermining their collective agreement. Situations when mediation may be particularly effective include conflicts between individuals, such as between two members of a nursing department, two nurse managers, or a nurse manager and a manager of a non-nursing department. The source of the disagreement may be related to different views on how work should be accomplished, or may be because of disrespectful communication between the two individuals. In these cases, mediation may lead to both parties agreeing on a solution, and their being able to work smoothly together and thus not impede efficient and effective client care.

DISRUPTIVE CLINICIAN BEHAVIOUR IN HEALTH CARE ORGANIZATIONS

Just as violence against women or children includes emotional as well as physical violence, the term "disruptive clinician behaviour" has been used to include physical violence in health care settings, as well as behaviours such as bullying, withholding information, and gossiping (Rogers-Clark, Pearce & Cameron, 2009). Others have defined dysfunctional workplace behaviours to include intimidation, bullying, and a reluctance to share information (Queensland Health, 2005) or defined victimizing behaviours to include belittling, punishing, excessive surveillance, and exclusion (Simons, 2006). There is no agreed upon definition of bullying (Roberts, 2009), and the terms "nurse-to-nurse hostility" or "nurse-to-nurse incivility" (Bartholomew, 2006), bullying, disruptive clinician behaviour, dysfunctional workplace behaviour, workplace incivility, and violence and aggression in the workplace seem to be used by different authors to describe the same phenomena. The term "incivility" has been used to describe behaviours that may be more subtle than other types of bullying, but are nevertheless disruptive ones that convey disrespect. Examples of incivility include being rude, sarcastic, late, rolling eyes, and belittling someone (Barker Caza & Cortina, 2007; Luparell, 2011; Marchiondo, Marchiondo, & Lasiter, 2010).

Nurses may not be aware that violence occurs in their workplace or that they are engaging in violence toward others at work. Physical violence or overt aggression is very visible. However, there are emotional and subtle types of violence that are also destructive. These more subtle types of aggression include withholding information, gossiping, intimidating, belittling achievements, excessive surveillance, and exclusion. Nurses who are aware that others gossip about them, scrutinize their work more than seems warranted, or exclude them from activities, such as going to coffee, perceive that they have been singled out, targeted, and victimized. Understandably, they experience stress, low job satisfaction, and higher absence from work, and may resign from the nursing department or organization. Nursing departments where there is a high incidence of bullying develop a reputation as a unit where many do not want to work or where "nurses eat their young." Ultimately, patient care suffers when nurses work on a unit where disruptive clinician behaviour has become part of the workplace culture.

Nursing students are not immune to violence, which can come from fellow students, instructors, or employees at clinical settings. A qualitative study of student nurses' lived experience of violence during clinical placements was performed in one province in Atlantic Canada (Churchill, 2014). One finding was that when the clinical instructor behaved with violence or incivility, students found this particularly hurtful because they expected their instructor to support them. As well, violence or incivility by their clinical instructor served to shake their feeling that they could provide competent care or become a good nurse.

Much of the literature on bullying in nursing has been descriptive, and there is a need for more research. There is evidence that supports that as disruptive clinician behaviours increase, so does nurses' intent to resign (O'Connell et al., 2000; Simmons, 2006). Additional negative outcomes for nurses associated with violence in the workplace include increased sick leave, use of alcohol and drugs, and burnout (O'Connell et al., 2000). Further, disruptive clinician behaviours are believed to jeopardize a culture of patient safety (Roberts, Demarco, & Griffin, 2008; Rosenstein & O'Daniel, 2005; The Joint Commission, 2008). In a survey of nurses and physicians, almost three-quarters of the 664 nurses who responded to the question "Have you ever witnessed disruptive behaviour from a nurse at your hospital?" said they had witnessed disruptive behaviour by nurses. Survey respondents also reported that **lateral violence** between or among nurses and physicians resulted in stress, reduced collaboration and communication, adverse events, and poorer patient outcomes (Rosenstein & O'Daniel, 2005).

Traditionally, nurses may have viewed bullying in the workplace as something that was done by managers to nurses who reported to them. This type of bullying has historically been referred to in the literature as Machiavellian leadership, which is characterized by unethical behaviours, including deceit, to obtain the outcomes desired by the leader. Regrettably, there are managers who misuse their power and abuse nurses. This type of violence is now referred to in the nursing literature as **vertical violence** and refers to emotional or physical violence from someone higher in the organization with the intent to harm a subordinate. The nurse who is abused by a manager, someone with power over the nurse, may feel reluctant to complain for fear of repercussions. If the manager is respected by others, the nurse may even feel no one will believe the complaint.

Horizontal violence or emotional or physical violence from a colleague generally with the intent to harm this colleague is also recognized as a significant problem. Similar to vertical violence, horizontal violence is a relatively new expression. Until the 1990s, this type of aggression was referred to as intragroup conflict when it was between members of the same work group and intergroup conflict when it was between members of different work groups (Duffy, 1995). Of course, intragroup and intergroup conflict includes not only horizontal violence, but also conflicts that may arise because of differing views about goals, how to attain goals, how scarce resources should be spent, and so on.

Horizontal violence may be overt or subtle (Hastie, 2002), but both types are harmful to the targeted nurse. Examples of overt violence include pushing, insulting, or using a derogatory name. Examples of subtle violence include gossiping about a nurse, ignoring issues important to the nurse, and excluding the nurse from conversations, or from joining others for breaks. Their subtle nature may result in the nurse only slowly becoming aware that she is targeted. Further, the subtle nature may make it difficult for a nurse manager to recognize that this type of violence is occurring. Even if this type of violence is reported to a nurse manager, he or she may have difficulty making an assessment of the situation, thereby hindering management of the violence.

We would add to vertical and horizontal violence an additional type of violence that we call **upward violence**. Upward violence occurs when a nurse is overtly or subtly violent toward his or her manager, or when a nursing student is similarly violent to a nursing teacher. Upward violence occurs when a nurse rolls his or her eyes when the manager is talking, informs colleagues that the manager has said something to him or her that is inaccurate, or sabotages initiatives led by the manager.

Separating an Aggressive Workplace from a Bad Day

There are many challenging moments in health care work because nurses work in emotionally charged patient care situations, workloads may be high, and patient care crises occur. It is only human when experiencing stress to occasionally respond angrily to others. We believe occasional incidents of violence need to be distinguished from horizontal, vertical, and upward violence in the workplace. Occasional incidents of violence are not a pattern of violence that is directed at a specific target, nor do they signify a culture of abuse. When a stressed nurse responds angrily or inappropriately but this is a rare incident, he or she is not singling out a target and intentionally acting to intimidate the other person. When the stressed nurse is calmer, he or she is likely to apologize for the behaviour, and others involved in the incident generally understand that the nurse's anger and inappropriate behaviour was related to the situation and because the nurse is human. This situation differs from a nurse showing a consistent pattern of disruptive behaviour that targets a particular nurse(s). The ongoing nature of pattern of disruptive behaviour that causes ongoing suffering of the person(s) targeted indicatives the workplace has a culture of abuse.

Another characteristic of disruptive clinician behaviour is that it may not be limited to one individual within a nursing department (Hutchinson et al., 2005). Instead, a number of nurses may group together and operate similarly to a gang. Together, they may operate to prevent changes on the unit and control the behaviours of persons new to this unit. Such gangs of clinicians suggest a culture of abuse on the unit. As well, gangs of clinicians who operate as bullies speak to the pervasiveness of abuse on the unit, and suggest why providing feedback to one nurse or dealing with one situation may be insufficient to deal with a pervasive situation of lateral violence.

RELATED RESEARCH

Outcomes from a Team-Building Intervention

The goal of this research study was to replicate the team-building intervention used in another study (DiMeglio et al., 2005) as well as to examine the effects of lateral violence on team cohesion. The study was implemented in a 247-bed, acute care hospital in Rhode Island. This hospital has magnet hospital status (see Chapter 9, Quality of Work Life Issues, for a discussion of magnet hospitals). Despite the magnet status of this hospital, the nurses on a unit within this hospital had low morale. Nurses new to this unit said they felt they were the targets of disruptive behaviour from other nurses. Therefore, a preliminary study was done on this unit. Team-building sessions were implemented to increase collaboration among team members. The results included an improvement in staff engagement, nurse satisfaction, and patient satisfaction.

Following this preliminary study, subsequent research was carried out to:

1. identify and improve nurse satisfaction and group cohesion among RNs on selected nursing units through planned unit-based interventions,

2. determine the effect of team-building intervention on cohesive team functioning, and

3. determine the effect of lateral violence training and communication style differences on improving team cohesion. (Barrett et al., 2009, p. 344)

RNs from four nursing units participated in the study. The four units were chosen because they had the lowest nurse–nurse interaction scores in the hospital, with cliques and scapegoating common. The nurse managers of the four units chose 20% of the nurses from their unit, or six to eight nurses from each unit, to participate in team-building.

The team-building intervention was implemented separately for each of the four units, and consisted of two, two-hour meetings led by a group facilitator and a nurse manager. During the first meeting, group members described their team and an ideal team. Information about lateral violence was presented and nurses discussed their experiences related to lateral violence. They also were provided with information about the Myer-Briggs Type

Indicator (MBTI), which is related to personality types, and started discussing the
differences in personalities among members of their work team. In the second
meeting, the participants considered their
discussion of MBTI differences and how this
was related to how they worked together.
Material related to giving and receiving
feedback and managing conflict was also
presented. The nurses used this information
to discuss some of the issues on their unit.
They were asked to discuss with the nurses
in their department what they had learned,
and "to function as 'champions' related
to creating cohesive work environments"
(Barrett et al., 2009, p. 345).

All nurses on the four units were
invited to complete a questionnaire prior
to the team-building intervention and

three months after the intervention.
Surveys were distributed to 145 nurses and
the response rate prior to the intervention was 41% (n = 59) and following the
intervention was 31% (n = 45). Findings
included that the questionnaire scores for
group cohesion was lower prior to the
intervention, and the nurse–nurse interaction improved following the intervention.
The authors conclude that the success of
the team building intervention depends
on the unit's manager's commitment to
spearheading and maintaining the change.

Source: Barrett, A., Piatek, C., Korber, S.,
& Padula, C. 2009. Lessons learned from a
lateral violence and team-building intervention. *Nursing Administration Quarterly, 33*(4),
342–351.

Reducing Disruptive Clinician Behaviour

A recent review of literature examined the evidence for interventions to reduce disruptive
clinician behaviour in nursing workplaces (Rogers-Clark, Pearce, & Cameron, 2009). Specifically, the authors searched for articles to answer the question, "What interventions are
successful in managing disruptive clinician behaviour in nursing workplaces?" The authors
located 23 articles that discussed interventions to reduce disruptive clinician behaviour.
However most of these articles were based on expert opinion with only nine of the articles
reporting research studies and only three of these (Boone et al., 2008; Griffin, 2004;
Taylor, 2001) assessing an intervention. While the authors of this literature review
acknowledge there is not enough evidence to answer their question, some of the articles
reviewed provide guidance for dealing with disruptive clinician behaviour and some
examples are summarized below.

One of the studies that assessed an intervention was a program that provided new
graduate nurses with education over a four-week period about lateral violence. This program targeted new nurses because earlier studies had found they are particularly sensitive
to horizontal violence (McKenna et al., 2003; Randle, 2003). The new nurses were provided with prescriptive responses (that is, a cognitive rehearsal intervention) for the ten
most common types of lateral violence. Study findings include that 75 percent of the
nurses confronted with their horizontal violence behaviour stopped this behaviour, and
the new nurses found this program beneficial and one that all nurses should attend.

A survey performed in the United Kingdom with 2,813 respondents included items about bullying and harassment (Ball & Pike, 2006). Nurses were asked what action they had taken when bullied and harassed and how effective this action was. Their responses are shown in Table 10.1.

Of interest is that 56% of those who had been bullied or harassed responded by telling their manager. However, for 63% of those who told a manager, the situation remained unchanged and for 10% the situation actually got worse. Similarly, 76% told a colleague of the abuse. However, for 81% of these persons the situation remained unchanged and for 5% the situation got worse. Only 38% spoke to the bully or harasser about the behaviour, and thus many bullies did not receive feedback about the impact of their behaviour. Also of interest is that 12% left their job, a high cost for the nursing department! Together, these findings suggest that to avoid losing nurses from the workplace, we need to educate nurses and nurse managers about the significance of bullying and how to respond when informed of a situation. Nurses may also benefit from education in how to confront abusers about their behaviour.

It is surprising that none of the articles located for this literature review (Rogers-Clark et al., 2009) focused on managing the behaviour of the person who was disruptive.

Table 10.1   Action Taken to Deal with Bullying/Harassment and How Situation Changed As a Result—Percentages

	Action taken %	How situation changed—%		
		Unchanged	Got worse	Improved
Told a colleague	76	81	5	14
Told manager	56	63	10	27
Told another more senior member of staff	47	64	8	29
Spoke to the bully/harasser about the problem	38	45	20	35
Sought help from the RCN	20	65	10	26
Made an informal complaint	29	59	15	26
Sought a change in work situation to get away from person causing problem	13	54	16	30
Resigned/left my job	30	34	11	55
Sought other support from employer	12	12	0	88
Sought other support from outside workplace	18	60	7	33
No action taken so far	30	55	5	40
Base n = 588	25	75	3	21

Instead, the focus was on approaches to help nurses who were affected by the aggressor. We believe it is timely to think of interventions to change the behaviours of aggressors, to make them accountable for changing their behaviour, rather than solely focusing on helping persons who have been targeted to deal with the aggression.

Interview

Linda Silas, RN, BScN

Linda Silas is the President of the Canadian Federation of Nurses Unions (CFNU). She is a proud New Brunswicker who throughout her nursing career has worked with or for nurses to defend nursing care and our public health care system. She works closely with many nurse researchers and believes in evidence-based decisions. CFNU's current research project is on how nurse staffing affects patient safety, and this research will be the main focus when meeting with federal and provincial elected representatives and policy makers.

Q: What advice would you give a nurse for how to proceed if he or she had a conflict with the nurse manager, for example, about the work schedule, the patient assignment, or overtime?

A: To take your time, assess the situation, think things through, and take notes. Emails and text messages can be the best and the worst tools. It is too easy to write a quick email which may not be thought through and which is based on raw emotion. Instead, take a step backward. Take notes about the situation and then set a meeting with the manager. Read your collective agreement and if you need advice or representation, call your union rep. At the meeting, propose a solution and take notes to protect yourself. Taking notes also helps to stay calm.

Q: Can you discuss an example when a dispute between nurses and management was successfully resolved? What helped to resolve this situation?

A: One example that happens in many work areas is related to the vacation schedule.

Today's nursing workforce has nurses from four generations, with nurses who are 60 to 65 years of age and older working with nurses who could be their grandchildren. These nurses have different values about work and family and we all need to understand each other's values. Vacation is given by seniority in most workplaces and therefore nurses with 35 years of seniority may get to take five or six weeks off in the summer while newer nurses are unable to take vacation in the summer. It is best for the nurses within a department to sit down and have a team discussion before they complete a form with their vacation requests.

For example, a new nurse may be planning to get married in July. Senior nurses may believe the nurse should not have planned her wedding for July, but there may be reasons, such as when family members can attend, that had to be considered. If the vacation schedule requests are just posted and then the manager posts the final schedule, it can be hard to change things after the fact. It is better for the nursing team to have a discussion, during which the vacation rules can be stated but each nurse can state what is important for him or her. For example, the new nurse who wants to get married in July may not be able to have two weeks off, but it may be possible to arrange for her to have a week off in July from Wednesday to Wednesday, and then take another week in September for the honeymoon. I always found that solutions can be found when everyone is working together and compromise is key.

(Continued)

Q: What do you see as current key issues related to managing conflict in the workplace?

A: Not only is workload at a dangerous limit, but there is role confusion throughout the health care system. Part of the role confusion may be caused by upper level managers who try and manage the system as cheaply as possible and may hire, for example, employees who are not licensed. As another example, in some jurisdictions, paramedics are working in emergency rooms where physicians may be talking with them rather than the nurse. Nurses obviously find this frustrating, and it can be a patient safety issue depending on the training and education levels. There may also be role confusion about the role of an aide, an LPN, or a nurse with a doctoral degree who specializes in wound care. Patients, family members, and even coworkers don't know who is in our fast-paced health care system. I always say there is enough work to go around for everyone. What we need is respect and knowledge of each other's qualifications, plus understanding our roles and having safe staffing models.

When you talk with nursing students about why they chose nursing, it is always because they want to work on a team and help others. They are good, nice people. When horizontal violence occurs, there is a tendency to blame the nurse manager for not preventing this, or to say this nurse is a real "pain." We forget that when we work under pressure, sooner or later everyone will explode. Workload is a huge problem. If you ask nurses today what they want, they talk about workload and work environment. With today's workload, nurses either explode or burn out. When the issue of horizontal violence is discussed, I think we are missing the big picture. Horizontal violence is not because of nurse managers (and there are not enough of them) or because nurses are bad, it is because anyone who works under pressure for too long will eventually explode or burn out. We need to fix the work environments in health care.

Q: Do you have suggestions for a nurse who is experiencing horizontal violence?

A: I would tell a nurse who is experiencing horizontal violence, again, to take a step back, assess the situation, and take notes. But do not let the situation continue too long, deal with it. Get help if you need it. The longer a situation such as horizontal violence lasts, the more it becomes the norm. New nurses who arrive in the department and see horizontal violence may think that this is just the way things are: "that's how colleagues treat each other on this unit." Therefore, it is important to stop horizontal violence right away and we all have a role to stop this, we can't say it is up to the nurse manager. There are resources available for the nurse who experiences horizontal violence, such as the union representative and counsellors within the organization, so use these resources.

Source: Interview with Linda Silas, President of the Canadian Federation of Nurses Unions. Reprinted by permission.

SUMMARY

Many health care organizations today are large, multi-site organizations. Care is increasingly complex not only in acute care settings but also in community and residential settings. At the same time, there are fewer nurse managers and educators to support the work of direct care nurses. Health care cutbacks in Canada and other countries have made resources scarcer, and scarce resources are always a recipe for conflict. Conflict is inevitable whenever human beings interact and work together. Yet most nurses work in groups, for example, nursing teams that provide nursing care in a nursing unit or a community agency, interdisciplinary teams, or research teams. Cohesive and effective health care teams are important for quality patient care, patient safety, nurse satisfaction, and the retention of nurses.

For teams to function smoothly, destructive conflict needs to be recognized and resolved, and constructive conflict that may lead to innovative approaches needs to be encouraged.

There is growing evidence that team building helps nursing teams to become more cohesive and effective. As the delivery of health care in Canada and elsewhere continues to evolve, nurses need to search for new strategies for nurses and nurse managers to work together effectively, for nurses to support each other rather than bully each other, and for destructive conflict in the workplace to be resolved.

Glossary of Terms

Arbitration A process for resolving a dispute between two parties, when a third party (the arbitrator) listens to evidence from the two disputing parties and makes a decision. Both parties agree prior to the arbitration that they will comply with the arbitrator's decision. In some cases, the decision may be legally binding.

Collocation The location of team members in the same physical space.

Grievance A complaint regarding something that has happened to a person that is wrong. In the case of a union grievance, the grievance is usually put in writing and submitted to management.

Groupthink Term used to describe the decision-making process that occurs when group members do not bring up dissenting points of view, and support a course of action without critical evaluation.

Horizontal leadership A style of leadership where the leader does not use his or her power to dominate members, but instead guides members to reach a consensus and to attain the group's goals.

Horizontal violence The physical or emotional abuse of someone toward a person in a similar position, generally with the

intent of harming this person. For example, the abuse among direct care nurses. Also referred to as **lateral violence**.

Mediation A process for resolving a dispute between two parties, when a third party (the mediator) helps the two disputing parties to identify and agree upon a solution.

Role bending When members are flexible about assuming another member's role if required.

Role overlap When roles are not exclusively held by one member, but different members share roles or aspects of the roles.

Team building The efforts of team members, team leaders, and/or staff developers to improve the smooth functioning and effectiveness of work teams.

Teamwork Teamwork in the workplace involves two or more employees working together to achieve a work-related goal that in many cases can only be achieved through teamwork or is achieved more effectively through teamwork.

Upward violence The emotional or physical abuse of a person in a lower position of power or authority toward someone in a higher position, generally with the intent of harming this person, for example, the abuse of a direct care nurse toward his or her manager. [Note: The term was developed by the authors of this book.]

Vertical leadership   A style of leadership where the leader uses his or her power to direct other group members, as opposed to all members sharing decision making.

Vertical violence   The emotional of physical abuse of a person in a higher position of power or authority toward someone in a lower position, generally with the intent of harming this person, for example, the abuse of a nurse manager toward a nurse who reports to the manager.

CASE

Bradley practised nursing in a rural, primary health care centre, and had health promotion as his mandate. The centre also employed two registered nurses, two licensed practical nurses, and several unregulated nursing personnel to provide home-care nursing. Primary health care clinics were staffed with a nurse practitioner, a part time pharmacist, and a part time physician. Kate was a social worker and the manager for this primary health care centre as well as three other centres and two nursing homes.

When Kate started in this management position six months ago, she said she expected two things from all of them. First, she expected all team members to work well together, and second, she expected them to work as an interprofessional team. She went on and said that by working well together, she meant that everyone should demonstrate respect for each other and their actions should promote the organization's goals. By interprofessional team, she meant that all of the health care providers should share information and determine which person(s) was the optimal one to work with a client. They should collaborate with each other to make sure the client benefited from all of their expertise, but they should work efficiently and not see the same client if the client's needs could be met by one health care provider. While Kate gave these expectations, she quickly became consumed with major issues in the nursing home, and for the past three months she had not even visited this primary care centre but instead, communicated with the staff through email.

Both of Kate's expectations required major changes in how the group had been working. There were many conflicts among group members. The home care nurses felt Bradley should help them because they had a heavy caseload. The licensed practical nurses felt the nurses were slow to transfer clients to them. The unregulated nursing personnel were allowed to attend case conferences, but they were also expected to stock supplies and prepare examination rooms, and found they had to stay late to do this if they attended a meeting. Also, they felt disrespected because they were generally not consulted for their opinion about a client situation. The nurses felt the nurse practitioner never asked their opinion. Since Kate had expressed her expectations to the work group, their conflicts had worsened.

Questions

1. Why do you think the conflict among group members increased after Kate expressed her expectations?

2. The work group is waiting for Kate to have time to meet with them. In the interim, how could they work to reduce conflict among members?

3. What suggestions do you have for the work group about how to develop as an interprofessional team and to work efficiently as team members, given the intergroup conflict and Kate's need to spend most of her time at the nursing home? How should they proceed?

4. How do you suggest the nurses deal with their conflict with the nurse practitioner?

5. The one thing that all team members agree on is that their manager should not be a social worker, because they do not feel a social worker understands the types of issues facing nurses, pharmacists, and physicians. What are the benefits and problems associated with their shared belief? How can the group move forward to work with Kate?

6. The nurses often go to a nearby restaurant for lunch on Friday, but do not invite Bradley or anyone else. When Bradley talks about health promotion projects he is thinking of initiating, the other nurses respond unenthusiastically, saying something like they doubt his program will make a difference. Bradley wrote a letter of complaint to Kate saying the other nurses are harassing him, and these nurses were shocked when they learned about this letter. Do you agree that this is harassment, and if not, what is it? If you were Bradley and felt the nurses were harassing you, how would you proceed?

Critical Thinking Questions and Activities

1. **a.** Describe an instance of horizontal violence that you have witnessed as a nursing student, either among other students or among nurses where you have done clinical work. What could you or others do to prevent this horizontal violence?

b. Describe an instance of upward violence that you have witnessed toward a nursing instructor, a nurse manager, or a health care administrator. What could you or others do to prevent this upward violence?

2. A preceptor is working with a nursing student and is concerned about her practice competencies. The preceptor feels accountable for the student's care and therefore is supervising her closely. The student feels the preceptor is using excessive surveillance, which she read during her nursing program was a type of workplace violence. The student is aware the preceptor is concerned about her practice competencies, but the student disagrees that this is an issue. How would you advise the preceptor to work with the student so she does not perceive she is harassed? What advice would you give the student?

3. Debate the statement: "If a nurse perceives he or she is bullied in the workplace, others have bullied him or her."

4. Think of the last time you disagreed with someone, for example, a classmate with whom you were working on a group project or a clinician when you were caring for clients in a clinical situation. Describe the conflict and how you dealt with it. Which of the five styles of dealing with conflict did you use? How could the outcome have differed if you used another style?

5. Debate the statement: "Transparency and participative democracy are possible in today's large health care organizations."

6. Identify a work team that you believe functions well, and relate how this team functions to the characteristics of successful teams described in this chapter.

7. Think about the last major disagreement you had with someone. Can you recall "I" or "you" or "you should" statements that either you or your adversary made?

Self-Quiz

1. Collaboration:
   a. May result in a win–win solution
   b. Should be used after trying accommodation
   c. Is the exact opposite of accommodation
   d. Is a time-efficient negotiation strategy

2. An example of groupthink is:
   a. A team meeting after an incident
   b. A meeting between union representatives and nurse managers
   c. A team agreeing to a nurse manager's plans without discussing concerns
   d. A meeting to brainstorm all possible strategies to implement change within a department

3. All of the following are true about horizontal violence except:
   a. It is sometimes referred to as lateral violence
   b. May include gossiping about a colleague
   c. Refers to patients and family members being rude to nurses
   d. A nurse demonstrating horizontal behaviours may not be aware that he/she is hurting a colleague

4. The nursing instructor asked her group of eight students what their plans were when they graduated. One of the students, Robert, responded that he wanted to work in the community doing health promotion, but eventually wanted to do this type of work in a developing country. Two of his fellow classmates, Cheryl and Kelly, looked at each other and then at him with an expression of disbelief. The term that best describes Cheryl's and Kelly's behaviour is:
   a. Vertical violence
   b. Passive aggressive behavior
   c. Incivility
   d. Sexual discrimination

5. Doreen, the nurse manager of a unit, is meeting with the nurses on her unit to encourage them to work on a project that, to date, they have adamantly refused to work on. Which of the following opening statements would be a good way for her to initiate this topic?
   a. You haven't been involved in projects recently, so you should consider this one.
   b. You should participate in this project because it will benefit clients.
   c. I would like you to consider working on this project because it is important for patient care on our unit.
   d. You have been refusing to work on this project, but keep in mind it is important to participate in group activities and I note this in your performance appraisals.

Useful Websites

CNA (Canadian Nurses' Association) and the Canadian Federation of Nurses Union joint position statement about workplace violence.
www2.cna-aiic.ca/CNA/documents/pdf/publications/JPS95_Workplace_Violence_e.pdf
or
www.nursesunions.ca/sites/default/files/workplace_violence_position_statement_cna-cfnu_0.pdf

Registered Nurses' Association of Ontario (2006). *Collaborative Practice Among Nursing Teams*. Toronto, Canada: Registered Nurses' Association of Ontario.
http://rnao.ca/sites/rnao-ca/files/Collaborative_Practice_Among_Nursing_Teams.pdf

Registered Nurses' Association of Ontario policy statement about violence against nurses and nursing students (revised 2008).
http://rnao.ca/policy/position-statements/violence-against-nurses

References

Baker, K. (1995). Improving staff nurse conflict resolution skills. *Nursing Economic$*, *13*, 295–317.

Ball, J., & Pike, G. (2006). *At breaking point? A survey of the wellbeing and working lives of nurses in 2005*. PTRC, University of Leeds.

Barker Caza, B., & Cortina, L. M. (2007). From insult to injury: Explaining the impact of incivility. *Basic and Applied Social Psychology*, *29*, 335–350.

Barrett, A., Piatek, C., Korber, S., & Padula, C. (2009). Lessons learned from a lateral violence and team-building intervention. *Nursing Administration Quarterly*, *33*(4), 342–351.

Bartholomew, K. (2006). *Ending nurse to nurse hostility: Why nurses eat their young and each other*. Marblehead, MA: HCPro Inc.

Boone, B., & King, M., et al. (2008). Conflict management training and nurse-physician collaborative behaviours. *Journal for Nurses in Staff Development*, *24*, 168–175.

Buckingham, M., & Clifton, D. (2001). *Now, discover your strengths*. New York, NY: Free Press.

Churchill, N. (2014). *Nursing students' lived experience of violence during clinical rotations: A phenomenological study*. MN thesis. St. John's, NL: Memorial University of Newfoundland.

Clark, P. (2009). Teamwork. Building healthier workplaces and providing safer patient care. *Critical Care Nursing Quarterly*, *32*(3), 221–231.

Cummings, T., & Worley, C. (2005). *Organization development and change*. 9th ed. Cincinnati, OH: South-Western College.

DiMeglio, K., Padula, C., Piatek, C., Korber, S., Barrett, A., Ducharme, M., et al. (2005). Group cohesion and nurse satisfaction. Examination of a team-building approach. *JONA*, *35*(3), 110–120.

Ducanis, A., & Golin, A. (19790. *The interdisciplinary healthcare team: A handbook*. Germantown, MD: Aspen Systems Corporation.

Duffy, E. (1995). Horizontal violence: a conundrum for nursing. *Collegian. Journal of the Royal College of Nursing Australia*. *2*(2), 5–17.

Eason, F., & Brown, S. (1999). Conflict management: Assessing educational needs. *Journal for Nurses in Staff Development*, *15*, 92–96.

Forman, H., & Merrick, F. (2003). Grievances and complaints. Valuable tools for management and for staff. *JONA*, *23*(3), 136–138.

Fry, R., Lech, B., & Rubin, I. (1974). Working with the primary care team: The first intervention. In: Wise, B., Beckhard, R., Rubin, I., & Kyte, A. (eds). *Making health teams work*. Cambridge, MA: Ballinger Publishing Co., 27–68.

Gilley, A., Gilley, J., McConnell, W., & Veliquette, A. (2010). The competencies used by effective managers to build teams: An empirical study. *Advances in Developing Human Resources*, *12*(1), 29–45.

Gilley, J., & Boughton, N. (1996). *Stop managing, start coaching: How performance coaching can enhance commitment and improve productivity.* New York, NY: McGraw-Hill.

Gilley, J., & Gilley, A. (2007). *Manager as coach.* Hartford, CT: Praeger.

Gilley, J., Morris, M., Waite, A., Coates, T., & Veliquette, A. (2010). Integrated theoretical model for building effective teams. *Advances in Developing Human Resources, 12*(1), 7–28.

Griffin, M. (2004). Teaching cognitive rehearsal as a shield for lateral violence: An intervention for newly licensed nurses. *Journal of Continuing Education in Nursing, 35*(6), 257–263.

Hall, W., Long, B., Bermbach, N., Jordan, S., & Patterson, K. (2005). Qualitative teamwork issues and strategies: coordination through mutual adjustment. *Qualitative Health Research, 15*, 394–410.

Hastie, C. (2002). Horizontal violence in the workplace. *Birth International.* Retrieved July 7, 2011, from www.birthinternational.com/articles/midwifery/69-horizontal-violence-in-the-workplace

Hutchinson, M., Vickers, M., Jackson, D, & Vickers, M. (2006). 'They stand you in a corner, you are not to speak': Nurses tell of abusive indoctrination in work teams dominated by bullies. *Contemporary Nurse, 21*, 228–238.

Janis, I. (1982). *Groupthink: Psychological studies of policy decisions and fiascos.* 2nd ed. Boston: Houghton Mifflin.

The Joint Commission (Issue 40). (July 9, 2008). Behaviours that undermine a culture of safety. Retrieved July 7, 2011, from www.jointcommission.org/assets/1/18/SEA_40.PDF

Klein, C., DiazGrandados, D., Salas, E., Le, H., Burke, C., Lyons, R., & Goodwin, G. (2009). Does team building work? *Small Group Research, 40*, 181–222.

Lavoie-Tremblay, M. (2004). Creating a healthy workplace: A participatory organizational intervention. *Journal of Nursing Administration, 34*, 469–474.

Lucas, M., Atwood, J., & Hagaman, R. (1993). Replication and validation of anticipated turnover model for urban registered nurses. *Nursing Research, 42*(1), 29–35.

Luparell, S. (2011). Incivility in nursing: The connection between academia and clinical settings. *Critical Care Nurse, 31*, 92–95.

Marchiondo, K., Marchiondo, L. A., & Lasiter, S. (2010). Faculty incivility: Effects on program satisfaction of BSN students. *Journal of Nursing Education, 49*, 608–614.

McKenna, B., Smith, N., Poole, S., & Coverdale, J. (2003). Horizontal violence: Experiences of registered nurses in their first year of practice. *Journal of Advanced Nursing, 42*(1), 90–96.

Molyneux, J. (2001). Interprofessional teamworking: What makes team work well? *Journal of Interprofesional Care, 15*, 29–35.

Northam, S. (2009). Conflict in the Workplace: Part 2. Strategies to resolve conflict and restore collegial working relationships. *AJN, 109*(7), 65–67.

O'Connell, B., Young, J., Brooks, J., Hutchings, J., & Lofthouse, J. (2000). Nurses perceptions of the nature and frequency of aggression in general ward settings and high-dependency areas. *Journal of Clinical Nursing, 9*(4), 602–610.

Parsons, M., Batres, C., & Golightly-Jenkins, C. (2006). Innovations in management: Establishing team behavioural norms for a health workplace. *Top Emerg Med, 28*, 113–119.

Pateman, C. (1970). *Participation and democratic theory.* Cambridge: Cambridge University Press.

Pellerin, C. (2009). *How NASA builds teams: Mission critical soft skills for scientists, engineers, and project managers.* Hoboken, NY: Wiley.

Porter-O'Grady, T., & Malloch, K. (2009). Leaders of innovation: Transforming postindustrial healthcare. *Journal of Nursing Administration, 39*(6), 245–248.

Queensland Health. (2005). *Queensland health systems review. Final report.* Retrieved on July 6, 2011, from www.health.qld.gov.au/health_sys_review/final/qhsr_final_report.pdf.

Rahim, M. (1986). *Managing conflict in organizations*. New York: Praeger Publishers.

Randle, J. (2003). Bullying in the nursing profession. *Journal of Advanced Nursing, 43*(3), 395–401.

Ridley-Duff, R., & Bennett, A. (2011). Towards mediation: Developing a theoretical framework to understand alternative dispute resolution. *Industrial Relations Journal, 42*(2), 106–123.

Roberts, S., Demarco, R., & Griffin, M. (2009). The effect of oppressed group behaviours on the culture of the nursing workplace: a review of the evidence and interventions for change. *Journal of Nursing Management, 17*, 288–293

Rogers-Clark, C., Pearce, S., & Cameron, M. (2009). Management of disruptive behaviour within nursing work environments: A comprehensive systematic review of the evidence. *JBI Library of Systematic Reviews, 7*(15), 615–678.

Rosenstein, A. & O'Daniel, M. (2005). Disruptive behaviour and clinical outcomes. *American Journal of Nursing, 105*, 54–64.

Shader, K., Broome, M., Broome, C., West, M., & Nash, M. (2001). Factors influencing satisfaction and anticipated turnover for nurses in an academic medical center. *Journal of Nursing Administration, 31*(4), 210–216.

Simons, S. (2006). Workplace bullying experienced by nurses newly licensed in Massachusetts. *Dissertation Abstracts International: Section B: The Science and Engineering, 67*, 3065.

Sportsman, S., & Hamilton, P. (2007). Conflict management styles in the health professions. *Journal of Professional Nursing, 23*(3), 157–166.

Stevens, M. & Campion, M. (1999). Staffing work teams: Development and validation of a selection test for teamwork skills. *Journal of Management, 25*, 207–228.

Taylor, B. (2001). Identifying and transforming dysfunctional nurse–nurse relationships through reflective practice and action research. *International Journal of Nursing Practice, 7*, 406–413

Thomas, K., & Kilmann, R. (1974). *Thomas-Kilmann conflict mode instrument*. Tuxedo, NY: XIDOM, Inc.

Thomas, K., & Kilmann, R. (1976). Conflict and conflict management. In M.D. Dunette (ed.), *Industrial and organizational psychology*. Chicago: Rand McNally.

Vivar, C. (2006). Putting conflict management into practice: A nursing case study. *Journal of Nursing Management, 14*, 201–206.

Wilmot, W., & Hocker, J. (2001). *Interpersonal conflict*. 6th ed. Boston: McGraw-Hill.

Chapter 11
Quality Improvement

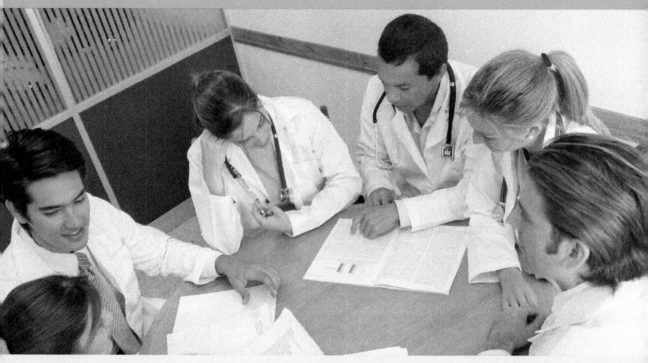

Andres Rodriguez/Fotolia

Learning Objectives

After reading, studying, and reflecting on this chapter's content, you will be able to:

1. Compare quality improvement, patient safety, and risk management programs
2. Debate the pros and cons of different quality improvement approaches such as structure, process and outcome indicators, Total Quality Management, root cause analysis, and nursing sensitive outcomes
3. Identify methods of communication to improve patient safety, including SBAR, huddles, checklists, briefings, time out, and handout process
4. Discuss how the accreditation of health care organizations can improve quality
5. Develop a quality improvement initiative to improve quality in your practice setting(s)

INTRODUCTION

The quality of care provided in Canadian health care organizations has been an important issue for health care workers and the public for decades. In 1958 the Canadian Council of Hospital Accreditation (now Accreditation Canada) was formed with the goal of setting and monitoring **standards of care** for hospitals. The accreditation standards included having a **quality assurance** program, and in later years this changed to **quality improvement** and **risk management** programs. In health care, the term "quality assurance" has been replaced by the term "quality improvement" because quality assurance suggests we can assure quality and, while we cannot do this, we can improve quality. Over time, Accreditation Canada expanded its accreditation process beyond hospitals, developing standards for other health care services including mental health hospitals, long-term care centres, rehabilitation facilities, and home care services.

While the accreditation of health care organizations is voluntary, the vast majority of hospitals in Canada are accredited. Perhaps that is one reason the findings of the American study, *To Err is Human* (Institute of Medicine Committee on Quality of Health Care in America, 1999), followed five year later by the findings of the Canadian study, *Adverse Events Study* (Baker et al., 2004), shocked both Canadian health care workers and the public. The 1999 American study reported that between 44,000 and 98,000 deaths occurred each year in the United States due to medical errors and the 2004 Canadian study reported that approximately 7.5% of hospitalized patients experienced an **adverse event**, approximately 21% of which resulted in unexpected death. A review of adverse events in hospitals around the world found almost one in ten admitted patients experienced an adverse event (DeVries et al., 2008), with adverse events defined as complications caused by care providers that result in a longer hospitalization, injury, or death.

Since the publication of *To Err is Human* and *Adverse Events Study*, there has been a great emphasis in Canada on patient safety. Funding agencies, including Canadian Institutes of Health Research and the Canadian Health Services Research Foundation, have supported research on patient safety, and there has been a marked increase in the number of patient safety organizations, initiatives, and programs across Canada. Canadian health care organizations now have quality improvement, risk management, and patient safety programs.

While patient safety has become a huge concern of the Canadian public, nurses have always been interested in patient safety and quality care. Florence Nightingale was the founder of modern nursing, but her research and advocacy work was in the area of quality improvement. Nightingale studied infection and mortality rates and corresponded with politicians and other decision makers to advocate for quality improvements. Nightingale studied statistics and used her mathematical knowledge to demonstrate the relationship between cleanliness and infections, and to advocate for reform (Kudzma, 2006). She also tried to improve patient care by looking at other patient outcomes, such as the mortality rates in different types of institutions, the incidence of mortality associated with childbirth, and the incidence of puerperal fever (Kudzma, 2006; McDonald, 2010).

As a direct care nurse, you will often hear about quality improvement, risk management, and patient safety programs. Each department within a health care organization often will have a quality improvement program, and the information in this chapter will help you understand this program and should facilitate your involvement if you become active in quality improvement initiatives at the level of the department or the organization. In this chapter you will also learn about Accreditation Canada's process for accrediting health care organizations. This will give you an understanding of the accreditation process and the value of knowing whether a health care organization is accredited and how it is working on accreditation recommendations. In this chapter you will also learn about methods used in quality improvement such as total quality management and root cause analysis.

QUALITY IMPROVEMENT IN HEALTH CARE

Quality improvement in health care encompasses all the programs and activities designed to monitor and improve the quality of health care. Methods that may be used in quality improvement programs include the use of **quality indicators** to measure the **structure**, **process**, and **outcome** dimensions of quality or to measure standards of care. **Total quality management** is a philosophy of management that includes continuous improvement of work processes and products (Deming, 1986). Risk management, patient safety programs, accreditation programs, clinical audits, and utilization reviews are other strategies for improving quality.

QUALITY MONITORING

Donabedian's Dimensions of Quality—Structure, Process, and Outcome

Donabedian's (1966) work in the quality of medical care laid the groundwork for understanding and measuring quality health care. His framework for assessing medical quality consisted of examining three dimensions: 1) structure, 2) process, and 3) outcomes. Today, this framework continues to be used not only for care provided by physicians but for all health care.

In Donabedian's (1966; 2005) framework, structure refers to the resources available in the setting such as human resources and their qualifications, system supports, administrative organization, and equipment and supplies. The presence of these resources in the clinical setting helps make quality care possible. The measurement of the structure dimension of quality often involves noting whether certain resources or characteristics are available.

The process dimension of quality refers to the procedures or activities that are implemented and how these are implemented. For example, process encompasses the actions that are taken when providing care and how accurately and completely these actions are followed. The measurement of the process dimension of quality often involves noting if different steps in a care procedure were implemented correctly.

The outcome dimension of quality refers to the end result of care, such as recovery, survival, changes in the health status of the patient, changes in health behaviours or attitudes, and satisfaction with care. The measurement of the outcome dimension of quality may simply involve noting the presence or absence of recovery or survival, or may involve using instruments that measure constructs such as quality of life, attitude toward health behaviours, or satisfaction with health care.

In Donabedian's framework of quality, structure or the presence of adequate resources in the environment helps to support quality processes. In turn, process leads to quality outcomes.

Structure → Process → Outcome

Measurement of quality

There are many aspects to quality and this makes the measurement of quality difficult. Therefore, persons responsible for measuring health care quality generally measure a number of different quality indicators to provide a partial picture of actual quality (Mainz, 2003). The term "quality indicator" refers to an aspect of quality that can be measured. Each indicator measures an aspect of the structure, process, or outcome dimension of quality. Examples of quality indicators that measure structure, process, or outcome are shown in Box 11.1.

Box 11.1

Examples of Quality Indicators That Measure Structure, Process, or Outcomes

Structure

- A copy of an updated hospital policy manual is available in the department.
- There are adequate supplies on the unit for dressing changes.
- A speech pathologist is available for consultations with persons who have had strokes.

Process

- Persons who are newly diagnosed with diabetes receive education.

- Patients requiring IV medications receive the right medication, the right dose, in the correct time frame.
- IM medications are administered in the correct site.
- Patient restraints are used correctly.

Outcomes

- Client is satisfied with care received.
- Client is knowledgeable about his or her health condition (for example, diabetes).
- Patient who had a cardiac arrhythmia has a normal heart rhythm.

Standards of care are standards that have been developed to express the best evidence we have about care. In some cases, the standards are based on research evidence. In instances where there is no or insufficient research, standards can be based on expert opinion. Many of the standards set by accreditation bodies such as Accreditation Canada or by health professionals who are monitoring quality within their health care setting are based on the beliefs of the persons who set the standards of care. Quality indicators can be developed to measure standards of care. Standards of care reflect structure and process dimensions of quality that should lead to the desired outcomes.

The measurement of quality indicators that are based on structure, process, and outcomes or on standards of care is done for a variety of reasons (Mainz, 2003). An important reason for measuring quality indicators is to examine how the quality of care in a health setting compares with the type of care that is desired. Further, by measuring the same indicators over time, you can document improvements or areas that are slipping in quality. Also, measuring quality indicators that are used by other settings can help settings compare how they are doing (Mainz, 2003). When the comparison is made with an organization(s) that is known to be performing very well, this comparison is referred to as **benchmarking**. Health professionals can look for a setting that scores higher than their setting on a quality indicator, and then examine how this setting achieves this high score.

NURSING SENSITIVE OUTCOMES AND INDICATORS

Nursing sensitive outcomes are outcomes that result from interventions that are within the domain of nursing practice and for which research evidence has demonstrated the link between the nursing interventions and the outcomes (Doran, 2003). Nursing sensitive outcomes are important for monitoring and improving nursing care. Nursing sensitive outcomes are also important as they can provide evidence of nursing's contributions to care (Albanese et al., 2010). Nurses know that the quality of nursing care affects patient outcomes, but there is an ongoing need to demonstrate this to health care administrators and the public to provide evidence of nursing staffing and education needs.

Nursing sensitive indicators refer to an aspect of a nursing sensitive outcome that can be measured (Maas, Johnson, & Morehead, 1996). Examples of nursing sensitive indicators are the prevalence of patient falls, or the prevalence of smokers hospitalized for pneumonia who receive counselling about smoking cessation (Kurtzman & Kizer, 2005). A recent Canadian report summarized several initiatives for nursing sensitive outcomes and indicators including, "the Health Outcomes for Better Information and Care project in Ontario (HOBIC), Canada-HOBIC (involving Saskatchewan and Manitoba), the National Database of Nursing Quality Indicators (NDNQI), the Collaborative Alliance for Nursing Outcomes California (CALNOC), the Military Nursing Outcomes Database (MilNOD), and the Veterans Affairs Nursing Outcomes Database (VANOD)" (Doran, Mildon, & Clarke, 2011, p. 3).

TOTAL QUALITY MANAGEMENT (TQM)

Total quality management (TQM) refers to W. Edward Deming's (1986) philosophy of management. Deming was an American, but he developed TQM in Japan after the Americans did not seem receptive to his ideas. He is credited with helping to build Japan's industrial success after World War II. TQM is not another quality improvement program; it is a management philosophy and as such it is a way of life in an organization. TQM differs from typical quality improvement programs in that quality improvement is seen as a way of life for all work teams and a way of managing an organization. With TQM, ongoing training of employees and managers is seen as important and includes everyone in the organization understanding the methods within TQM for continuous quality improvement (Deming, 1986; Scholtes, 2003).

Deming developed his management philosophy on the ideas that production and services must be based on customer needs, and that quality is a continuous process. Further, teamwork is required for continuous improvement of products and/or services and **work processes** to satisfy customers. In health care, services such as medical and nursing procedures are provided. A work process consists of all the steps required to complete a work-related activity. For example, the work process of obtaining a scan on a hospitalized patient may involve the physician ordering the scan, the unit clerk transferring this order to the radiology department, the scheduling of the scan, notification of the unit and the patient about the time of this scan, sending the patient to the radiology department, doing the scan, developing a report, and sending the report to the physician. As you can see, this work process has a number of steps, and mistakes can occur at any step in a work process.

Total quality improvement (TQM) requires data collection that is performed by all or many employees, not by a quality improvement team or department. These data are used to reduce variability in production and work processes. Trained as a statistician, Deming taught statistical process control (known as SPC) as a way to decrease variation in work processes (Deming, 1986; Scholtes, 2003). For example, to improve the work process of obtaining a scan on a hospitalized patient, the team could start by listing the steps in this process. Next, they could identify at which steps errors could occur and what these errors might be. Following this, a plan to reduce these errors is developed and implemented. The more steps there are in a work process, the more chances there are for errors to occur. Therefore, the team would also discuss if any of the steps in the work process could be eliminated. For example, steps 1 and 2 are the physician ordering the scan and the unit clerk transferring the order. If instead the physician orders the scan on the hospital's intranet and the radiology department receives the order from the intranet, the two steps have been reduced to only one step and so fewer errors might occur.

Deming (1986) developed 14 points for organizations to follow when using TQM and these points are summarized in Box 11.2.

Box 11.2

Summary of Deming's 14 Points for Organizations Following Total Quality Management (TQM)

1. Create constancy of purpose toward improvement of product and service.... (p. 23)
2. Adapt the new philosophy ... (p. 23)
3. Cease dependence on inspection to achieve quality. Eliminate the need for inspection on a mass basis by building quality into the product in the first place. (p. 23)

4. End the practice of awarding business on the basis of price tag. Instead, minimize total cost. Move toward a single supplier for any one item, on a long-term relationship of loyalty and trust. (p. 23)
5. Improve constantly and forever the system of production and service, to improve quality and productivity,

(Continued)

Box 11.2 *(Cont.)*

and thus constantly decrease costs. (p. 23)

6. Institute training on the job. (p. 23)

7. Institute leadership ... The aim of supervision should be to help people and machines and gadgets to do a better job.... (p. 23)

8. Drive out fear, so that everyone may work effectively for the company.... (p. 23)

9. Break down barriers between departments.... (p. 24)

10. Eliminate slogans, exhortations, and targets for the work force asking for zero defects and new levels of productivity.... (p. 24)

11. a. Eliminate work standards (quotas) on the factory floor. Substitute leadership. (p. 24)

    b. Eliminate management by objective. Eliminate management by numbers, numerical goals. Substitute leadership. (p. 24)

12. a. Remove barriers that rob the hourly worker of his right to pride of workmanship. The responsibility of supervisors must be changed from sheer numbers to quality. (p. 24)

    b. Remove barriers that rob people in management and in engineering of their right to pride of workmanship. This means, *inter alia*, [Latin for "among other things"] abolishment of the annual or merit rating and of management by objective.... (p. 24).

13. Institute a vigorous program of education and self-improvement. (p. 24)

14. Put everybody in the company to work to accomplish the transformation. The transformation is everybody's job. (p. 24)

Source: Deming, *Out of the Crisis,* Copyright © 1974, the MIT Press. Reprinted by permission.

Common Methods used in TQM

Common methods used in TQM to improve work processes are:

1. identifying customers,

2. identifying customer needs,

3. reducing errors,

4. reducing steps (streamlining the process),

5. reducing waste, and

6. reducing variation (**statistical process control**).

A key component of TQM is the emphasis on customers, and each work process has customers. Employees need to determine who their customers are for an identified work process, assess the needs of their customers, and work to meet these needs. Each employee may have customers who are internal or external to the organization. Employees participate in numerous work processes, and each work process may have different customers.

For example, in a hospital, the work process of consulting an external agency for home care services has internal customers such as the person who takes the consult and notifies others of the consult, and external customers such as the person who receives the consult.

As another example, consider the work process of obtaining medications to administer to patients. In this work process, obvious customers are the patients; however, other customers are the employees in the pharmacy department because employees on patient care units supply them with requests for medications. Pharmacy department employees have needs related to how they receive requests for medications. For the same work process, nurses are also customers of pharmacy employees in that nurses have needs related to the provision of medications on the unit. To illustrate another example of customers, we will look at the work process of change-of-shift report in a nursing department. In this work process, the nurse receiving the report is a customer and has needs, for example, related to the type of information he or she receives, when this is received, and how long it takes (Deming, 1986; Scholtes, 2003).

After identifying the customers for a work process, one of the first steps in TQM to improve quality is to find out what the customers' needs are and what makes them satisfied. A TQM approach to quality improvement includes meeting with customers to discuss their needs in order to be able to supply what will satisfy the customers.

To improve a work process, typical errors that might occur during the work process need to be identified and reduced. Errors can occur at any step in a work process, and therefore, the more steps a work process has, the more likely that errors and hence delays may occur. Reducing the number of steps in a work process, or streamlining the work process, reduces the chance for error and delays. To improve work processes, work teams can list the steps in a work process and then consider if there are any steps that can be eliminated or if there is a different way of doing the process that would require fewer steps.

As an example of streamlining a work process, consider the work process of a physician requesting that a consultant see a patient. The steps in this procedure may be handwriting this order in the patient's chart, transcribing the order, telephoning the consultant's office and leaving a message, and informing the consultant. Errors or delays can occur at any of these steps. If the health setting has a system where physicians request a consultation on a hospital computer that then immediately sends an email to the consultant's smartphone, the work process has been streamlined and we can anticipate fewer errors or delays in notifying the consultant.

Reducing waste is another TQM method to improve a work process. There is a wide variety of sources of waste in an organization (Scholtes, 2003), including but not limited to waste of materials, supplies, and human resources, waste of time, and waste of movement. Supplies are wasted if more costly, sterile supplies are used for a procedure that only requires clean supplies. Human resources are wasted if health professionals' knowledge of how to improve work processes is not used. When patients are scheduled for appointments and have to wait a long time, their time is wasted and staff time is also wasted while they explain the delays and deal with patient complaints. If a nurse has to gather supplies for a procedure from several locations within the department, his or her movements are wasted.

Another method used in TQM to improve a work process is reducing variation within a work process. This is referred to in TQM as bringing the work process under statistical process control. The variation is measured and studied to determine causes of the variation. Next, a plan to reduce variation is developed and implemented. Charts or graphs are often kept to measure the variation and improvements.

Patients who are triaged in the emergency room as not urgent sometimes take more than 12 hours to be assessed by a physician. This is an example of how statistical process control can improve the work process of non-urgent patients being seen by a physician. It is probable that some, if not all, of the patients who wait 12 or more hours are not satisfied with service, and although there may be alternative settings the patients could be encouraged to go to, this may not always be the case. The variation can be monitored by keeping a chart of the time patients arrived; the time the patient is seen by a physician; the date, time, number of physicians in the department, number of nurses in the department, and any other variable that the team believes may have an impact on the time it takes for the patient to be seen. Next, the files of patients who are not seen for an extreme length of time can be reviewed to see if there are any particular reasons. Some of these patients may not have family physicians and if there are family physicians who are accepting new patients, these patients can be referred to them. However, monitoring the time it takes patients to be seen may lead to discovering a source of the variation that can be changed. For example, it may be the delays are due to too few nurses available at certain days or times, or there are too few physicians at some times but too many at other times, or patients with certain non-urgent diagnoses are never seen until all other non-urgent diagnoses are seen.

When mistakes are made, TQM focuses on improving the work process rather than blaming an individual (Deming, 1986; Scholtes, 2003). For example, when an error is made in administering a medication, the process of administering medications is examined to see if the process can be improved.

TQM and Performance Appraisals

Performance appraisal of individuals is *not* a focus of TQM (Deming, 1986; Scholtes, 2003). Performance appraisals are seen as focusing on individuals, and although individuals are important, the performance of the entire team is what needs to be evaluated. In addition, performance appraisals can lead to individuals focusing on ensuring their own work is seen rather than helping the team with its goals. Performance appraisals can lead to employees feeling fearful, particularly when negative feedback is documented. This may in turn lead to employees not speaking out about potential problems or making innovative suggestions. In Chapter 7, Motivation and Performance, we discuss the pros and cons of performance appraisals in more detail.

TQM and Organizational Structure

An important aspect of TQM is the reduction of barriers between departments. To continuously improve quality, members of different work groups need to be able to talk with each other. This way of working can be at odds with the way health care organizations have been structured, with a vertical hierarchy that may require first talking with the department head before moving an issue forward. See Chapter 5, Decision-making and

Management of Workflow, for more information about how health care organizations are structured.

Value of TQM in Improving Health Care

Unfortunately, a number of Canadian health care organizations implemented TQM around the time of downsizing in the early 1990s. When implemented during downsizing, streamlining procedures can be seen as a way of reducing staff rather than as a way to reduce errors in procedures. This is because, as procedures are simplified or steps in work processes are reduced, it is possible that the same work can be done with fewer employees.

TQM is a useful approach to continuously improving quality through continuously improving work processes. We also believe TQM is a valuable management philosophy for health care as many of Deming's 14 points include premises that are important for health professionals. For example, Deming's points include an organizational culture that supports quality and an emphasis on employee involvement in quality improvement. Health professionals want to work in a setting in which the culture promotes quality and they can be involved in quality initiatives related to the care they provide. Deming's points also include an emphasis on employee learning and as professionals, health care workers value learning. Further, Deming's points include modern methods of leadership and emphasize employees feeling free to talk about problems within the organization. Highly educated health professionals expect their leaders to demonstrate modern methods of leadership and they expect the freedom to debate and critique issues within the health care setting with the objective of creating a culture of quality. Health care professionals value being able to provide good care and they need to be able to talk about situations where changes are required so they can implement the kind of care they believe should be implemented. Additional relevant points within Deming's framework are minimizing barriers between departments and the importance of teamwork. There is an increasing realization that health professionals work on interdisciplinary teams and members of these teams need to communicate and work well together in order to provide safe care.

If you decide to initiate the use of TQM in your health setting to improve a work process, start by selecting a work process that you believe you can improve and that will make a visible difference to others when it is improved. This will help the work team to feel they can affect improvements in the organization and will help validate the usefulness of TQM methods. In Chapter 4, Change and Culture, we discuss other strategies for implementing change successfully.

RISK MANAGEMENT PROGRAMS

Risk management programs identify potential risks to patients, staff, or property such as injuries, loss, or damage. Once potential risks are identified, actions are taken to reduce the risks. Patient injury, employee injury, and property loss or damage can all result in financial costs to the organization. Thus, reducing financial risk is a major goal of risk management programs. Potential risks that might be identified by a risk management program include patient falls, fire, theft of patient valuables, and injury to staff or patients from faulty equipment.

Many potential risks such as fire and theft of patient valuables are known, and therefore health care organizations have well-established policies to reduce the occurrence of these risks. Occasionally an incident happens that exposes a risk, and following this incident the health care setting usually develops a policy to reduce harmful outcomes in the future. For example, a radio station in a Canadian city announced a large prize to a caller who phoned at a specific time. Many phone calls were made at the same time from a large, multi-site hospital, with the result that the telephone system ceased to function and no one could phone into the hospital, including ambulances. One can expect that this hospital will develop a risk management plan to prevent this type of occurrence in the future.

An important purpose of risk management programs in health care settings is to avoid **sentinel events**. A sentinel event is an undesirable occurrence that requires investigation (Mainz, 2003), such as an unexpected death, wrong site surgery, or a fire in an operating room. Such events may have negative outcomes for the patient and/or the health setting including patient morbidity or mortality, lawsuits, loss of the health setting's reputation, and high financial costs. Sentinel indicators measure the presence of a sentinel event (Mainz, 2003).

Another important purpose of risk management programs is to reduce incidents and **near misses**. Therefore, a key activity of risk management programs is the investigation of actual or near-miss incidents involving patients, visitors, employees, or the organization's building or grounds. Most health care organizations have developed an incident report form and employees are required to complete the form when there is an actual incident or a near miss. Examples of an actual incident are medication errors, equipment failures, patient falls, nosocomial infections, pressure ulcers, aggression of a patient or employee toward another person at the health care setting, employee injuries, theft, and vandalism. Examples of near misses are the wrong medication ordered or delivered for a patient but noted prior to administration.

Root Cause Analysis

Root cause analysis originated in total quality management and has been adapted for use in health care. Health care teams use root cause analysis to investigate the causes of near misses, incidents, and sentinel events. After the incident to be analyzed has been identified, a team of people who have relevant knowledge is assembled to review how the incident occurred and to take action. A variety of techniques can be used when doing root cause analysis such as timelines, cause and effect charts, brainstorming, and re-enactment of the incident (Woloshynowych et al., 2005). Through the use of root cause analysis, the underlying causes of incidents can be identified, allowing the team to learn from the incident and take actions to avoid similar incidents. For example, after a serious incident such as giving a client who is allergic to eggs an immunization that is contraindicated in persons with this allergy, a community health team might meet to determine the underlying cause(s) for this mistake. As another example, after a patient who needed a left hip replacement was operated on for a right hip replacement instead, the surgical team would meet to review the underlying cause(s) for this error.

Researchers have identified difficulties that health care teams can encounter when using root cause analysis (Nicolini et al., 2011a; 2011b). For example, root cause analysis requires a number of meetings and therefore the time required is a barrier to its use. In some cases, the persons with the relevant knowledge do not agree to be part of the root cause analysis team, and in other cases some persons might dominate the discussion or intimidate others from participating. While root cause analysis consists of a variety of methods, health care teams frequently only use a timeline, walking through the incident as it may have occurred (2011a; 2011b). Teams that have to write a final report that includes their action plan, may limit themselves to a plan that they believe is possible for them to implement, rather than what is really required, or limit their plan of action to their team when it may be required throughout the organization (2011a; 2011b). Teams that consist of persons who were involved in the incident may be anxious to complete the root cause analysis quickly (2011a). In addition, the process of assembling a different team for each incident, near miss, or sentinel event may limit the different teams from identifying patterns across events (2011a).

An important underlying or root cause of sentinel events is faulty communication. Box 11.3 shows the top three causes of recent sentinel events reviewed by The Joint Commission. Note that while most sentinel events have more than one root cause reported, communication is in the top three root causes for the sentinel events shown in Box 11.3.

Box 11.3

Top Three Causes for Different Sentinel Events That Resulted in Death or Permanent Loss of Function Reviewed by The Joint Commission during 2004 through Third Quarter 2011

Fall-related events (N = 538)

1. Assessment – 400
2. Leadership – 309
3. Communication – 299

Elopement-related events (N = 79)

1. Communication – 57
2. Assessment – 54
3. Physical Environment – 52

Delay in treatment events (N = 790)

1. Communication – 634
2. Assessment – 619
3. Human Factors – 545

Infection-related events (N =153)

1. Leadership – 75
2. Surveillance, Prevention & Control of Infection – 66

3. Communication – 63

Infection-related events (N =153)

4. Leadership – 75
5. Surveillance, Prevention & Control of Infection – 66
6. Communication – 63

Restraint-related events (N = 117)

1. Human Factors – 94
2. Communication – 81
3. Assessment – 74

Source: The Joint Commission. Sentinel Event Data Root Causes by Event Type 2004-2012. Downloaded July 25, 2013 from: http://www.jointcommission.org/Sentinel_Event_Statistics/.

PATIENT SAFETY PROGRAMS

Karl (2010) compares safety practices related to the work of pilots and surgeons and describes differences that we should find shocking. Techniques such as simulator training, briefings, and checklists are habitually used in aviation but the use of these or other routine safety procedures have been alarmingly absent in health care. The focus of checklists in aviation is to work through steps verbally, with steps often shown sequentially on a monitor and no documentation required. In contrast, the focus of checklists in health care is documentation for the health record.

Karl (2010) notes differences in hiring practices of pilots and surgeons; pilots are often asked to participate in a simulated "cockpit trainer" while surgeons are hired following an unstructured interview and going to out to dinner. Further, newly hired pilots are provided six to eight weeks of orientation to their airline's policies and procedures while surgeons may operate on their first day of work, often with unfamiliar equipment and with team members who are not familiar with the new surgeon's procedures. Pilots return to simulator training on a regular basis while surgeons are expected to keep themselves up to date. Pilots are randomly checked for use of drugs and alcohol and the number of hours they can work before a rest period is set. Surgeons are assumed not to work while using substances, and with the exception of the recent trend to reduce the worked hours of medical residents, the hours surgeons work are not monitored. When flying below 3 kilometres, pilots can only have discussions related to the flight, while conversations in operating rooms can distract other members of the team.

Although Karl (2010) compares safety practices related to the work of pilots and surgeons, we believe that comparing safety practices for pilots and nurses suggests changes that need to be made if the public is to experience the same level of safety when they enter a health care setting as when they board a plane. Nursing schools across Canada are developing simulation labs, but equipment is expensive and many have insufficient budgets to create simulation labs where students have frequent access to simulation scenarios. Further, practising nurses, like pilots, could benefit from semi-annual participation in simulation scenarios, but most do not work for organizations that have access to simulation labs.

Unlike pilots, many nurses are not provided with a long orientation when they are new to the health organization or department—lengthy orientations are often limited to nurses going into specialty units such as intensive care. However, in today's health care environment, nursing care in any setting is complex. Further, nurses may be asked to move without orientation to a department that is short staffed. While nursing professional associations may require evidence of continuing education, they do not directly observe the practice of nurses. Nurses would not get in a plane if they knew a pilot had recently been drinking, yet they may have difficulty reporting a colleague who they suspect is dependent on alcohol or drugs. Twelve-hour shifts are the norm in many health care settings, and nurses are sometimes asked to do overtime after completing a shift. While more research is needed to see the relationship between the number of hours worked and patient safety, there is some evidence that adverse work schedules are associated with patient mortality (Trinkoff et al., 2011).

Methods of Communication to Improve Patient Safety

Given that communication is an important root cause of many sentinel events, in recent years there have been renewed efforts to improve communication among health professionals. The Canadian Patient Safety Institute set up a working group to prepare a document on the importance of communication and teamwork in patient safety (Teamwork and Communication Working Group, 2011). In their report they emphasize the importance of communication and teamwork for reducing patient safety incidents, improving the quality of care and creating a **culture of safety**. The goal of their document is "…to provide a framework for organizations to understand and convey to their teams the importance and impact of teamwork and communication in healthcare, and to select appropriate training tools to improve this" (p. 2).

One tool noted by the Teamwork and Communication Working Group (2011) is including a patient and his or her family as members of the health care team and the importance not only of health professionals in communicating well with the patient and family but the patient and family communicating well with the health team. For example, to receive safe care the patient (or family member or caregiver if the patient is unable to provide information) needs to inform the health team of medications they have been prescribed and how they are using these medications. Their report summarizes structured communication approaches in a table, which we have reproduced as Table 11.1, and includes briefings, debriefings, assertive language such as the CUS guideline, and critical language such as **SBAR** that we discuss on page 338 along with some other communication strategies for patient safety.

Briefings and Debriefings

Briefings are brief updates that are given at specified times during a procedure. They are used regularly in aviation, for example prior to the flight, prior to taking off, on approach to the landing, and post-flight as well as at other times. These briefings are expected and their content follows a set pattern (Karl, 2010). In general, briefings are not part of the way that health care professionals practise, although one exception is the use of preoperative briefings that were introduced at John Hopkins in the United States and resulted in 36 percent fewer unexpected delays in surgery (Nundy et al., 2008).

We believe that briefings could have benefits in some patient care situations because they could help refocus health professionals on a particular health care situation. Nurses are frequently interrupted while they work, as shown in a Canadian study that found medical and surgical nurses were interrupted frequently and concluded that the majority of these interruptions had the potential to have a negative impact on patient care (Hall, Pederson, & Fairley, 2010). Communication techniques such as briefings may be able to help nurses recall what they were doing prior to the interruption.

Handout Process

Clinical handover, for example at the change of shift, involves communication that can affect patient safety (Shendell-Falik, 2007). Accreditation Canada (2008) includes safe

Table 11.1   Communication Techniques, Tools, and Strategies

Communication Techniques, Tools and Strategies	Characteristics
Briefings	▪ Set the tone for team interaction.
	▪ Ensure that care providers have a shared mental model of what is going to happen during a process to identify any risk points and plan for contingencies.
	▪ Can establish predictability, reduce interruptions, prevent delays and build social relationships for future interactions.[*]
Debriefings	▪ Used to identify what happened in a particular circumstance, what was learned, and what can be done better next time.
	▪ Allows the team to determine how members are feeling about processes and recognises opportunities for improvement and further education.
	▪ The effectiveness of a debriefing is dependent on the quality of the briefing.[†]
Assertive Language	▪ Effective assertion is persistent, polite, timely, clear, and solution focused. The two-challenge rule, where a concern is stated at least two times to ensure it has been heard, is a form of assertive language.
	▪ Using "CUS" as a guideline—"I'm **C**oncerned," "I'm **U**ncomfortable," "This is a **S**afety issue"—allows for succinct escalation of a concern.
Critical Language	▪ A strategy to get another's attention.
	▪ Flags the immediacy of a concern to members of the team.[‡]
	▪ Ensures that specific, relevant, critical information is communicated each time a patient is discussed. (Eg. SBAR – Situation, Background Assessment, and Recommendation) is used in clinical handovers and is valuable within nurse–physician communication.[§]
Common Language	▪ Agreed upon method of communicating critical issues on concerns.[‡]
Closed Communication Loop	▪ Receiver of communication restates what was said to the sender to ensure correct understanding of a message.
Active Listening	▪ Entails listening completely, maintaining eye contact and body language, and repeating back what was said to confirm understanding.
Call Outs	▪ Used particularly in the OR to confirm the phase of a process.

* Makary, M., Holzmueller, C., Thompson, D., Rowen, L., Heitmiller, E., Maley, W., et al. (2006). Operating room briefings: Working on the same page. *Joint Commission Journal on Quality and Patient Safety, 32*, 351–355.

† Frankel, A., & Leonard, M. (2008). Essential components for patient safety strategy. *Perioperative Nursing Clinics, 3*, 263–276.

‡ Frankel, A., Leonard, M., Simmonds, R., Haraden, C., & Vega, K. (2009). *Essential guide for patient safety officers.* Oakbrook Terrace, IL: Joint Commission Resources.

§ Raines, M., & Mull, A. (2007). Give it to me: The development of a tool for shift change report in a level I trauma center. *Journal of Emergency Nursing, 33*, 358–360.

Teamwork and Communication Working Group, 2011.

Source: *Improving Patient Safety with Effective Teamwork and Communication: Literature Review Needs Assessment, Evaluation of Training Tools and Expert Consultations.* From the Canadian Patient Safety Institute. Reprinted with permission.

clinical handover as a **required organizational practice** for safe patient care. Accreditation Canada developed the term "Required Organizational Practice," also known as ROP, to identify practices that are essential for safe patient care.

Box 11.4

Patient Safety Area 2: Communication

Goal: Improve the effectiveness and coordination of communication among care/service providers and with the recipients of care/service across the continuum.

ROP: The team transfers information effectively among providers at transition points.

Test(s) for compliance
- The team uses mechanisms for timely transfer of information at transition points (e.g. transfer forms, checklists) that result in proper information transfer.
- Staff is aware of the organizational mechanisms used to transfer information.
- There is documented evidence that timely transfer of information has occurred.

© Accreditation Canada

Source: From Accreditation Canada. Reprinted by permission.

Checklists

The goal of checklists is to help ensure safe procedures are implemented. Pre-operative checklists, for example, have been used in nursing for many years. However, in health care settings the checklists were often completed rapidly, for example as the patient is leaving for surgery or at the end of a shift, or the checklists were left in the patient's chart only partly completed or not completed at all. In contrast, airline employees have been diligent in using checklists.

One recent example of a checklist designed to improve patient safety is the WHO surgical checklist (Mahajan, 2011). This checklist was developed by the World Health Organization as part of their *Safe Surgery Saves Lives* initiative and is shown in Figure 11.1. The WHO piloted this checklist in a number of countries, including at the Toronto General Hospital in Canada, and the checklist is now used widely throughout Canada

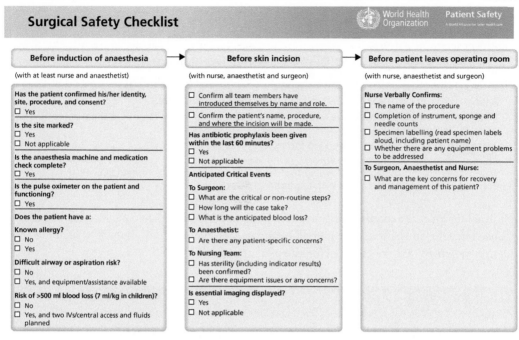

Surgical Safety Checklist

World Health Organization — Patient Safety — A World Alliance for Safer Health Care

Before induction of anaesthesia	Before skin incision	Before patient leaves operating room
(with at least nurse and anaesthetist)	(with nurse, anaesthetist and surgeon)	(with nurse, anaesthetist and surgeon)

Before induction of anaesthesia
(with at least nurse and anaesthetist)

Has the patient confirmed his/her identity, site, procedure, and consent?
☐ Yes

Is the site marked?
☐ Yes
☐ Not applicable

Is the anaesthesia machine and medication check complete?
☐ Yes

Is the pulse oximeter on the patient and functioning?
☐ Yes

Does the patient have a:

Known allergy?
☐ No
☐ Yes

Difficult airway or aspiration risk?
☐ No
☐ Yes, and equipment/assistance available

Risk of >500 ml blood loss (7 ml/kg in children)?
☐ No
☐ Yes, and two IVs/central access and fluids planned

Before skin incision
(with nurse, anaesthetist and surgeon)

☐ Confirm all team members have introduced themselves by name and role.
☐ Confirm the patient's name, procedure, and where the incision will be made.

Has antibiotic prophylaxis been given within the last 60 minutes?
☐ Yes
☐ Not applicable

Anticipated Critical Events

To Surgeon:
☐ What are the critical or non-routine steps?
☐ How long will the case take?
☐ What is the anticipated blood loss?

To Anaesthetist:
☐ Are there any patient-specific concerns?

To Nursing Team:
☐ Has sterility (including indicator results) been confirmed?
☐ Are there equipment issues or any concerns?

Is essential imaging displayed?
☐ Yes
☐ Not applicable

Before patient leaves operating room
(with nurse, anaesthetist and surgeon)

Nurse Verbally Confirms:
☐ The name of the procedure
☐ Completion of instrument, sponge and needle counts
☐ Specimen labelling (read specimen labels aloud, including patient name)
☐ Whether there are any equipment problems to be addressed

To Surgeon, Anaesthetist and Nurse:
☐ What are the key concerns for recovery and management of this patient?

Figure 11.1 The WHO Surgical Checklist

Source: The World Health Organization Surgical Check List. Reprinted by permission of the World Health Organization.

(Information and Privacy Commissioner of Ontario, 2009) and the world, It has been shown to reduce morbidity and mortality (Gawande, 2010; Haynes et al., 2009; De Vries et al., 2010).

SBAR

SBAR stands for Situation, Background, Assessment, and Recommendation (see Box 11.4). SBAR is a communication strategy that was designed by the military, adapted by the aviation industry, and more recently by health care (Thomas et al., 2009). Essentially, SBAR can serve as a checklist for nurses when they are communicating important information about a patient. The recommendation step in the communication forces the nurse to tell another nurse, a physician, or another health professional what he or she feels should be done (Dunsford, 2009).

Here is an example of a SBAR communication:

"My name is Tom McDonald, I am a nurse on 4 East who is caring for Mrs. Henderson, a 76-year-old patient who was admitted yesterday with pneumonia and a history of COPD **(Background)**. I am calling because she fell out of bed approximately 10 minutes ago **(Situation)**. She has a laceration about 2 cm long and a hematoma above her left eye. Her pulse is 102, PB 135/85, RR 28 **(Assessment)**. I am calling to request a CT scan of her head" **(Recommendation)**.

Nurses and physicians are socialized to use different communication styles (Arford, 2005). Nurses learn to describe situations in detail but to not medically diagnose, while physicians learn to briefly state facts leading to a diagnosis. These different communication styles can lead to frustration when members from each professional group communicate with each other. When nurses communicate with a physician using SBAR, they present a concise description of the situation, provide their assessment, and end by saying what they want the physician to do. We note that SBAR promotes nurses to communicate like physicians, and leave the reader to reflect on the pros and cons of changing nurses' communication styles.

SBAR Communication Strategy

Situation   **Assessment**
Background   **Recommendation**

Some studies have looked at the effectiveness of SBAR in reducing adverse events as well as for improving communication; however, more research is needed before we can conclude that the introduction of SBAR is an important practice that reduces adverse events. One study combined training in SBAR with learning about teambuilding, collaborative and other communication styles and techniques, and problem-solving strategies in one American hospital (Beclett & Kipnis, 2009). They found participants reported improved communication and patient safety; however, this study is limited in that adverse events were not measured. Another study implemented SBAR in a nursing home, and this study is described in the Related Research box in this chapter (Field et al., 2011).

RELATED RESEARCH

A Study of the Effectiveness of SBAR Communication

Patient safety problems are associated with the use of warfarin in nursing homes and are often related to errors in monitoring the residents and adjusting dosages. In nursing homes, the communication between nurses and physicians related to warfarin is frequently done on the telephone.

This study involved a randomized clinical trial in 26 nursing homes in one state in the United States. The nursing homes were randomly assigned to either the intervention group where SBAR training for telephone communication related to warfarin was implemented, or the control group.

Two outcomes were measured to assess if the use of SBAR for telephone communications related to warfarin improved the quality of care:

1. the percentage of time that residents' blood work was within the therapeutic range, and

2. the percentage of patients with blood work above the therapeutic range identified within three days.

These outcomes were measured for one year after the SBAR training. There was a statistically higher number of days that residents in the SBAR intervention nursing homes were within the therapeutic range. However, there was no significant

(Continued)

difference in the percentage of patients with blood work above the therapeutic range identified within three days, nor was there a significant difference in the number of warfarin-related incidents.

The authors conclude that the SBAR warfarin-related telephone communica-

tion led to a modest improvement in care. Do you agree with this conclusion?

Source: Field, T., et al. (2011). Randomized trial of a warfarin communication protocol for nursing homes: an SBAR-based approach. *The American Journal of Medicine, 124*, 179. e1(2)–179e7.

CUS guideline

CUS stands for "I'm concerned," "I'm uncomfortable," "this is unsafe" (Leonard, Graham, & Bonacum, 2004). When communicating using the CUS guideline, the person includes the words "I'm **C**oncerned," "I'm **U**ncomfortable," "this is unsafe" or "this is a **S**afety issue." The use of the word "I" in two of the statements promotes assertive communication. As well, the guidelines promote saying the concern three times, which surpasses using the "two-challenge rule" that promotes assertive communication by saying the concern twice.

Huddles

In a huddle, all team members come together for a short, structured communication to review what their next steps should be. The name of this communication technique probably comes from the huddle used by football teams (Stewart, 2007). In health care settings, a huddle can be used for all team members to update the rest of the team about what they have assessed and implemented, and to have input into the next course of action, or for brief discussions or problem solving about other work related issues. Huddles can be used at routine times, such as at the beginning of a shift, or when team members feel they need to regroup to think about an issue or a patient. Given the importance for patient safety of communicating with the patient and his or her family members and including them on the team, we recommend including them on the team's huddle.

For examples of how huddles may be used in health care, watch the utube video at: www.youtube.com/watch?v=VxdG2_nZ2fc or at: http://www.youtube.com/watch?v=dJr ORZEiXpo&feature=related.

The Health Care Organization's Role in Promoting Nurses' Voice

The discussion on pages 335–40 identifies the key role of communication for patient safety and a number of tools or strategies to improve communication. While the communication strategies of individual nurses are important, the organization also has a role to play in creating structures and processes whereby nurses' views related to patient safety are heard.

To illustrate what can happen when nurses' complaints are ignored, we will use an infamous Canadian example. In 1994, 12 babies and children died during or shortly after surgery at the Winnipeg Health Sciences Centre (HSC) in Manitoba and the following year the province's Chief Medical Examiner ordered a public inquiry into these deaths. The report from this public inquiry noted that nurses had voiced concerns about the quality of the cardiac surgery program but their concerns were dismissed (Sinclair, 2000). Associate Chief Judge Murray Sinclair's report included the following recommendations:

> **It is recommended that:** The HSC restructure its Nursing Council to allow nurses to select its membership and to give it responsibility for nursing issues within the hospital. The Nursing Council should have representation on the hospital's governing body and be responsible for monitoring, evaluating, and making recommendations pertaining to the nursing profession within the hospital and for nursing care. The Council should also serve as a vehicle through which nurses could report incidents, issues, and concerns without risk of professional reprisal.
>
> **It is recommended that:** The HSC establish a clear policy on how staff is to report concerns about risks for patients. This policy must ensure that there is no risk to the person who is making the report. It should be clear to every staff member to whom they are to present such reports.
>
> **It is recommended that:** The Province of Manitoba consider passing 'whistle blowing' legislation to protect nurses and other professionals from reprisals stemming from their disclosure of information arising from a legitimately and reasonably held concern over the medical treatment of patients. (Sinclair, 2000, pp. 478–479)

The recommendations that nurses within the hospital elect a nursing representative who can bring issues of concern directly to the board of directors, that the hospital have a clear policy on how to bring concerns forward, and that the provinces have whistle blowing legislation to protect nurses who bring concerns forward have implications for all health settings and jurisdictions. Quebec has legislation that requires nurses to elect a council that meets regularly with the executive director and nursing director and reports to the board of directors (Éditeur officiel du Québec, 2012).

Health care organizations that have councils of nursing and/or a committee structure, such as used with shared governance, provide the structure for nurses to bring their concerns forward. It is expected that professionals bring their concerns to their administrators or their professional associations as outlined in the policies or guidelines of these organizations. However, health settings that have councils of nursing and/or committee structures for nursing practice provide the structure for nurses to have a voice in patient safety and quality issues. In Chapter 5, Decision-Making and Management of Workflow, we discuss shared governance and other organizational structures in more detail.

CORONERS OR MEDICAL EXAMINERS AND PUBLIC INQUIRIES

The discussion of the public inquiry into the unexpected deaths of 12 babies and children at the Winnipeg Health Sciences Centre can be used to illustrate the role of coroners or medical examiners, the chief coroner or chief medical examiner, and public inquiries.

Coroners, also known as medical examiners in some Canadian provinces, examine deaths when a person dies unexpectedly or from unknown causes or from violence or negligence. Each Canadian province has a Chief Coroner or a Chief Medical Examiner. The Chief Coroner (or Chief Medical Examiner) can call for a public inquiry, which is a public review requested by government of a situation with important outcomes for the public. Public inquiries are lengthy and costly and while special interest groups frequently call for a public inquiry, relatively few are approved.

ACCREDITATION OF HEALTH CARE PROGRAMS

Accreditation is an external peer review process whereby an organization or service is reviewed to see how it compares with developed standards for similar organizations or services. For example, the Canadian Association of Schools of Nursing (CASN) accredits schools of nursing across Canada and, since 2011, internationally with the University of Calgary–Qatar being the first program that operates outside of Canada to receive accreditation. Accreditation Canada, formerly known as the Canadian Council of Hospital Accreditation, accredits health care organizations and programs in Canada. It is a not-for-profit, independent organization. Health professionals and administrators from across Canada are trained by Accreditation Canada in how to conduct an accreditation review and serve as peer reviewers for other health care organizations or services. The Joint Commission is a not-for-profit, independent organization that accredits health care organizations and programs in the United States. Like CASN, both Accreditation Canada and the Joint Commission also accredit international health care organizations and programs upon request.

The accreditation of health care organizations or programs is believed to improve the quality of patient care because, to receive accreditation, the organization or program works to achieve specified standards. But is accreditation effective? A study that examined the performance related to 16 quality indicators of accredited and non-accredited hospitals in rural United States found that accredited hospitals performed significantly better for 4 of the 16 indicators (Lutfiyya et al., 2009). In another research study, quality indicators were measured the year prior to accreditation and one to two years following accreditation in a hospital in Saudi Arabia that underwent a review by Accreditation Canada (Awa et al., 2011). Significant improvements were found for the data collected one to two years following accreditation when compared with the data collected the year prior to accreditation for 21 of the 81 clinical indicators studied.

CULTURES OF QUALITY AND PATIENT SAFETY

Teamwork and communication are important components of a culture of safety (Teamwork and Communication Working Group, 2011). The Teamwork and Communication Working Group (2011) developed a number of recommendations for Canadian health care organizations to help them improve patient safety and some of these are shown in Box 11.5. The recommendations emphasize the importance of funding education programs that help

Recommendations for Supporting Communication and Teamwork

Leaders and Decision-makers

- Actively promote, fund and evaluate integration of team work and communication training and education programs within organizations and pre-practice settings.

Middle Managers

- Establish formalized training in effective teamwork and communication as part of the core education and continuing education requirements within healthcare organizations with a particular focus on everyday practice and crisis situations.

- Standardize (as much as possible) general approaches to teamwork and communication training across organizations.

- Consider incorporating one of the recommended training approaches contained within this summary document.

Front-line Healthcare Providers

- Actively incorporate patients and family members as full members of the healthcare team ensuring all opportunities are sought and created to solicit information for healthcare decisions.

- Actively engage and participate in training opportunities for improved teamwork and communication and commit to integrating this knowledge into practice.

Source: *Improving Patient Safety with Effective Teamwork and Communication: Literature Review Needs Assessment, Evaluation of Training Tools and Expert Consultations*. From the Canadian Patient Safety Institute. Reprinted with permission.

teams become effective and improve communication, and standardizing approaches to teamwork and communication throughout a health care organization.

One of the recommendations encourages direct care providers to seek information from patients and families and work with them as full members of the team. At a recent presentation by a manager at a large health care facility in Canada, a member of the audience asked if, given the Teamwork and Communication Working Group's (2011) recommendation to include patients and families as team members to ensure patient safety, was practised at the manager's place of work. The response was that some teams include the patient and family, but the reality is that physicians are still the head of the team and some physicians do not want to work that way. It is this type of thinking that has to change; we would not accept that airline safety was second to pilots' preferences, and we cannot allow health care organizations to take safety less seriously than airlines.

For a culture of quality and patient safety, health professionals need to feel their leaders encourage them to discuss actual or potential incidents rather than blaming them for any errors they made. In a culture of quality and patient safety, health care professionals and their managers embrace the opportunity to discuss patient safety as they continuously seek to improve the quality of care.

Leading Health Care Example

Guelph General Hospital has an interdisciplinary Healthy Hospital Human Resources Quality Team (HHHRQT) with the mandate to develop and implement strategies that will help recruit and retain staff. When this committee was formed in 2005, they began by surveying staff about their safety concerns. The registered nurses, nurse practitioners, and registered practical nurses who responded to this survey identified safety concerns, including lack of knowledge about what security workers could do, parking lot security, insufficient communication about patients with a history of violence, need for more security for nurses working in isolated sections of the hospital, and sections of work areas where public could enter. As well, reported experiences of verbal harassment (48%), disrespectful behaviour (84%), and physical abuse (20%) were reported.

THE HHHRQT worked with other departments on a number of initiatives to improve safety concerns such as clarifying the role of security workers, implementing a system of electronic monitoring to ensure security rounds were done, and adding a security worker to the emergency department on evenings and nights to help control access of the public to areas where they should not have access. As well, public access was controlled by installing doors that opened only with employee identification cards and units were provided with locks that they could use to prevent access during a security alert. Nurses working in isolated sections of the hospital were given personal alarms.

Best practices were examined to investigate how a process could be developed to communicate about patients with a history of violence, and while the HHHRQT decided to refer this complex problem to the professional practice committee, they implemented a one-day workshop for all employees to attend, to learn strategies to de-escalate aggressive persons. The HHHRQT reviewed all of the hospital's policies related to respectful workplaces and while they found them adequate, they consolidated the policies into a single document for easier access by employees.

In 2009 they again surveyed hospital employees and found the nurses felt safer in the workplace but the area of nurses' harassment experiences still needed improvement. The HHHRQT is continuing with their quality improvement efforts and repeated the survey in May 2012.

Source: Guelph General Hospital's HHHRQT. *The Canadian Nurse, 108(4), 20-21.* Reprinted by permission of the Canadian Nurses Association.

Interview

Wendy Nicklin is the President and Chief Executive Officer of Accreditation Canada. She has worked as a nurse in several emergency and critical care departments, as a clinical nurse specialist and educator, and has taught nursing at Queen's and Ottawa universities. She has held a variety of nursing leadership roles as well as senior administration roles. She was a member of the National Steering Committee on Patient Safety that led to the development of Canada's Patient Safety Institute, on which she was a founding board member, recently completing an eight-year term.

Q: In terms of quality improvement, what does Accreditation Canada look for in a health organization?

A: The name of Accreditation Canada's accreditation program is Qmentum. The program is built on standards and supported by survey tools and other instruments. There are standards for governance, leadership, and client care delivery, such as critical care, cancer care, home care, hospice palliative care, and so on. Each organization is encouraged to use the standards and tools on an ongoing basis as an integral component of their quality improvement program.

The standards are standards of *excellence*. It would be unrealistic for any organization to "check them all off" and say all were met. The purpose of the standards is for an organization to use them to identify areas where they are doing well and areas within which they can improve. This self-assessment is a key component of the program.

In addition to standards, the Qmentum program includes Required Organizational Practices (ROPs). ROPs are evidence-based practices—patients are at risk if these practices are not in place.

Accreditation Canada also provides access to survey tools, as I mentioned earlier. Survey tools include a patient safety culture survey, a survey focusing on quality of work life, and a survey for board members to examine their governance practices.

Q: What advice would you give nurses about the accreditation process?

A: Accreditation should not be a project that is conducted every few years. Accreditation should be part of the organization's quality improvement program, and the accreditation components (standards and ROPs, surveys) should be used on an ongoing basis. The on-site accreditation survey visit takes place every four years. It should not be considered a major event if the organization is continually doing quality improvement. The purpose of the accreditation survey is not to audit the standards but to look at the degree to which the standards are being achieved, and provide feedback and recommendations that will help the organization strengthen and prepare for the future.

Accreditation Canada looks for commitment to quality improvement from everyone in the organization, from board members to front-line employees. Commitment does not mean conducting a few fragmented projects, but instead having an ongoing coordinated quality plan with numerous interdisciplinary initiatives underway or completed, and once implemented, are sustained. A commitment to quality must be part of the organization's culture.

There is no one way to address quality improvement; an organization must develop and adapt their approach based on what works for them and their reality, whatever the scope (stand-alone organization or region).

Sometimes nurses are afraid of the accreditation process. They should not be. It is a tool to enable quality improvement, to help improve care. Accreditation is not a test, but a process to suggest how to move forward in the future.

Q: Including the patient and family as team members can improve communication and patient safety. While it is common for specialty services such as oncology, mental health, and pediatrics to include the patient and family as team members, this is not the way that other specialties have traditionally practised. What do you think would help all teams to include the patient and family as team members?

A: This to me is a no brainer. The patient *is* the centre of the team, and this is fundamental throughout the Accreditation Canada accreditation program. Care must be organized with the patient/client at the centre, not passively at the centre but as an active partner in the care. We cannot expect patients to manage their own care when they are discharged from the program/organization (for example, whether home care or acute care) if they have not been actively involved previously. Within the current process of the accreditation on-site survey, the surveyors do not interview the team; instead they trace the path of a patient's care, including noting the degree to which the patient and family are involved.

(Continued)

We need to be sensitive when talking about the family as a team member. For a child, family involvement is essential. For an independent person it depends—if this person wants a family member present/involved, that is his or her decision.

Q: Can you discuss a specific example of how the accreditation process led to improved quality care in a health care setting?

A: In the past, concentrated electrolytes were stock medication on hospital care units. Too many adverse events occurred, and research findings suggested they be stored in the pharmacy department. A survey in Ontario in the early 2000s showed that approximately 50% of hospitals were not following this recommendation. An ROP (Required Organizational Practice) that focused on this problem was developed—requiring that concentrated electrolytes (such as potassium chloride, potassium phosphate, and sodium chloride >0.9%) should *not* be stock medication. This was one of the first 21 ROPs developed by Accreditation Canada. With this ROP in effect, there has been a dramatic increase in compliance with this requirement.

Q: What suggestions do you have for nurses who have identified an aspect of client care that they would like to improve?

A: All nurses have a professional responsibility to take action if they identify an aspect of client care that requires improvement. Whether they mention it to the manager or to someone else, the issue needs to be brought forward. When nurses are oriented to a new health care organization or unit, they should be informed as to who to approach and the process to bring issues forward. If they are not informed about this, they should ask.

Nurses are the core of health care; we are in a position to identify care issues requiring improvement. Health care is continually changing and so there will continually be practices and procedures that need to improve. When patient care issues are improved, this not only improves patient outcomes but also improves efficiency. Poor quality care increases length of stay, may increase infection rates, and so on. Poor care costs money. Each and every one of us has an important responsibility and contribution to make in improving the quality of care.

SUMMARY

Patient safety is forefront in the minds of health care providers, health care regulators and policy makers, and consumers. We need to operate health care organizations with the same emphasis on safety that is used in the airline industry. To do this, all members of the health care team including patients and families need to be engaged in patient safety. We need to involve patients, residents, clients, and their families in work on patient safety. Their view of patient safety needs to be included in patient safety research.

To improve the quality of patient, client, or resident care, we need to have active quality improvement, risk management, patient safety, and accreditation programs. We also need to challenge the ingrained, traditional ways of operating in health care organizations and professional groups. For example, if we know that the patient and his or her family members need to be active members of the team for patient safety, it is no longer acceptable that this does not happen in all teams because some physicians or other team members do not like to work this way. When we know a way of operating saves lives, we owe it to the public to implement this practice, even if it calls for a paradigm shift in health care delivery.

Glossary of Terms

Adverse event An event caused by health care providers that led to a longer hospitalization, injury, or death.

Benchmarking The process of comparing an organization's performance with other organizations. Generally, the comparison is made with an organization that is performing higher, with the goal of trying to establish what the organization is doing differently. The best performance becomes known as the benchmark.

Culture of safety An organization is where safety is valued and incorporated into its culture is said to have a culture of safety. Similarly, an organization where quality is valued and incorporated into its culture is said to have a culture of quality, and an organization where employees are blamed for errors is said to have a culture of blame.

Near miss An event when an incident almost occurred but was prevented.

Nursing sensitive indicators An aspect of a nursing sensitive outcome that can be measured.

Nursing sensitive outcomes Outcomes that result from interventions that are within the domain of nursing practice and for which research evidence has demonstrated the link between the nursing interventions and outcomes (Doran, 2003).

Outcome The outcome dimension of quality refers to the end result of care, such as recovery, survival, changes in the health status of the patient, changes in health behaviours or attitudes, and satisfaction with care.

Process The process dimension of quality refers to the procedures or activities that are implemented and how these are implemented.

Quality assurance The process of setting standards and surveying or measuring to see if the standards have been met. This term has generally been replaced by the term "quality improvement" in health care quality programs because we cannot assure quality, but we can improve it.

Quality improvement The process of measuring quality indicators and based on the findings, developing and implementing strategies to improve quality.

Quality indicators Refers to an aspect of structure, process, or outcome that can be measured.

Required Organizational Practice (ROP) A term developed by Accreditation Canada for practices identified as essential for safe patient care.

Risk management Involves the identification of potential risks to the organization, such as patient injury, employee injury, property loss or damage, and developing and implementing a plan to reduce these risks.

SBAR Stands for Situation, Background, Assessment, and Recommendation and is a guideline developed in the aviation industry for communicating information that has in turn been adapted for use in health care organizations.

Sentinel event An undesirable occurrence that requires investigation.

Standards of care Standards that are developed to state the best evidence we have about care.

Statistical process control Statistical process control (known as SPC) is a method used in Total Quality Management (known as TQM) to reduce variation in work processes. The variation is measured, studied to determine causes of variation, a plan to reduce variation is then developed and implemented.

Structure The structure dimension of quality refers to the resources available in the setting such as human resources and their qualifications, system supports, administrative organization, equipment, and supplies.

Total quality management   Total quality management (TQM) refers to W. Edward Deming's (1986) philosophy of management that includes continuous improvement of work processes and products. TQM is not another quality improvement program; it is a way of life in an organization.

Work process   All the steps required to complete a work related activity.

CASE

Every week, several patients who were discharged from The Sunnyside Hospital ended up having their follow-up care "fall through the cracks." The Sunnyside Hospital was located in a large town and had the mandate to provide acute care services to the population that lived in the small towns and rural areas of a region that covered approximately about 130 square kilometres. When a patient who needed nursing care either in the home or at the community services centre was discharged, the hospital nurse was responsible for faxing a request to community services. If this person needed to be seen the day after discharge, community services required the fax by 12 noon the day before in order to place the person on their home care client list or phone the person to tell them what time to come to their clinic.

Not only were the forms not always sent, but also the forms sometimes were late, and other times information about what services were required was lacking. The community home care nurses were particularly frustrated when the hospital nurses forgot to interview the patient about potential risks for the nurse visiting, such as if there was a dog not on a leash, and who else lived with the client. Nurses and clerical staff at the community services centre were upset when patients presented and expected to be seen, and the staff had not realized the patient was coming, or could not figure out from the referral what care was required.

The manager of the community services centre often phoned the patient care coordinator of the acute care unit where a person with an incorrect referral had been hospitalized, but the situation continued. This past week there had been more persons than usual who had inadequate referrals, and the community nurses told their manager they were sick of the lack of consideration by the hospital nurses. This manager was angry that she had called patient care coordinators on numerous occasions, and while these coordinators reported to division managers who reported to a vice president for patient services, the manager decided to phone the CEO of the hospital to complain. The CEO then spoke to the vice president who was unaware of this situation, as were the division managers, and informed them this matter had to be fixed immediately.

Questions

1. Put together a quality improvement team to work on improving the referral system. Who should be on the team? How often should they meet? Where should they meet?

2. Considering the referral process as a work process, what are the steps in this work process?

3. What are the possible errors that can occur at each step? Suggest strategies for decreasing each of the errors you identify.

4. The community nurses complained to their manager and their manager complained to various patient care coordinators, but nothing changed. What could the manager of the community services department have done differently that may have resolved this problem earlier?

5. Instead of phoning the CEO, how could the community services manager have approached this issue differently? Given the CEO response when he learned of the situation, do you think the community services manager did the right thing by going to the CEO?

6. Do you think that either the hospital or the community services centre had a culture of safety or a culture of quality? Discuss your reasons.

7. To what extent does the CEO's reaction help create a culture of quality or a culture of blame? Discuss your reasons.

Critical Thinking Questions and Activities

1. Identify quality indicators in clinical nursing for a clinical setting where you have practised. Discuss how you could monitor these quality indicators.

2. Provide examples of structure, process, and outcome standards in a clinical setting where you have practised. Suggest how you would measure performance related to these standards.

3. Think of a health care setting where you have practised. Discuss what this setting should put in place before implementing total quality management (TQM). Refer to Deming's (1986) 14 points for organizations.

4. The Association of Registered Nurses of Newfoundland and Labrador has published a document recommending how nurses should proceed when they have a concern about the quality of care. This document is entitled "Registered Nurses' Professional Duty to Address Unsafe and Unethical Situations" and is located on their website at www.arnnl.ca/documents/pages/RN_Professional_Duty_to_Address_Unsafe_and_Unethical_Situations_Jan_08.pdf. In which situations do you feel nurses who have a concern about quality would feel comfortable proceeding as outlined in this document? Are there barriers to proceeding as outlined in this document?

5. Identify your internal customers in a clinical setting where you have practised. Also, identify the persons in this setting for whom you are a supplier.

6. Think of a work process in a clinical setting. What are the steps involved in this work process? What are the internal and external customers for this process? What are their needs? How satisfied are they with the work process? How could this work process be streamlined? How could variation in this work process be monitored and reduced?

7. Legislation for the province of Quebec includes the requirement that nurses elect a council that meets regularly with the executive director and nursing director and to report to the board of directors (see Box 11.5). Does the jurisdiction where you live have similar legislation?

Self-Quiz

1. An example of the structure dimension in Donabedian's framework is:
   a. The number of nosocomial infections per month
   b. The cost of IV solutions
   c. The streamlining of steps required to obtain medications
   d. The availability of the health care setting's policy manual within the department

2. Risk management programs:
   a. Study sentinel events
   b. Implement total quality management
   c. Focus on structure, process, and outcome
   d. Are not suitable for community health care settings

3. An example of benchmarking is:
   a. Developing a chart to show trends in patient falls
   b. Holding a brief meeting to discuss an incident
   c. Comparing the rate of restraining elderly patients with the rate of a residential setting recognized for excellent care
   d. Organizing a quality committee to review the length of stay in a hospital's emergency department

4. Which of the following is a good way to promote a culture of safety?
   a. After an incident the work group meets to discuss how to improve the work process to prevent a similar occurrence.
   b. After an incident the person responsible completes an incident report and meets with his or her supervisor.
   c. One member from each department is made accountable for filling out documents for the accreditation review.
   d. Senior administrators inform departmental managers that they are accountable for safety in their departments.

Useful Websites

Accreditation Canada
www.accreditation.ca/en/default.aspx

Canadian Patient Safety Institute
www.patientsafetyinstitute.ca/English/Pages/default.aspx

Donabedian's (1966) landmark article on how to assess the quality of medical care
www.milbank.org/quarterly/830416donabedian.pdf

The Institute for Safe Medication Practices Canada
www.ismp-canada.org/

The Joint Commission (accredits health care organizations and programs in the United States)
www.jointcommission.org/

Institute for Healthcare Improvement (United States). Website includes learning resources such as videos and improvement stories.
www.ihi.org/Pages/default.aspx

National Patient Safety Agency (United Kingdom)
http://npsa.nhs.uk/

Safer Healthcare Now!
www.saferhealthcarenow.ca/EN/Pages/default.aspx

Videos on patient safety
www.bing.com/search?q=national+patient+safety+UK+videos&src=IE-SearchBox&Form=IE8SRC

WHO global safe surgery program and safe surgery checklist
www.who.int/patientsafety/safesurgery/en/

References

Accreditation Canada. (2008). Patient Safety Area 2: Communication. Retrieved January 25, 2012, from www.accreditation.ca/uploadedFiles/information%20transfer.pdf?n=1212

Albanese, M., Evans, D., Schantz, C., Bowen, M., Moffa, J., Piesieski, P., & Polomano, R. (2010). Engaging clinical nurses in quality and performance improvement activities. *Nursing Administrative Quarterly, 34*(3), 226–245.

Awa, B., De Wever, A., Almazrooa, A., Habib, H., Al-Noury, K., et al. (2011). The impact of accreditation on patient safety and quality of care indicators at King Abdulaziz University Hospital in Saudi Arabia. *Research Journal of Medical Sciences, 5*(1), 43–51.

Baker, G., Norton, P., Flintoft, B., et al. (2004). The Canadian Adverse Events Study: the incidence of adverse events among hospital patients in Canada. *Canadian Medical Association Journal, 170,* 1678–1686.

Beckett, C., & Kipnis, G. (2009. Collaborative communication: Integrating SBAR to improve quality/patient safety outcomes. *Journal for Healthcare Quality, 31*(5), 19–28.

Bott, M., & Suk-Patrick, K. (2012). Guelph General Hospital's HHHRQT. *The Canadian Nurse, 108*(4), 20–21.

Deming, W.E. (1986). *Out of the crisis.* Cambridge, MA: Massachusetts Institute of Technology Center for Advanced Engineering Study.

de Vries, E., Prins, H., Crolla, R., et al. (2010). Effect of a comprehensive surgical safety system on patient outcomes. *New England Journal of Medicine, 363,* 491–499.

de Vries, E., Ramrattan, M., Smorenburg, S., Gouma, D., & Boermeester, M. (2008) The incidence and nature of in-hospital adverse effects: A systematic review. *Quality and Safety in Health Care, 17,* 216–223. Retrieved January 20, 2012, from www.ncbi.nlm.nih.gov/pmc/articles/PMC2569153/

Donabedian, A. (1966). Evaluating the quality of medical care. *The Milbank Quarterly, 44*(Supplement, 3), 166–203.

Donabedian, A. (2005). Evaluating the quality of medical care. *The Milbank Quarterly, 83,* 4, 691–729. (Note: This is a reprint of Donabedian's 1966 article.)

Doran, D. (2003). Preface. In: *Nursing sensitive outcomes: State of the science.* Sudbury, MA: Jones and Bartlett.

Doran, D., Mildon, B., & Clarke, S. (2011). *Toward a national report card in nursing: a knowledge synthesis.* Prepared for the Planning Committee - Toward a National Report Card for Nursing. Retrieved January 31, 2012, from www.nhsru.com/wp-content/uploads/Knowledge-Synthesis-Toward-a-National-Nursing-Report-Card-March_11-_2_.pdf

Dunsford, J. (2009). Structured communication. Improving patient safety with SBAR. *AWHONN, 13,* 384–390.

Éditeur officiel du Québec. (2012). An Act Respecting Health Services and Social Services. Quebec. Retrieved January 29, 2012, from www2.publicationsduquebec.gouv.qc.ca/dynamicSearch/telecharge.php?type=2&file=/S_4_2/S4_2_A.html

Field, T., Tjia, J., Mazor, K., Donovan, J., et al. (2011). Randomized trial of a warfarin communication protocol for nursing homes: an SBAR-based approach. *The American Journal of Medicine, 124,* 179.e1(2)–179e7.

Haynes, A., Weiser, T., Berry, W., et al. (2009). A surgical safety checklist to reduce morbidity and mortality in a global population. *New England Journal of Medicine, 360,* 491–499. Retrieved January 20, 2012, from www.nejm.org/doi/full/10.1056/NEJMsa0810119#t=articleTop

Gawande, A. (2010). *The checklist manifesto.* New York, NY: Metropolitan Books, Henry Holt and Company.

Hall, L., Pederson, C., & Fairley, L. (2010). Losing the moment: Understanding interruptions to nurses' work. *Journal of Nursing Administration, 14*(4): 169–176.

Information and Privacy Commissioner of Ontario. (2009). *The surgical safety checklist: A must for hospitals performing surgery.* Retrieved January 20, 2012, from www.ipc.on.ca/images/Resources/surgicalsafety.pdf.

Institute of Medicine Committee on Quality of Health Care in America. (1999). *To err is human: building a safer health system.* Washington, DC: National Academy Press.

The Joint Commission. (2011). *Sentinel Event Data Root Causes by Event Type* 2004–Third Quarter 2011. Retrieved January 20, 2012, from www.jointcommission.org/assets/1/18/Root_Causes_Event_Type_2004-3Q2011.pdf.

Karl, R. (2010). Briefings, checklists, geese, and surgical safety. *Annuals of Surgical Oncology, 17,* 8–10.

Kudzma, E. (2006). Florence Nightingale and healthcare reform. *Nursing Science Quarterly, 19*(1), 61–64.

Kurtzman, E., & Kizer, K. (2005). Evaluating the performance and contribution of nurses to achieve an environment of safety. *Nursing Administrative Quarterly, 29*(1), 14–23.

Leonard, M., Graham, S., & Bonacum, D. (2004). The human factor. The critical importance of effective teamwork and communication in providing safe care. *Quality and Safety in Health Care, 13*(Supplement), 85–90.

Lutfiyya, M., Sikka, A., Mehta, S., & Lipsky, M. (2009). Comparison of US accredited and non-accredited rural critical access hospitals. *International Journal for Quality in Health Care, 21*(2), 112–118.

Maas, M., Johnson, M., & Moorehead, S. (1996). Classifying nursing-sensitive patient outcomes. *Journal of Nursing Scholarship, 28*(4), 295–301.

Mahajan, R. (2011). The WHO surgical checklist. *Best Practice & Research Clinical Anaesthesiology, 25,* 161–168.

Mainz, J. (2003). Defining and classifying clinical indicators for quality improvement. *International Journal for Quality in Health Care, 15*(6), 523–530.

McDonald, L. (2010). Florence Nightingale. Passionate statistician. *Journal of Holistic Nursing, 28*(1), 92–98,

Nicolini, D., Waring, J., & Mengis, J. (2011a). The challenges of undertaking root cause analysis in health care: a qualitative study. *Journal of Health Services Research & Policy, 16*(Suppl 1), 34–41.

Nicolini, D., Waring, J., & Mengis, J. (2011b). Policy and practice in the use of root cause analysis to investigate clinical adverse events: Mind the gap. *Social Science & Medicine, 73,* 217–225.

Nundy, S., Mukherjee, A., Sexton, J., et al. (2008). Impact of preoperative briefings on operating room delays. *Archives of Surgery, 143,* 1068–1072.

Scholtes, P., Joiner, B., Streibel, B. (2003). *The team handbook.* 3rd ed. Madison, WI: Oriel Incorporated.

Sinclair, C.M. (2000). Report of the Manitoba pediatric cardiac surgery inquest. Retrieved January 26, 2012, from www.pediatriccardiacinquest.mb.ca/pdf/

Stewart, E., & Johnson, B. (2007). Huddles: Improve office efficiency in mere minutes. *Family Practice Management, 14,* 27–29.

Teamwork and Communication Working Group. (2011). Improving patient safety with effective teamwork and communication: Literature review needs assessment, evaluation of training tools and expert consultations. Edmonton (AB): Canadian Patient Safety Institute. Retrieved January 22, 2012, from www.patientsafetyinstitute.ca/English/toolsResources/teamworkCommunication/Documents/Canadian%20Framework%20for%20Teamwork%20and%20Communications.pdf

Thomas, C., Bertram, E., & Johnson, D. (2009). The SBAR communication technique. Teaching nursing students professional communication skills. *Nurse Educator, 34*(4), 176–180.

Trinkoff, A., Johantgen, M, Storr, C., Gurses, A., Liang, Y., & Han, K. (2011). Nurses' work schedule characteristics, nurse staffing, and patient mortality. *Nursing Research*, 60(1), 1–8.

Woloshynowych, M., Rogers, S., Taylor-Adams, S., & Vincent, C. (2005). The investigation and analysis of critical incidents and adverse events in healthcare. *Health Technology Assessment*, 9(19), 1–162. Retrieved January 31, 2012, from www.hta.ac.uk/fullmono/mon919.pdf

World Health Organization. *Safe surgery saves lives*. Retrieved January 20, 2012, from www.who.int/patientsafety/safesurgery/en/

Chapter 12
Diversity in Health Care Organizations

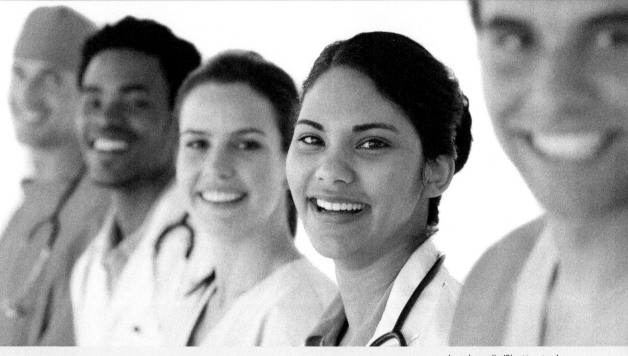

wavebreakmedia/Shutterstock

Learning Objectives

After reading, studying, and reflecting on this chapter's content, you will be able to:

1. Discuss cultural diversity and the ways in which the people you work with may differ from you and from each other
2. Discuss the implications of diversity in health care organizations for nursing staff members, clients/patients, visitors and family members, and nurse leaders
3. Examine your attitudes and experiences in working with others who differ in age, culture, gender, profession, experience, education, and hierarchical position
4. Identify the continuum of cultural competence in an organization and characteristics of organizations that embrace diversity in the workforce
5. Describe the role of individual team members in a health care workplace with respect to cultural diversity
6. Describe responsibilities of nurse mangers and health care organizations with respect to diversity in health care organizations

INTRODUCTION

Diversity refers to variation in some characteristic or attribute that makes one individual seem different from another. Increased diversity is a global reality; not only has migration of people increased over time, but also more and more organizations have become multi-national in character so that more people work across cultures. While the ethnic origin of populations has become more diverse in many countries in Western Europe, North America, and Australia, in the Western world, Canada is among the most ethnically and/or culturally diverse (Fearon, 2003). Indeed, multiculturalism has been the official policy in Canada for many decades and such diversity is considered a characteristic of Canadian society. This characteristic is most evident in large metropolitan areas of the country—the greatest ethnic diversity can be found in the cities of Toronto, Montreal, and Vancouver (Statistics Canada, 2010). You may have grown up in a community that was culturally very homogeneous and nursing school may be your first experience in a group and surrounding community that is diverse. In Canada however, the general population is increasingly diverse in colour, ethnic origin, religion, and culture (Clark, 1998; Statistics Canada, 2008a).

Although ethnocultural origin or heritage is one component of diversity in the larger population, there are many ways in which there is diversity in the population and in health care organizations. In this chapter we use the term **cultural diversity** to refer to a range of ways in which people vary: age, gender, origin, race, ability, religion, beliefs, sexual orientation, socio-economic status, experience, education, and so on (Gardenswartz & Rowe, 1998; Registered Nurses Association of Ontario [RNAO], 2007). Societal changes have brought about greater social diversity. For example, the nature of families has changed over time, with more people living alone, smaller families, more single-parent families, more blended families with step-children, and more same-sex couples with children (Statistics Canada, 2012). Also in Canada, the proportion of non-Christians has increased as well as the proportion of people reporting no religion (Statistics Canada, 2010). Since the 1950s, there has been a steadily increasing proportion of women in the labour market and shifts in the traditional proportion of men and women in specific jobs and professions. Such changes bring greater diversity to the workplace.

In your nursing courses you likely have encountered the terms "cultural diversity" and **"cultural competence"** as you have learned to care for individuals who range in age, socio-economic status, language, religion, ethnic origin, and cultural beliefs about health and illness. In this chapter, we do not focus on clinical care of diverse groups, but rather on what it means to work in and manage nursing care in diverse health care organizations. Health care organizations may provide health care services to a diverse population of patients/clients receiving, and those individuals who work in the organization, such as medical staff, volunteers, and employees may also be diverse. We will discuss why attention to diversity in the workplace matters, the kinds of diversity you are likely to encounter during your career as a nurse, and how organizations are, and sometimes fail to, address the reality of diversity.

CULTURAL DIVERSITY

There are many dimensions to cultural diversity in the health care workplace. Gardenswartz and Rowe (1998) developed a framework that they use to look at the many factors involved in differences among people in health care settings—clients/patients, visitors, employees, and non-employee health professionals. They describe "four layers of diversity," each with numerous factors that are ways in which individuals can differ. They identify four dimensions: personality (individual differences), internal dimensions (such as race, age, gender, sexual orientation and physical ability), external dimensions (such as income, education level, religion, work experience), and organizational dimensions (such as management status, union membership, seniority). These dimensions and aspects provide a way for you to systematically consider the diversity in your professional setting—do you work with clients and colleagues who vary in terms of race, age, gender, ethnicity, physical ability, and sexual orientation? How great is the diversity along these internal dimensions? What about the external and organizational dimensions?

There was a time when patients, staff, visitors, and health professionals within many Canadian health care organizations shared many of the attributes reflected in the dimensions of diversity. Increasing diversity in Canada, however, means that fewer assumptions can be made about expectations, values, preferences, beliefs, and health care choices of those we care for and those we work with than in earlier times. For the most part, we will discuss cultural diversity in broad terms, although we will highlight some kinds of diversity that have received recent research attention in nursing, such as differences among **generations**.

Why Does Diversity in Organizations Matter?

A number of reasons have been given to argue that organizations ought to pay attention to diversity, and these reasons have changed and evolved over time. According to Jonsen, Maznevski, and Schneider (2011), the original interest in workplace diversity in organizations, at least in North America, was a result of the civil rights movement of the 1960s in the United States. Legislation followed that resulted in equal opportunity policies aimed at ensuring access to interviews and equal hiring treatment and equality of pay, training, promotions, and other employment matters. Later, affirmative action programs developed, involving practices such as setting quotas for hiring to increase the proportion of minorities and compensate for past discrimination. These notions of justice and fairness drove the diversity agenda in those earlier decades. However, now the driving forces as well as the perspective on workplace diversity have changed. Now, the growing reality of global diversity has brought about an emphasis on the "business case" for increasing ethnic and gender diversity. Business organizations in particular make the case that there is a "diversity advantage" for an organization in that diversity in employees brings about better decisions, due to a wider range of perspectives, and a diverse workforce better understands a diverse customer base (Cox, 1991; Cox & Blake, 1991). Some of the arguments that have been made for a diverse organizational workforce are highlighted in Table 12.1. It should be noted that there may be differences from one country to another in how they view organizational diversity and the degree to which diverse views might be embraced or

Table 12.1 Arguments Supporting a Diverse Workforce

Focus of Argument	Aspects of Argument
Justice and Fairness	Fairness in hiring, compensation, promotion, etc., based on merit, performance
	Representation of full range of groups in society
	Equality of individuals
	Improvement of delivery of culturally competent care in health care
Business Case or Competitive Advantage	Attract, obtain, and retain the best organizational members when drawing from the full talent pool
	Diverse workforce understands the diverse market or client base, so better marketing
	Diverse perspectives in decision making result in attracting and retaining diverse client or customer base
Improved Decision Making	Broader range of perspectives, knowledge, experience, and skills
	Less "groupthink"
	Broader range of options and solutions considered so better problem solving
	More creativity in decisions

Sources: Based on Baxter (2001), Cox & Blake (1991), Jonsen, Maznevski, & Schneider (2011); Gardenswartz & Rowe (1998); RNAO (2007); Yang and Konrad (2011).

considered desirable. For example, Jonsen, Maznevski, and Schneider (2011) note that cultures that think in terms of the collective, as opposed to the individual, may encourage conformity and regard deviations from norms as unacceptable.

The idea of adding value to an organization with a diverse workforce and treating differences in an organization as an asset, as opposed to a legislated requirement, also makes sense in health care (Baxter, 2001). Diverse employees are likely to be more effective when serving diverse populations, and bring cultural sensitivities to clients or customers who are diverse.

In health care, the motivation to diversify the health care workforce may vary by country. Kalra, Abel, and Esmail (2009) note that the National Health Service (NHS) in the United Kingdom has a legal responsibility to achieve such public policy goals as equality and diversity of the workforce. In New Zealand, a consultant noted that an ethnically diverse workforce was one way to reduce health inequalities and ensure culturally appropriate care (DeSouza, 2008).

While the positive side given for a diverse workforce is that it brings more perspectives to decisions and improves decision making, there is also concern about that there is a downside to diversity, unless diversity is managed effectively. Some concerns are that diversity in an organization may bring with it miscommunication, conflict due to misunderstandings, and differing values and beliefs that affect team functioning. For that reason, a great deal of attention has been given to **diversity management** in organizations, and the argument has been made that a diverse workforce is an advantage to an organization, but only if it is managed and when managers are culturally competent.

Cultural Competence

Cultural competence is a focus of discussion both at the level of the individual nurse and at the level of the health care organizations in which nurses practise. For the purposes of this chapter we give most of the attention to organizational aspects of cultural diversity and competence, as more on this topic is addressed in other courses you will complete on clinical care.

Cultural Competence of Individual Nurses

Cultural competence refers to knowledge, skills, and attitudes that are needed by nurses to provide quality nursing care to individuals, and this is likely a topic that you encounter across nursing courses as you deal with individuals who differ in age, income, culture, sexual orientation, experience, and so on. The work of Madeline Leininger (1995), who developed the concept of cultural competence in nursing and others, has been an important source for curriculum development for nursing schools on the topic of diversity. Nursing theory and practice courses that focus on clinical care usually draw on one or more models such as one by Campinha-Bacote (1994) that describes cultural competence components of cultural awareness, cultural knowledge, cultural skill, and cultural encounter.

There is evidence to indicate that those with cultural competence training are more apt to engage in culturally competent behaviours (Schim, Doorenbos, & Borse, 2005). In health care, much attention has focused on fairness in access to care, equitable treatment, and the provision of culturally competent care by individual providers, and organizational supports for training for cultural competence (Gardenswartz & Rowe, 1998; Spector, 2004; Hart-Wasekeesikaw, 2009). Schim, Doorenbos, and Borse (2005) studied a convenience sample of hospital-based providers in Ontario (N = 71) and Michigan (N = 74) who completed a survey that included an instrument to assess cultural competence. A majority of the respondents were nurses, but other professions and workers were also represented. They found that providers on both sides of the border were generally culturally aware and sensitive, but that overall, culture competence behaviour was associated with prior cultural training and higher educational attainment by the respondents.

The Registered Nurses Association of Ontario (RNAO) (2007) has published a set of recommendations on developing cultural competence in a best practice guideline that is aimed at individuals. Their recommendations, as well as the anticipated outcomes of these, are reproduced in Table 12.2.

Cultural Competence of Organizations

Organizational cultural competence refers to attitudes, structures, policies, and practices that combine to enable employees to work constructively in a diverse organization (Olavarria, et al., 2009). A number of models of cultural competence have been developed that address individual behaviour, but for the purposes of this chapter, we focus on those that focus on what organizations would do.

Table 12.2   Individual Recommendations to Develop Cultural Competencies and Behaviours

Recommendation

1. Self Awareness – To learn to embrace diversity in individuals:

1. Perform self-reflection of one's own values/beliefs, incorporating feedback from peers.
2. Express an awareness of one's own views of differences among people (e.g. different opinions, different world views, different races, different values, different views of society).
3. State and continually explore, through reflection and feedback, how one's own biases, personal values, and beliefs affect others.
4. Identify cultural differences among clients and colleagues in the practice setting.
5. Acknowledge one's own feelings and behaviours toward working with clients, families, and colleagues who have different cultural backgrounds, health behaviours, belief systems, and work practices.
6. Explore one's strategies for resolving conflicts that arise between self and colleagues and/or clients from diverse groups.
7. Identify and seek guidance, support, knowledge, and skills from role models who demonstrate cultural proficiency.
8. Recognize and address inequitable, discriminatory, and/or racist behaviours or institutional practices when they occur.
9. Acknowledge the presence or absence of individuals from diverse cultural backgrounds at all levels in the workplace, reflecting the cultural makeup of the clients or community being served.
10. Reflect and act on ways to be inclusive in all aspects of one's practice.

2. Communication – To develop communication skills that promote culturally diverse settings:

1. Are aware of different communication styles and the influence of culture on communication.
2. Are aware of one's preferred communication style, its strengths and limitations, and how it affects colleagues and recipients of care.
3. Seek feedback from clients and colleagues, and participate in communication validation exercises (e.g. role-playing exercises, case studies).
4. Use a range of communication skills to effectively communicate with clients and colleagues (e.g. empathetic listening, reflecting, non-judgmental open-ended questioning).
5. Seek and participate in learning opportunities that include a focus on communication and diversity.

In many of the models of organizational cultural competence, this competence is seen as a developmental process that occurs along a continuum. In an early model, the structures of an organization were shown as ranging from cultural destructiveness to the other end of the continuum at which point the organization could be characterized as culturally proficient (Cross, et al., 1989). Organizations that wish to move along the continuum to become culturally proficient must work on three aspects: attitudes, policies, and practices. There must be congruence between valuing differences, and the policies and practices that reflect such values.

In the development of best practice guidelines related to cultural competence practices, the RNAO included a set of recommendations aimed at employers and unions in health care. These recommendations are to promote **cultural safety** in organizations as well as the recruitment and retention of a culturally diverse nursing workforce. These recommendations focus on nurses and other employees feeling culturally safe and working in organizations where diversity is "embraced." This set of recommendations for best practice is presented in Table 12.3.

Olavarria, Beaulac, Bélanger, Young, and Aubry (2009) carried out a project to identify standards of cultural competence and tools that could be used by a Canadian community-based health centre to evaluate its organizational cultural competence. Using an extensive review of published and grey literature as well as documents from governments and social organizations relevant to the U.S. and Canadian contexts, they identified five key categories for consideration of standards of cultural competence: organizational norms, principles, and policies; asset and need identification; human resources and management; services and service delivery; and community consultation, partnership, and information exchange. Someone in the organization could use these standards and indicators to conduct a self-assessment for the organization and rate how it measures in terms of performance. For example, a standard related to organizational policies is that cultural competence is an item in the organization's budget. An indicator that this standard is met would be that the annual budget contains funding for activities related to cultural competency. Another category would be services: a standard would relate to interpretation and translation services and a related indicator of that standard would be evidence of the availability of interpreters for various cultural groups. You might use such standards to evaluate how the organization in which you work incorporates the idea of cultural competency. For example, does the organization spend money on assessing the cultural competency of staff and allocate funds for training and continuing education in cultural competence?

Although an organization might use such evaluation tools, not everyone believes that self-assessment is the best approach. The assessment may be flawed if the rater has a low level of cultural awareness, and the approach may be biased unless the rater is comparing the organization's practices to established benchmarks (Bowen, 2008). In searching for benchmarks, Bowen identified dimensions of organizational philosophy in addressing issues of diversity that are worth noting. She describes three types of philosophical approaches to addressing issues: multi-cultural, which tends to focus on new immigrants who come from ethnic or cultural groups who differ from the dominant societal group;

Table 12.3 **Recommendations for Best Cultural Competence Practices for Employers and Unions**

Recommendation

1. **Workplace policies and procedures – To move forward on environment of cultural safety organizations:**

   1. Articulate, implement, and evaluate the effectiveness of a mission statement, values and corporate strategic plans that emphasize the value of cultural diversity and competence.

   2. Dedicate funding in the budget, including funding for human resources and expertise to plan, implement and evaluate strategies to strengthen diversity in the workplace.

   3. Integrate cultural competence into the organization's Code of Conduct and enforce the code. (Codes of conduct implemented in work settings must reflect the principles of the existing Canadian Charter of Rights and Freedoms, and be consistent with provincial/territorial human rights codes.)

   4. Develop policies, guidelines and processes to address change and conflict.

   5. Implement, evaluate and adapt policies and guidelines that are respectful of cultural diversity, integrate cultural competence and eliminate discriminatory practices.

   6. Implement and evaluate strategies to develop leadership skills for succession planning that target under-represented populations to address the organization's identified gaps and inequalities.

2. **Recruitment – To recruit a diverse nursing workforce, employers and unions:**

   1. Identify and monitor the cultural, ethnoracial, linguistic and demographic profile of the workforce in the organization and in the communities it serves on a systematic basis.

   2. Identify gaps by asking. "Who is not here who should be here?" (e.g. men, First Nations people, other ethnic groups) and develop a plan to address the gaps.

   3. Establish outreach processes in collaboration with cultural communities and other organizations to recruit a culturally diverse population for the workforce.

   4. Purposefully seek applications from qualified professionals of diverse cultural backgrounds to recruit to all levels of the organization, including leadership roles so that the organization is reflective of the communities served.

   5. Review and amend all steps in recruitment processes (e.g. wording of job advertisements, role profiles, credentials required) to assess cultural competence and remove systemic biases in the selection process.

3. **Retention – To retain a diverse nursing workforce, employers and unions:**

   1. Plan employee orientation and continuing education programs, based on culturally sensitive preferred learning styles, assumptions and behaviours within culturally diverse groups.

   2. Develop educational strategies to address the diversity of preferred learning styles and behaviours within employee groups.

(Continued)

3. Follow a cultural diversity model in implementing education and training for cultural competence.

4. Provide employees with ongoing continuing education on concepts and skills related to diversity and cultural including:

    ■ Communication

    ■ Cultural conflict

    ■ Competence models

    ■ Culturally-appropriate assessments

5. Allocate fiscal and human resources, as part of the operating budget for educational strategies to promote cultural competence.

6. Evaluate the results of cultural competence education and adapt strategies as appropriate.

7. Work with national and jurisdictional organizations to collectively monitor the diversity of the workforce and the extent that diverse cultural and linguistic communities, ethnoracial groups, and demographic characteristic are represented.

8. Work with national and jurisdictional organizations to collectively establish mechanisms to address barriers to the recruitment and retention of under-represented groups within the workforce.

4. Internationally educated nurses – To better support internationally educated nurses:

1. Assess the unique learning needs of internationally educated nurses and the staff who will work with them.

2. Establish support and monitoring programs for internationally educated nurses and the existing members of the workforce who will work with them.

3. Implement and promote programs to help internationally educated nurses transition successfully into Canadian practice settings.

4. Establish competency-based orientation and continuing education for internationally educated nurses, with a focus on:

    ■ Introduction to Canadian multicultural society, the health care system, and nursing as a profession in Canada

    ■ Language nuances and social norms

    ■ Psychosocial skills

    ■ Human rights

    ■ Employer and employee expectations, rights, and responsibilities

    ■ Mentoring

anti-racist, which tends to focus on racial minorities; and equity, which tends to focus on groups who may have problems accessing health care or with greater health problems. An example of how the approach an organization takes may affect access to care or cultural competence is the situation in which a multicultural approach may only focus on visible differences. With this approach, Bowen notes that "gay, lesbian, bisexual, and transgendered persons, for example, may experience less sensitivity and appropriate care … as may persons with disabilities" (p. 9). As there are limitations with each approach, plans to strengthen a health care organization in terms of cultural responsiveness benefits from a consideration of the strengths and limitations of all three approaches.

Ethnic and Racial Diversity

As mentioned earlier, there is considerable diversity in the Canadian population, with 20% of the population foreign-born in 2006 and the expectation that this would rise to as much as 28% by 2031. By that time, 63% of the population of Toronto would belong to **visible minority** groups, 59% in Vancouver, and 31% in Montreal (Statistics Canada, 2010). Since the mid-1990s, approximately 225,000 immigrants have been admitted to Canada each year (Statistics Canada, 2008b). The 2006 Census identified more than 200 different ethnic origins, a list that includes Canada's Aboriginal peoples as well as those who came to settle in Canada over many centuries (Statistics Canada, 2008a). In the Canadian census, ethnic origin refers to the cultural origin of a census responder's ancestors. It does not refer to nationality or birthplace. There are approximately one million Aboriginal people in Canada, almost 4 percent of the population and it represents a growing group with a young population compared to non-Aboriginal people (Statistics Canada, 2009).

While the terms **race** and racial groups are used in literature and in research as a way to identify population groups, Hyman (2009) reminds us that race is a social construct, and the idea that humans can be categorized into discrete groups in some scientific way, be it genetic or social sciences, no longer has currency. **Racism**, the belief that members of such groups have inherent characteristics and abilities and that some groups are superior to others, is based on a concept of race that is essentially socially constructed rather than "natural." The beliefs lead to attitudes and actions that are abusive, discriminatory, harmful, and oppressive. Racism occurs at the level of individuals, but also a more subtle form is systemic or **institutional racism** whereby organizations and society fail to provide service because of colour, culture, or ethnic origin. The idea of **racialization** arises from the concept of race and the reality of racism (Hyman). Racialization is the process whereby groups become designated as "different" and are treated unequally, marginalized, and excluded. This process and experience means that the group becomes racialized, and many authors prefer to use this term **racialized group** rather than *racial group* because it underscores two key points: race is a social construct rather than a biological reality, and such groups are exposed to racism.

National data on diversity within the nursing workforce or nursing school enrolments and graduations do not exist in Canada, so information on diversity, other than in terms of gender or age, is very limited. Prior to the 1940s in Canada, we know that black women and women of colour were excluded from nursing schools (Flynn, 2009), and current reports suggest that numbers of black and Aboriginal students are low in nursing schools, so that the diversity of specific communities or Canadian society in general is unlikely to be reflected in nursing school enrolments (Etowa, et al., 2005; RNAO, 2007). We know from historical studies and from anecdotal reports that nurses from minority groups have been subject to discrimination and feel uncomfortable in some workplaces (Flynn, 2009: RNAO, 2007). You are even less likely to find numbers of nurses from ethnocultural groups in specialist and management positions in nursing, proportionate to their representation in the population.

Gender Diversity

Although the participation of men in nursing has been documented as far back as the fourth and fifth centuries, continuing through the period of the Crusades and up to the present day, persistent stereotypes and a view of nursing as a feminine profession have been important factors in the low percentage of men currently working as nurses (Evans, 2004). This situation is almost universal, and Purnell (2007) found that, while international data were difficult to obtain for many countries, participation of men only seemed to reach 50% in francophone Africa, with countries more typically reporting a range from 2% in Nicaragua to 25% in the Philippines. Most other countries fell in between these points, as does Canada. The Canadian data on men working in nursing show a very gradual increase between 2005 and 2010 (see Table 12.4).

Table 12.4   Registered Nursing Workforce in Canada, by Sex, 2005–2010

Sex	Year	Count	Percent Distribution
Female	2005	237,257	94.4
	2006	239,520	94.4
	2007	246,268	93.8
	2008	249,866	94
	2009	249,866	93.8
	2010	251,349	93.6
Male	2005	13,985	5.6
	2006	14,299	5.6
	2007	15,002	5.8
	2008	15,621	6
	2009	16,475	6.2
	2010	17,163	6.4

Sources: The Canadian Institute for Health Information © 2010.

The call for greater gender diversity in nursing in Canada was renewed during the most recent shortages in nursing following cutbacks in the 1990s and attention was given to the importance of recruiting more men into the profession (Meadus, 2000). Some of the barriers to men entering the profession include ridicule from family, friends, and peers who see nursing as a female profession; stereotyping of men who are nurses as feminine or gay; lack of role models in the media and in the profession; isolation in nursing; and in some countries in particular the low status of nursing (Bartfay, 2007; Keogh & O'Lynn, 2007; Purnell, 2007).

There is a long history of discrimination against men in nursing. In Canada, it was not possible to enter nursing schools or be licensed in some jurisdictions for many decades (LaRocco, 2007). In Chapter 6, we discussed some of the research related to men in nursing and the difficulties they encounter in nursing school and practice settings. Despite sporadic efforts to recruit more men into the profession in Canada, the increase in recent years has been quite small and far from reaching levels that have been attained in recruiting women into traditionally male-dominated professions. Those who do enter nursing may find that it is not a comfortable place to be and that an "old girls club" operates to exclude them, that they may be a "token male" on a nursing committee, or subject to reverse discrimination (Porter-O'Grady, 2007). Some have noted that men in nursing, unlike women in male-dominated professions, however, have advantages that promote their careers. Despite the historic difficulty men had in entering the profession, a number of authors have noted that they have had an advantage in obtaining management jobs and progressing in their careers, although the employment advantage may be subtle (Lane, 2000) and explained in part by men's greater interest in personal and professional power (Kleinman, 2004). Kleinman believes that these benefits could facilitate the recruitment of more men into the profession.

Generational Diversity

In Chapter 9, some of the differences between nurses of different generations were discussed relative to their expectations of the workplace. Generation cohort theory proposes "that a generation is a social construction in which individuals born during a similar time period experience, and are influenced by, historic and social contexts in such a way that these experiences differentiate one generational cohort form another" (Lester, et al., 2012, p. 342). Different authors give slightly different dates and names to the current generations in the workforce. At the time of writing, there are four generations in the Canadian labour force, although probably most in the oldest group, traditionalists (born before 1946), have retired and the boomers (born between 1946 and 1964) have now started to retire (Lester et al., 2012; Spinks & Moore, 2006; Wortsman & Crupi, 2009). Members of generation X (born between 1965 and 1981), generation Y (born between 1982 and 2000), and boomers will continue to share the workplace over the next several decades. Many have proposed that these generations have differing attitudes to work and have had different experiences in entering the nursing workforce than previous generations. These and other generational perspectives shape their approach to work. We are just beginning to understand what the differences are between generations that share a workplace and the implications of those differences. However, it is important to avoid stereotyping nurses from different generations, as individuals may not share the attitudes of their generation.

Table 12.5　Four Generations in the Workplace

Generation	History	Preferences/Beliefs/ Expectations re Work
Traditionalists or Veterans	Born prior to 1946	Adhere to rules
	Most now in 60s and 70s	Respectful of authority
	Grew up during less affluent times, WWII, and Cold War	Disciplined work habits
		Risk averse
	Entered a predictable workplace—nurses had positive work outlook	Comfortable with hierarchy, structure
		Expect clear roles, responsibilities
		Expect rewards with seniority
Boomers or baby boomers	Born between 1946 and 1964	Consensus seekers, value collaboration
	Raised during a period of growing post-war prosperity	Competitive
	Hard work to "stand out" and be recognized	Moderate level of disrespect for authority
	Leadership and formal authority were synonymous in workplace	"whatever it takes" approach to work
	Part of dominant group entering workforce, favoured by public policies, period of grown and expansion—nurses entered an expanding job market with medicare	Will work long hours and hard for rewards, somewhat materialistic
		Like somewhat formal workplace and moderate pace in workplace
		Define themselves through work, work a priority over non-work life
		Like formal feedback, promotion
Generation X, gen X, or the nexus generation	Born between 1965 and 1981	Somewhat cynical and skeptical
	Brought up with two working parents, so learned to be self-reliant, independent	Prefer relatively informal work climate
	Exposure to technological developments in early learning years	Weaker work ethic than boomers
	Leadership based on competency	Challenge authority
		Autonomy and independence very important

	Many entered labour force at a difficult time with hospital restructuring and layoffs in the 1990s. Some left the country, held several part time jobs, or left the profession	Seek work-life balance, personal activity takes priority
		Prefer technology-based interaction, dislike unnecessary face-to-face meetings
		Strongly motivated by intangibles like autonomy, flexibility in work
		Value direct communication and feedback from leaders
Generation Y, gen Y, millennials, or net generation	Born between 1982 and 2000	Self-confident, well educated
	Grew up in a digital world and an era of instant gratification through technology	Technology savvy, multitaskers
		Committed to culturally sensitive, upbeat, and fun workplace
	Raised to express their feelings and ideas, to challenge, to negotiate for what they want or think they deserve	Prefer clear expectations, instant access to information
	Educated to work in teams/groups, problem-solve, and collaborate	Like teamwork environment, interaction, less formality, non-hierarchical environment, bosses who value input and give feedback, provide positive encouragement
	Scrutinize workplaces for what they want and gen Y nurses are entering the workplace looking for organized units with teams, respect, and recognition for their contribution	Seek balance between work and play, prioritize time with family and friends over work commitments

Sources: Based on Lester, S.W., Standifer, R.L., Schultz, N.J. & Windsor, J.M. (2012). Actual versus perceived generational differences at work: An empirical examination. *Journal of Leadership & Organizational Studies, 19*(3), 341–354.; Wortsman, A. & Crupi, A. (2009). From *textbooks to texting. Addressing issues of intergenerational diversity in the nursing workplace*. Ottawa: Canadian Federation of Nurses Unions.

People born at the beginning or end of a generation (known as *cuspers*) may have attitudes that include those of both generations (Wilson, et al., 2008). Table 12.5 outlines four generations that currently work alongside each other, how their generational histories differ, and their preferences or expectations of work and the workplace.

We work on multigenerational teams and individual nurses, nurse leaders and managers, and health care organizations must deal with this reality. The concern is that differences often give rise to misunderstandings, misperceptions, and conflict, which results in an unhealthy workplace climate, low job satisfaction, and turnover. Lavoie-Tremblay, O'Brien-Pallas, Gélinas, Desforges, and Marchionni (2008) found that an imbalance between level of effort and workplace reward contributed to a high reported intent to leave a nursing job among Quebec nexter nurses, members of a generation that is said to expect frequent praise and consistent rewards. The research example at the end of this chapter highlights some of the differences in job satisfaction among generations of nurses and how job satisfaction of younger generations might be enhanced. However, it is important to avoid stereotyping individuals who belong to a particular age cohort, as one cannot assume that any individual nurse shares the characteristics of the group.

The research findings on generational differences in the workplace are mixed and so the evidence on whether different generations are really looking for different things from the workplace is limited (Lester, et al., 2012). In Lester et al.'s study of employees from all levels in a U.S. organization, 263 employees responded to a survey about their personal values and about their perception of how different generations valued the same thing. They compared boomers, generation X, and generation Y respondents who rated how they valued 15 items ("I Value") and their perception of how the other generations would rate them. Of the 45 potential value differences, the researchers found 8 *actual* differences across generations relating to 5 of the value items. However, the researchers found 27 out of 45 *perceived* value differences pertaining to the 15 items that were statistically significant. They suggest that, in the workplace, perceived generational differences outnumber actual differences. In this research study, some of the actual differences were:

- Generation Y reported valuing email communication more than boomers
- Generation Y reported valuing social media more than generation X
- Generation Y reported valuing fun at work more than generation X and more than boomers
- Generation Y reported valuing continuous learning more than boomers
- Boomers reported valuing professionalism more than generation X.

Given the results of their study, Lester et al. suggest that managers should educate employees about the actual differences in generational values, but more importantly, highlight for employees the many commonalities across the generations. For example, all generations in this study valued face-to-face communication, despite generational preferences in use of technology in communication.

MANAGING DIVERSITY

As an individual nurse in a health care organization, you can review the recommendations shown in Table 12.2 to consider how you embrace diversity in your workplace. In assessing your self-awareness and identifying cultural differences among clients and colleagues, you may become aware of practices that are unfair, discriminatory, or even racist. You may want to develop your communication skills and knowledge of cultural norms and you may also need to seek assistance and support in speaking up or addressing conflicts and issues that you identify in the workplace. When you are new to a workplace, you may look with "fresh eyes" at a practice or issue that others have missed. In this way, you can contribute to improvements in the management of diversity in your workplace.

Definitions and meanings

Jonsen, Maznevski, and Schneider (2011) define diversity management as "a set of managerial actions aimed at either increasing diversity, and/or promoting amicable, productive working relationships" (p. 36). Some definitions refer to managers in organizations taking strategic decisions and actions to create a positive environment that not only acknowledges, but also embraces differences in age, skin colour, gender, ability, ethnicity, and work experience (Baxter, 2001). The management of diversity implies a move beyond earlier eras of business or health care management in which the emphasis was on compliance with equal opportunity legislation or affirmative action orders and non-discriminatory human resource practices and policies.

One of the challenges of a diverse workforce is that of cross-cultural conflicts and management of these in the workforce (Beberi, 2009). Such conflicts can heighten stress and lower productivity in the workplace and result in high turnover. Beberi looked at the effect of cultural diversity on interaction among nursing staff in a U.S. healthcare organization and the sensitivity of RNs who work in a diverse organization. Her study looked at diversity in terms of race-ethnicity, education, age, and years of experience, and interaction with other colleagues in the organization or workgroup. Using a survey, she examined cultural inclusion/exclusion, which was the ability/inabilty to engage with others in the workgroup; valuing differences, which meant ability to acknowledge, appreciate, and admire different values and beliefs; trust or the ability to rely on colleagues; adaptation or the ability to adjust to an attribute of another culture. Based on a sample of 194 RNs in departments of a community hospital, 81 percent of the nurses reported being satisfied with their current job. Most were not planning to leave their current job, but 28 percent had such plans. Beberi found that nursing education level was significantly related to cultural group inclusion/exclusion and trust, with the masters group scoring significantly higher on level of trust with other diverse cultural groups. Job satisfaction was associated with valuing differences and with trust, and those planning to stay at their current job scored higher on levels of trust with diverse groups. Overall, educational level affected the nurses' cultural group inclusion/exclusion and trust level as those with higher education seemed more open and involved with other cultural groups and more likely to build trusting relationships. The researcher suggests that, at a time of shortage of nurses, there is a need to foster an organizational climate that supports interaction among groups and that nurses with higher education might be more open and talented in mentoring interpersonal and intercultural communication. Creating a work environment of **inclusion** is critical in a multicultural society such as that in Canada.

In a review of the literature on embracing cultural diversity, Pearson et al. (2007) examined a number of topics, including managing diversity in healthcare. Most of the literature was not researched-based, although they identified one U.S. study that suggested that a health care organization than is focused on its external world is more apt to engage in active management of diversity than organizations that are more internally focused. A major topic in the diversity management literature involved conflict behaviours and how to manage these so that a diverse health care team can work together to achieve goals. Managers must build and maintain an inclusive culture in which employees feel they are heard, can participate in decisions, and can succeed. The idea of inclusion goes beyond recruiting a diverse workforce—it means building a workplace culture that values differences, something that means rethinking management practices to incorporate diverse views, promote respectful dialogue about differences, and promote supportive relationships among employees (Chavez & Weisinger, 2008). An organization that is inclusive is one that values the unique abilities of individuals and believes that they "add value" to the organization (Scott, Heathcote, & Gruman, 2011).

Frusti, Niesen, and Campion (2003) describe how a diversity competency model was used to assess two acute care hospitals that were part of the Mayo Clinic in the United States as they sought to build a nursing diversity framework throughout the organization. The elements of the model were:

- drivers (how the organization leads, sets diversity direction, and plans),
- linkages (how diversity is integrated throughout all levels and guiding documents of the organization),
- culture (how the organization creates a work environment from recruitment to development of diverse teams and education/training for diversity and development of respect), and
- measurements (how the organization evaluates and seeks to improve diversity performance).

One of the approaches used with respect to culture for example, was Diversity Dialogue sessions used first in the nursing administrative leadership group and gradually expanded to nursing unit council meetings. These sessions occurred in a safe environment, initially with trained facilitators, with the goal of understanding differences. Participants engage in "deep listening" without thinking of a response. Gradually, all staff begin to discuss how differences in gender, race, and sexual orientation play out in the organization.

Diversifying the Nursing Workforce

Professional organizations in both Canada (National Expert Commission, 2012) and the United States (American Nurses Association, 2009) have indicated in their publications that the nursing workforce in their respective countries should be more diverse and reflect the societies in which they practise. Among the ways of diversifying the workforce are those aimed at increasing enrolments in nursing schools from diverse groups and approaches have focused on student recruitment strategies, such as making recruitment materials more diverse, increasing the diversity of faculty members, and enhancing the cultural competence of faculty with respect to minority and international students (Etowa, et al., 2005; Wilson, Sanner, & McAllister, 2010). Another approach is recruiting and retaining nurses from diverse groups, including internationally educated nurses (Baumann & Blythe, 2012; Frusti, Niesen, & Campion, 2003).

Mentoring Program for Minority and International Students

Wilson, Sanner, and McAllister (2010) describe a mentoring program in a university in the southern United States with considerable student diversity among minority and English as a second language (ESL) groups. Many of these students had difficulties with test performance, and high attrition from the program among these students was a problem. The program involved students and their faculty mentors exploring reasons for difficulties and developing strategies to address problems. A major aspect of the program was the development of cultural competence among faculty members, some of whom had demonstrated judgmental and insensitive behaviour. Training workshops with testing before and after were used to improve the level of cultural competence; training for mentorship was a subsequent step. As part of a larger program to increase minority and disadvantaged student success, the mentoring component was a major strategy to improve retention in the program. Focus groups were used to evaluate perceptions of the mentoring program, and the authors concluded that a formal mentoring program assists disadvantaged students to be successful and that administrative support is essential to facilitate mentor development.

Facilitating Integration of Internationally Educated Nurses (IENs)

One of the groups in Canada that has had difficulty entering the workforce is internationally educated health professionals. In recent years, much more attention has been given to how to integrate nurses who were educated abroad into the Canadian workforce. Baumann and Blythe (2012) describe a three-year project involving six hospitals and a cancer centre that was aimed at fully integrating and retaining 60 RNs and RPNs (LPNs outside of Ontario), either internationally educated nurses (IENs) or English as a second language (ESL) nurses, into the workforce. A key aspect of the project was to prepare staff nurses, clinical educators, and clinical managers as "clinical integrators" who mentored and coached IEN/ESL nurses in the organizations. Interventions in the project included workplace communication courses, skill labs, job coaching and mock interviews, workshops on cultural competency, networking, and websites. The project was successful and all targets were exceeded: 132 participants accessed at least two of the seven interventions available, 81 either became or remained employed during the project, and 40 nurses were trained as cultural integrators in the organizations involved.

Job Satisfaction

Job satisfaction among a multigenerational nursing workforce (2008)

Researchers from the University of Toronto were interested in examining differences in overall job satisfaction among the generations of nurses in acute care settings as well as exploring components of their job satisfaction. As job satisfaction had been shown to be a significant factor in retention in a current job, the researchers thought it was important for employers of nurses to understand how different generations of nurses might evaluate their satisfaction in order to retain nursing staff, particularly during periods of nurse shortage. Data for the study came from the Ontario Nurse Survey of 2003 that was sent to registered nurses (RNs) and registered practical nurses (RPNs) who worked in Ontario's 75 acute care hospitals in medical, surgical, or critical care areas. The study focused on a subset of that survey (N = 6,541) in that it looked only at RNs and the youngest three generations. Veteran or traditionalist generation nurses were not included as they were preparing for retirement at the time of the study. The sample was made up of 3,043 baby boomers, 2,898 generation X members, and 600 generation Y members. The average age of each group was 51, 37, and 26 years respectively.

Job satisfaction was measured using the McCloskey Mueller Satisfaction Scale, an instrument with 31 items that addressed eight aspects of job satisfaction: extrinsic rewards, scheduling, family-work balance, co-worker interaction, other interaction opportunities, professional opportunities, praise and recognition, and control and responsibility. Only the family-work balance subscale was not used in the study due to low reliability coefficients found in previous work. The overall score and subscores were standardized to 100, so that the theoretical range was 0 to 100. Multivariate analysis was used to look at how the generations differed in overall job satisfaction and satisfaction in the subcomponents measured in the study. (Multivariate analysis allows the researchers to look at more than one variable at a time and control the effects of several variables while examining the effects of a variable on an outcome.)

The researchers found that baby boomers were significantly more satisfied than generation X and Y members, but the difference between generation X and Y members was not statistically significant for overall job satisfaction. These overall scores by generation were 54, 51, and 52 respectively. They also found that baby boomers were significantly more satisfied than the other two generations with the following components: pay and benefits, and scheduling. Baby boomers were significantly more satisfied than generation X nurses with the following components, but did not differ significantly from generation Y in these: professional opportunities, praise and recognition, and control and responsibility. Generation X and generation Y did not differ significantly on overall job satisfaction or any subcomponent of job satisfaction. Of note was that no significant differences were found across the three generations in satisfaction with co-worker relationships and other opportunities for interaction.

Noting that nurses in the two younger generations were less satisfied with their job than baby boomers, the researchers discussed ways to improve job satisfaction so as to retain these younger nurses in the nursing workforce. Baby boomers were more satisfied with pay, benefits, and scheduling than younger nurses, items that are generally linked to seniority as part of collective agreements in unionized settings. However, the researchers indicate that managers may be able to increase opportunities for self-scheduling within collective agreement parameters and increase satisfaction of younger nurses. (See Chapter 8 for a discussion of scheduling). They also suggest that job sharing opportunities may increase satisfaction for younger nurses, as it could increase control over work hours. Baby boomers reported higher satisfaction with professional opportunities, praise and recognition, and control and responsibility than generation X nurses, a generation that is considered to highly value self-directed recognition and professional activity.

Support for education and career development and recognition programs may be key ways that managers could increase satisfaction for younger generations. Providing more opportunities for generation X and generation Y members to engage in decision making through shared governance structures could increase a sense of autonomy and control over practice. Unit councils, organization-wide committees, and other empowerment practices are suggested by the researchers as ways to increase job satisfaction among younger nurses.

Source: Based on, "Job satisfaction among a multigenerational nursing workforce," in the *Journal of Nursing Management*, 16, 716, 723. John Wiley and Sons.

Leading Health Care Example

Integrating Internationally Educated Nurses (IENs) into the Healthcare Workforce

The Hamilton Health Sciences (HHS), composed of six hospitals and a cancer centre, is carrying out a project with support of four partners—the Centre for Internationally Educated Nurses in Ontario, Mohawk College Institute for Applied Health Sciences, Hamilton Centre for Civic Inclusion Ontario Hospital Association (OHA) and the Nursing Health Services Research Unit of McMaster University. The project is underway between 2012 and 2015 and in an interim report, Baumann and Blythe (May 2013) describe some of the activities in this project which was designed to support the integration of

internationally educated nurses (IENs) into HHS and other Ontario health care organizations. The project involves the development of tools and processes for new hiring of IENs and the development of clinical managers, educators and RNs as mentors and coaches for these new employees. Interventions used in the project included a course in language communication for nurses (with such skills as giving and receiving verbal reports); clinical skills laboratory simulations; a training workshop for IENs, staff nurses, and managers on cultural awareness; job coaching and practice interviews for IENs; learning plan review materials, a website providing resources for IENs; networking support; and

(Continued)

workplace experiences (such as general nursing orientation and job shadowing). A total of 166 new participants entered the program in the first year and those exiting the program indicated that they had increased their nursing skills and awareness of Canadian work. As the project continues, new components, such as on-line modules, are added to the interventions and material available to assist with the integration of IENs.

Source: Baumann, A. & Blythe, J. (May, 2013). Hamilton Health Sciences, Internationally Educated Nurse (IEN) and English as a Second Language (ESL) Nurse Integration Project 2012–2015. Interim Report. Series Report 37.

Interview

Dr. Mary Ferguson-Paré

Dr. Mary Ferguson-Paré has extensive experience as a nurse leader and nurse executive in health care. Most recently, she was Vice-President, Professional Affairs and Chief Nurse Executive at University Health Network in Toronto and is currently President and Chair of the Board of the Canadian Nurses' Protective Society. She is a Member of the Order of Canada and the recipient of the Queen Elizabeth II Diamond Jubilee Medal and has received numerous awards for her leadership roles in nursing and health care.

Q: What do you see as the benefits of cultural diversity in health care organizations? What kinds of problems have you seen arise when there is cultural diversity?

A: There are tremendous benefits to diversity of all types—the more perspectives we have, the stronger the whole. Simply being able to relate to the people we serve is very important and we need diversity among staff to serve our community. In my leadership team at work, I always had the greatest amount of diversity as possible in my team, because we make stronger decisions as a result. That does require acceptance, a non-judgmental approach with each other, and being prepared to listen to each other.

The other part of this question is about the kinds of problems that arise and I have seen tremendous number of problems—both overt and covert ones. The overt type can be easier to address than the covert problems. One example is gender and the clear and solid glass ceiling that exists for women in advancing in health care or, for nurses, in particular, who are mostly women. We also need to find a way to show men that this is a positive career option for them and that if they join it, they will be respected. It is very hard for men because in nursing, it is always about the women. We need to have equal opportunity for women and men in nursing in the health care workplace.

Another area is racial issues. I've had very troubling experiences with staff fighting with each other and threatening each other, discrimination related to race, and people not being able to respect one another. Also there is not enough representation of people from ethnic groups in leadership positions. I've witnessed several incidents involving a lack of respect for and discrimination against those whose sexual orientation is not heterosexual, even at the executive level. And after 9/11, religion actually cropped up more visibly with regard to Muslim staff. There have been some issues between patients and staff with regard to gender, race, and religion. All members of our staff are valued and it can only be addressed by getting people together, understanding the values and perspectives, and talking it through openly, working it though. It takes time to work it through, but it certainly cannot be ignored—it has to be openly addressed.

Q: You have worked in different kinds of health care organizations in culturally diverse settings—acute care most recently, but also in long-term care, etc. Are there differences from one kind of organizations to another?

A: In long-term settings, a larger proportion of caregivers are unregulated, many are immigrants, and there is greater cultural diversity of staff, particularly in large cities. There is very little representation of this group at the leadership/management level. Another issue that arises is ageism. In acute care, for example, elderly people are not afforded the same level of respect or access to treatment or consultations, they are frequently dismissed, frequently restrained, and things go on that really demonstrate that there is a lack of respect for elderly people. There is an issue of bullying, not to say that bullying isn't a problem for all ages, but elder abuse is alive and well. And for nursing, long-term care is a place where nurses can shine, where nurses can lead, and it is a tremendously rewarding area of practice, working with elderly people. Here's the irony—people in acute care may say they don't want to be looking after old people, but that is who is in acute care! The complexity of the care required by elderly persons is not seen as a positive challenge. The complexity of gerontology and of mental health care are not acknowledged—bias in both cases is rampant and so much needs to be done.

Q: What do you think a nurse who has limited experience with cultural diversity should do when she is considering, or has accepted a position, in a new setting that is very diverse in terms of co-workers and clients/patients/residents? What should a nurse look for in terms of organizational policies and practices? How would they recognize a well-organized workplace in this regard?

A: The first thing I would say is: know yourself. It really requires people to think about this and to look inside because we all have our biases and our areas of discrimination and beliefs. Try to understand what the organization is about and what does the organization say it stands for. Look at the leader who you're going to work for—what do they stand for? In the vision or values of the organization, there should be something about respect. Ask yourself: Can I give the gift of respect—regardless of who another person is or where they came from? I think going in to a diverse environment when you have come from one with very little diversity, you have to do your homework. Get the support of the leader; seek advice; and look at the policies, services, and educational programs offered. Look at the organizational values and the policies and practices related to diversity. Organizations that are doing a good job in this area are ones that are showing that they value people from all backgrounds in their policies, but also in the practices and in their education and promotion of staff-career development for everyone.

Q: There is a great deal of discussion of the multigenerational workplace and the challenges of diversity when there are three, even four, generations working together. What has been your experience?

A: At University Health Network, nursing staff was made up of about 50 percent novice nurses or new graduates. And there have been some tensions around the new grad group, the mid-career, and late-career group. Really more with the mid-career group because the late career group are saying, "You know, I'm retiring in a few years." We had to really work to helping the generations to understand each other. The new grads couldn't understand, for example, why things were happening in practice, why experienced nurses were so cranky to them, or why they couldn't get time off like the experienced nurses could. Seniority is one of the issues, and we had to develop educational programs for all of the groups.

Source: Interview with Dr. Mary Ferguson-Paré. Reprinted with permission.

SUMMARY

Thinking about diversity in the workplace has moved from programs that focus on equal opportunity for minority groups and eliminating discriminatory practices to embracing and celebrating diversity, and recognizing the benefits that diversity in the workforce brings to decision making and organizational performance. The approach of organizations and their managers is to value differences in the workplace, to consider multiple perspectives and incorporate them into every aspect of organizational structure and function in order to benefit from the full range of talent and creativity that is possible with a diverse workforce. The benefits to health care include a diverse workforce that brings a wealth of ideas, cultural knowledge, and talent to provide culturally appropriate and high quality care to a diverse Canadian population.

Glossary of Terms

Cultural competence refers to the knowledge, skills, and attitudes that are needed by nurses to provide quality care to patients/clients or by nurse managers to manage diversity in the workplace.

Cultural diversity refers to the range of ways that people differ from each other including gender, age, race, ethnic background, sexual orientation, ability, education, socio-economic status, beliefs and values, religion, language, appearance.

Cultural safety refers to an environment in which there is the ability to act, to advocate, and to redress inequities and in which power differentials are recognized and challenged.

Diversity management refers to management practices or actions that are aimed at promoting positive working relationships amid differences and/or increasing diversity of the workforce in an organization. This approach goes beyond the traditional equal opportunity or affirmative action approaches.

Generation as used here, and in social science, the term refers to a group within a population that were born within a specified range of years and that share a common social history or cultural experience. Social generation is sometimes also known as a birth cohort.

Inclusion refers to valuing differences in an organization and incorporating differing perspectives in all aspects of organizational life.

Institutional or **systemic racism** whereby organizations and society fail to provide service because of colour, culture, or ethnic origin.

Organizational cultural competence refers to attitudes, structures, policies, and practices that combine to enable those who work in organizations to work constructively in a diverse organization.

Race has been defined as groups of persons connected by common descent or of distinct ethic stock (Fowler & Fowler, 1964). It should be noted that the terms race and racism are based on social constructs, rather than actual genetically discrete categories.

Racialized groups refers to those groups who have been racialized, a social process that designates some group as "different" and exposes the members to experiences of unequal treatment, lack of access to services, and other forms of discrimination. The use of this term rather than racial group underscores the idea of a social process of designating a group, rather than any scientific or biological basis to the categorization of a group.

Racism is an attitude and resulting actions based on the belief that race is a key determinant of human abilities and characteristics and that some races are inherently superior to others. These attitudes and actions harm and oppress others.

Visible minority as used in some government documents in Canada refers to non-Caucasian race or non-white in colour. This term is losing its meaning and will likely change over time because non-Caucasians in some population areas are not in the minority.

CASE

Tamara lives in a large multicultural city in Canada and has worked for several years in a nursing home/long-term care facility located a suburb of the city that has a middle-class population that is predominantly Canadian-born with a European heritage. Most of the residents in the facility reflect this cultural background, with about 20 percent of the residents having immigrated to Canada 40 to 50 years earlier from Italy, Portugal, Germany, and other European countries. The staff in the facility consist of seven RNs, five who are full-time or part-time nurses in charge on all shifts, one who is a staff educator, and one who is a nurse practitioner providing primary health care services; 12 LPNs/RPNs who act as team leaders, and 35 unregulated health care workers who form the largest number of care providers. Although the RNs and RPNs are almost exclusively from the majority, white Canadian population, most of the unregulated workers who provide direct care to clients are new immigrants from the Middle East, Africa, and Southeast Asia. Tamara has recently accepted a position of Director of Care for the facility, which is a position that reports to the Administrator and has management responsibilities, as well as professional leadership responsibilities, for nursing in the facility. She is aware of tensions between regulated and unregulated workers and believes that the facility needs to pay more attention to these tensions and to management of diversity.

Questions

1. What do you think Tamara's challenges will be with respect to diversity management in her new position?

2. What kind of information do you think she might begin to collect in order to address the topic of diversity management?

3. What resources might be available to Tamara to assist her with thinking about and addressing the topic?

4. What strategies might Tamara use to begin to deal with the diverse workforce?

5. What are the potential benefits to the organization that Tamara can highlight to support addressing the topic of diversity?

6. What kinds of supports might Tamara seek from her organization to facilitate her work on managing diversity?

7. Assume that Tamara is an immigrant from India. How do you think Tamara's experience might differ if she was of Indian background, but born in Canada or a Canadian with European heritage?

Critical Thinking Questions and Activities

1. Working with another student or nurse who is in your current organization, discuss whether or not you can identify the philosophical approach the agency takes to cultural diversity.

2. Reflect on your learning in nursing courses to date that contributes to the development of develop cultural competence. Search for a cultural competency assessment tool in the literature and conduct a self-assessment.

3. Organize a small group meeting or use a clinical group that works in the same clinical setting. Using what you have learned about organizational cultural competence, collect as much information from documents and/or staff and managers as possible to find indicators of competence.

4. You have moved to a large Canadian city with a multicultural population and work in a community hospital. The community hospital is located in a suburb of the city with a large Caribbean population. What would you expect in terms of mission statement, human resources management, and community consultation in this organization with respect to culture?

5. Review RNAO's recommendations for individuals with respect to cultural competence in Table 12.2. Develop a plan to implement these recommendations for your current workplace.

6. Search the website of the regulatory body/organization for nursing in your province or territory and search for information and guidance regarding cultural competence or diversity. Use any guidelines or recommendations for your jurisdiction with respect to cultural competence, cultural diversity, or self-assessment regarding these topics.

Self-Quiz

1. An early step in embracing diversity in your workplace as an individual nurse would be to:
   a. Attend learning sessions that focus on communication and diversity.
   b. Develop knowledge about cultural norms and beliefs relevant to client groups.
   c. Explore how your biases affect others in your workplace.
   d. Find and use cultural resources in the community.

2. A health care organization that would be considered to have cultural blindness has which of the following characteristics:
   a. Seeks cultural assimilation of clients and employees.
   b. Adopts policies that destroy cultural links.
   c. Supports staff to express differing perspectives and beliefs.
   d. Seeks consultation from cultural groups.

3. One of the challenges in managing diversity when working with several generations is that:
   a. Older nurses are less respectful of authority.
   b. Younger nurses are more competitive than older nurses.
   c. Generations vary in what they find satisfying about a job.
   d. Baby boomers are dominant in the nursing workforce.

4. Managing diversity in the workplace goes beyond recruitment and retention of diverse employees in that it includes:
   a. Reducing conflicts between individuals with different views.
   b. Ensuring equal treatment of all employees.
   c. Assessing job satisfaction of nursing staff.
   d. Building a culture that values differences.

Useful Websites

The Academy of Canadian Executive Nurses
www.acen.ca

Canadian Centre for Diversity
http://centrefordiversity.ca

Canadian Nurses Association
www.cna-aiic.ca

Canadian Association of Schools of Nursing
www.casn.ca

CARE Centre for Internationally Educated Nurses (CARE)
www.care4nurses.org/

Diversity in the Workplace
http://diversityintheworkplace.ca

International Council of Nurses
www.icn.ch

Statistics Canada
www.statcan.gc.ca/start-debut-eng.html

Registered Nurses Association of Ontario
www.rnao.org

Nurse One Portal
www.nurseone.ca

References

American Nurses Assocation. (2009). *Nursing administration: Scope and standards of practice.* Silver Springs, Maryland: ANA.

Bartfay, W.J. (2007). Men in nursing in Canada: Past, present, and future perspectives. In C. E. O'Lynn & R. E. Tranbarger (Eds.). (2007). *Men in nursing. History, challenges, and opportunities.* pp. 205–218. New York: Springer.

Baumann, A., & Blythe, J. (May, 2013). Hamilton Health Sciences, Internationally Educated Nurse (IEN) and English as a Second Language (ESL) Nurse Integration Project 2012-2015. Interim Report. Series Report 37. Downloaded September 3, 2013 from http://nhsru.com/publications/series-report-37-hamilton-health-sciences-internationally-educated-nurse-ien-and-english-as-a-second-language-esl-nurse-integration-project-2012-2015.

Baumann, A., & Blythe, J. (May, 2012). *Community collaboration for IEN/ESL employment: Bridging the gap. A descriptive evaluation. Health human resources series 32.* Hamilton, Ontario: Nursing Health Services Research Unit, McMaster University.

Baxter, C. (Ed.) (2001). *Managing diversity & inequality in health care.* London: Balliere Tindall.

Beberi, W.H. (2009). Diversity within nursing. Effects on nurse-nurse interaction, job satisfaction, and turnover. *Nursing Administration Quarterly, 33*(3), 216–226.

Bowen, S. (2008). Beyond self-assessment—Assessing organizational cultural responsiveness. *Journal of Cultural Diversity, 15*(1), 7–15.

Campinha-Bacote, J., 1994. Cultural competence in psychiatric mental health nursing. *Nursing Clinics of North America 29*(1), 1–8.

Canadian Institute for Health Information (CIHI). (2009). *Regulated nurses: Canadian trends, 2005 to 2009.* Ottawa: CIHI.

Canadian Institute for Health Information (CIHI). (2010). *Regulated nurses: Canadian trends, 2006 to 20010.* Ottawa: CIHI.

Chavez, C.I., & Weisinger, J.Y. (2008). Beyond diversity training: A social infusion for cultural inclusion. *Human Resource Management, 47*(2), 331–350.

Clark, W. (1998). Religious observance. Marriage and family. *Canadian Social Trends,*

Autumn 1998, 2–7. Catalogue 11-0080XPE Statistics Canada.

Cox, T. (1991). The multicultural organization. *Academy of Management Executive*, 5(2), 34–47.

Cox, T., & Blake, S. (1991). Managing cultural diversity: implications for organizational competitiveness. *Academy of Management Executive*, 5(3), 45–56.

Cross, T., Bazron, B., Dennis, K., & Issacs, M. (1989). *Towards a culturally competent system of care, Volume 1.* Washington, DC: CASSP Tehnical Assistance Center, Centre for Child Health and Mental Health Policy, Georgetown University Child Development Center. Downloaded from http://archive.org/details/towardscultural-l00un

DeSouza, R. (2008). Developing diversity in the workforce. *Kai Tiaki Nursing New Zealand*, 14(10), 23.

Etowa, J. B., Foster, S., Vukic, A. R., Wittistock, L., & Youden, S. (2005). Recuritment and retention of minority students: Diversity in nursing education. *International Journal of Nursing Education Scholarship*, 2(1), 1–10.

Evans, J. (2004). Men nurses: a historical and feminist perspective. *Journal of Advanced Nursing*, 47(3), 321–328.

Fearon, J.D. (2003). Ethnic and cultural diversity by country. *Journal of Economic Growth*, 8, 195–222.

Flynn, K. (2009). Beyond the glass wall: Black Canadian nurses, 1940–1970. *Nursing History Review*, 17, 129–152.

Fowler, H.W., & Fowler, F.G. (eds.) (1964). *The concise Oxford dictionary of current English*, 5th ed. Toronto: Oxford University Press.

Frusti, D.K., Niesen, K.M., & Campion, J.K. (2003). Creating a culturally competent organization. Use of the Diversity Competency Model. *Journal of Nursing Administration*, 33(1), 31–38.

Gardenswartz, L., & Rowe, A. (1998). *Managing diversity in health care*. San Francisco: Jossey-Bass.

Hart-Wasekeesikaw, F. (2009). *Cultural competence and cultural safety in nursing education. A Framework for First Nations, Inuit and Métis nursing. Making it happen: Strengthening First Nation, Inuit and Métis health human resources*. Ottawa: Aboriginal Nurses Assocaition of Canada.

Hyman, I. (2009). *Racism as a determinant of immigrant health. Policy brief commissioned and funded by the Strategic Initiatives and Innovations Directorate (SIID) of the Public Health Agency of Canada*. Submitted March 30, 2009. Downloaded November 2, 2012, from http://canada.metropolis.net/pdfs/racism_policy_brief_e.pdf

Jonsen, K., Maznevski, M.L., & Schneider, S.C. (2011). Diversity and its not so diverse literature: An international perspective. *International Journal of Cross Cultural Management*, 11(1), 35–62.

Kalra, V.S., Abel, P., & Esmail, A. (2009). Developing leadership interventions for Black and minority ethnic staff. A case study of the National Health Service (NHS) in the UK. *Journal of Health Organization and Management*. 23(1), 103–118.

King, E.B., Dawson, J.F., West, M.A., Gilrane, V.L., Peddie, C.I., & Bastin, L. (2011). Why organizational and community diversity matter: Representativeness and the emergence of incivility and organizational performance. *Academy of Management Journal*, 54(6), 1103–1118.

Keogh, B.J., & O'Lynn, C.E. (2007). Gender-based barriers for male student nurses in general nursing education programs: An Irish perspective. In C.E. O'Lynn & R.E. Tranbarger (Eds.). (2007). *Men in nursing. History, challenges, and opportunities*. pp. 193–204. New York: Springer.

Kleinman, C.S. (2004). Understanding and capitalizing on men's advantages in nursing. *Journal of Nursing Administration*, 34(2), 78–82.

Lane, N. (2000). The management implications of women's employment disadvantage in a female-dominated profession: A study of NHS nursing. *Journal of Management Studies*, 34, 705-731.

LaRocco, S.A. (2007). Recruitment and retention of men in nursing. In C.E. O'Lynn

& R.E. Tranbarger (Eds.). (2007). *Men in nursing. History, challenges, and opportunities.* pp. 241–253. New York: Springer.

Lavoie-Tremblay, M., O'Brien-Pallas, L., Gélinas, C., Desforges, N., & Marchionni, C. (2008). Addressing the turnover issue among new nurses from a generational viewpoint. *Journal of Nursing Management, 16,* 724–33.

Leininger, M. (1995). Cultural care theory, research, and practice. *Nursing Science Quarterly, 9*(2), 71–74.

Lester, S.W., Standifer, R.L., Schultz, N.J., & Windsor, J.M. (2012). Actual versus perceived generational differences at work: An empirical examination. *Journal of Leadership & Organizational Studies, 19*(3), 341–354.

Meadus, R. J. (2000). Men in nursing: Barriers to recruitment. *Nursing Forum, 35,* 5–12.

National Expert Commission. (2012). *A nursing call to action. The health of our nation, the future of our health system.* Ottawa: Canadian Nurses Association.

Olavarria, M., Beaulac, J., Bélanger, A., Young, M., & Aubry, T. (2009). Organizational cultural competence in community health and social service organizations: How to conduct a self-assessment. *Journal of Cultural Diversity, 16*(4), 140–150.

Pearson, A., Srivasatava, R., Craig, D., Tucker, D., Grinspun, D., Bajnok, I., Griffin, P., Long, L., Porritt, K., Han, T., & Gi, A.A. (2007). Systematic review on embracing cultural diversity for developing and sustaining a healthy work environment in healthcare. *International Journal of Evidence Based Healthcare, 5,* 54–91.

Porter-O'Grady, T. (2007). Reverse discrimination in nursing leadership: hitting the concrete ceiling. In C.E. O'Lynn & R.E. Tranbarger (eds.). (2007). *Men in nursing. History, challenges, and opportunities.* pp. 143–151. New York: Springer.

Purnell, L.D. (2007). Men in nursing: An international perspective. In C.E. O'Lynn & R.E. Tranbarger (eds.). (2007). *Men in nursing. History, challenges, and opportunities.* pp. 219–235. New York: Springer.

Registered Nurses Association of Ontario. (2007). *Healthy work environments best practice guidelines. Embracing cultural diversity in health care: Developing cultural competence.* Toronto: RNAO.

Schim, S.M., Doorenbos, A.Z., & Borse, N.N. (2005). Cultural competence among Ontario and Michigan healthcare providers. *Journal of Nursing Scholarship, 37*(4), 354–360.

Scott, K.A., Heathcote, J.M., & Gruman, J.A. (2011). The diverse organization: Finding gold at the end of the rainbow. *Human Resource Management, 50*(6), 735–755.

Spector, R.E. (2004). *Cultural diversity in health & illness.* 6th ed. Upper Saddle River, New Jersey: Pearson.

Spinks, N., & Moore, C. (2007). The changing workforce, workplace and nature of work: Implications for health human resource management. *Nursing Leadership, 20*(3), 26–41.

Statistics Canada. (2008a). *Canada's ethnocultural mosaic, 2006 census. Catalogue number 97-562-X.* Ottawa: Ministry of Industry.

Statistics Canada. (2008b). *Demographics at a glance. Catalogue number 91-003-X.* Ottawa: Ministry of Industry.

Statistics Canada. (2009). *Aboriginal peoples in Canada in 2006: Inuit, Métis and First Nations, 2006 census: Findings.* Ottawa: Author. Available from www.statcan.ca

Statistics Canada. (2010). Study: Projections of the diversity of the Canadian population 2006 to 2031. *The Daily,* March 9, 2010. Available from www.statcan.ca

Statistics Canada. (2012). *Fifty years of families in Canada: 1961 to 2011. Families, households and marital status, 2011 census of population. Catalogue no. 98-312-X2011003.* Available from www.statcan.ca

Wilson, A.H., Sanner, S., & McAllister, L.E. (2010). An evaluation study of a mentoring program to increase the diversity of the nursing workforce. *Journal of Cultural Diversity, 17*(4), 144–150.

Wilson, B., Squires, M., Widger, K., Cranley, L., & Tourangeau, A. (2008). Job satisfaction among a multigenerational nursing workforce. *Journal of Nursing Management, 16,* 716, 723.

Wortsman, A., & Crupi, A. (2009). *From textbooks to texting. Addressing issues of intergenerational diversity in the nursing workplace*. Ottawa: Canadian Federation of Nurses Unions.

Yang, Y., & Konrad, A.M. (2011). Understanding diversity management practices: Implications of institutional theory and resource-based theory. *Group and Organizational Management, 36*(1), 6–38.

Chapter 13
Financial Leadership and Accountability in Nursing

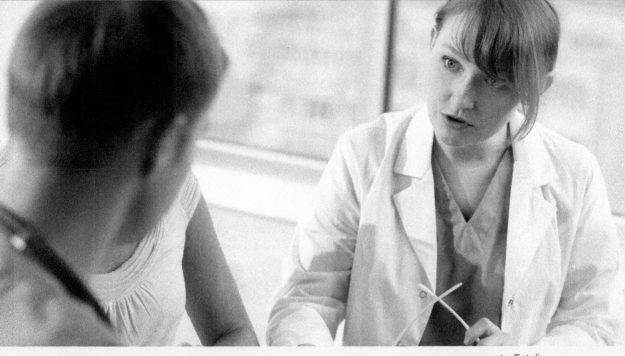

pressmaster/Fotolia

Learning Objectives

After reading, studying, and reflecting on this chapter's content, you will be able to:

1. Discuss the meaning of accountability and the types of accountabilities that health professionals and health care organizations have
2. Describe the responsibilities that nurse leaders have in managing resources of all types
3. Differentiate between operating budgets and capital budgets, and identify different approaches to budgeting
4. Differentiate between and identify fixed, variable, direct, and indirect costs in your workplace
5. Describe the process of operational budgeting in a health care organization
6. Discuss the challenge of balancing financial performance and quality improvement in nursing

INTRODUCTION

Nurses, no matter where they work in a health care organization, are accountable for their actions. In this chapter we begin with a broad discussion of accountability and what it means to be accountable, followed by a focus on accountability in health care and in nursing. During your work in health care, you will also have some financial accountability, and we identify some beginning-level financial competencies before focusing on those of nurse managers and executives. Because you will work with those who bear primary responsibility for the financial aspects of nursing care, you will feel the effects of their leadership and management ability. To support and assist nurse leaders in the workplace, you should understand some of the basics of budgeting and finance, as well as what it means to be accountable for these aspects of nursing services. Nurse managers must not only exhibit financial leadership, they must also account for nursing performance and clinical care within the organization. Balancing cost and quality is a challenge that requires leadership, managerial knowledge and skill, and an understanding of how to use clinical and financial data to make decisions and account for performance. In the following sections you will be introduced to some financial and performance accountability terms that will assist you in understanding this aspect of nurse leadership.

THE CONCEPT OF ACCOUNTABILITY

In democratic countries, **accountability** is often discussed in terms of governments being accountable or answerable to citizens. In recent decades, there has been much discussion of the accountability of health care systems to citizens and the meaning of such accountability (Fooks & Maslove, 2004; Macdonald, 1999). In an analysis of the concept, Fooks and Maslove identified the following six elements of accountability:

- Establishment of a relationship—a relationship between those making decisions and those affected—is required
- Agreed-upon defined responsibility—defined responsibilities are decided between parties (individual or organization) so that decisions and actions can be taken by the one accountable
- Delegate or confer authority—those with the authority to take action can delegate to others; for example, a provincial government can delegate to a regional authority or a health agency
- Answerability—those who are accountable, answer for decisions and actions, justify and explain them, and these answers may be public ones
- Performance—refers to the requirement to account for action, which involves a judgment about performance
- Sanction/correction—refers to the requirement for correcting for unmet standard of performance

Accountability in Health Care

Types of accountability within health care include financial accountability (by those who receive public resources for health care), managerial accountability (for effective and efficient use of resources), political accountability (elected officials need to respond to citizens and make good on commitments), and professional accountability (for maintaining professional standards) (Fooks & Maslove, 2004). Throughout your program, you have learned about your accountability as a health care professional—as a member of a self-regulating profession, you will be accountable to your licensing/registering body for your professional practice. If you are employed as a health care professional by an organization, you will also be accountable to that organization for the responsible use of organizational resources. For example, as a staff nurse in the immunization program of a public health unit, you are responsible for the appropriate use of resources, such as vaccines and supplies, and thus have financial accountability to the public health unit.

In health care, nurse executives and managers have financial, managerial, and professional accountability. Using the elements listed on page 384, you can see that when a nurse executive assumes a position within a health care organization, a relationship is established between that nurse and the organization. The employing institution defines the responsibilities and the nurse agrees to these when the appointment is accepted, thus enabling the nurse to make decisions and take actions appropriate for the scope of the responsibilities of the position. The nurse executive may delegate authority to nurse managers and others in the organization, but is answerable to higher authorities (vertical) for decisions and actions that are taken. While managerial accountability involves delegation of authority and activities to others, accountability is not delegated. Part of the nurse executive's accountability involves reporting on decisions, actions, and results so that performance can be judged and corrective actions can be taken, if necessary. These performance and financial reports form part of the information material that is given regularly to the governing board of a health organization, for example, the board of directors of a public hospital.

Accountabilities in health care, including the accountabilities of health professionals, are summarized in Table 13.1.

Accountability in Nursing

Porter-O'Grady and Malloch (2013) identify accountability and ownership as the centrepiece of professional practice. They consider the professionalization of nursing in the twentieth century as "the path to accountability" and a path that began with Florence Nightingale, whom they describe as "the original accountability-based nurse leader" (p. 489). They do not use the terms *responsibility* and *accountability* interchangeably (although many authors do), as they believe that the term accountability is a more modern one that is results-focused or outcome-oriented and that would reflect the difference between someone who viewed his or her work as a professional role, rather than a job. In Table 13.2 you will see the ways in which they distinguish responsibility from accountability.

Table 13.1   Health Care Accountability

Actor	Primary Accountability	Type of Accountability	Direction of Accountability	Accountability Mechanism
Government	Citizens	Financial	Vertical	Citizen Governance
				Public Reporting
		Managerial	Vertical	Citizen Governance
				Public Reporting
		Political	Vertical	Citizen Governance
Regulators	Government	Financial	Vertical	Citizen Governance
				Public Reporting
		Managerial	Vertical	Citizen Governance
				Public Reporting
Quality Agencies	Government	Financial	Horizontal	Citizen Governance
				Public Reporting
		Managerial	Horizontal	Citizen Governance
				Public Reporting
RHAs	Government	Financial	Vertical	Citizen Governance
				Public Reporting
		Managerial	Vertical	Citizen Governance
				Public Reporting
	Citizens	Financial	Vertical	Citizen Governance
				Public Reporting
		Managerial	Vertical	Citizen Governance
				Public Reporting
				Citizen Engagement*
Health Care Facilities	Government	Financial	Vertical	Citizen Governance
				Public Reporting
		Managerial	Vertical	Citizen Governance
				Public Reporting
		Patients	Vertical	Legal
Health Professionals	Patients	Professional	Vertical	Legal
	Facilities (if employees)	Financial	Vertical	Legal
		Managerial	Vertical	Legal
	Regulators	Professional	Vertical	Legal

* RHAs in some provinces have begun to engage their communities in needs assessments or some form of community consultation about priorities.

Table 13.2 Responsibility Versus Accountability

Responsibility (20th Century)	Accountability (21st Century)
Process	Product
Action	Result
Work	Outcome
Do	Accomplish
Task	Difference
Function	Fit
Job	Role
Incremental	Sustainable
Externally generated	Internally generated
Quality effort	Quality impact

Source: O'Grady, Tim Porter, Malloch, Kathy, Leadership in nursing practice: Changing the landscape of health care, Jones and Bartlett Learning, © 2013. Reprinted with permission of Jones and Bartlett Learning.

Dohmann and Hahn (2011) also distinguish between accountability and responsibility, and they emphasize the meaning of accountability as a commitment to deliver and report on or explain a result. Financial accountability refers to the wise use of financial resources (Macdonald, 1999), and although all nurses have the responsibility not to waste or misuse health care resources, such as supplies and equipment, nursing management is answerable for the effective use of resources in a health care organization. For example, a nurse manager who has made a commitment to reduce the **staffing budget** for a clinical unit by a specific amount is accountable when he or she takes specific action to accomplish that goal, reports regularly on the results of the plan, and explains how and why it did or did not achieve the intended financial outcomes. Therefore, it would not be accountable for the manager to simply say: "I succeeded in reducing the budget for staffing as promised, but I have no idea how." A nurse manager might not achieve the results desired, but is still accountable, in that the manager "owns" the results and develops new plans to achieve improvements in performance. Similarly, a nurse practitioner in a small primary health care organization is accountable for meeting the needs of clients while using diagnostic equipment and supplies appropriately.

The International Council of Nurses (ICN) (2008) makes the point that knowledge and skills on financial management are required by nurses who have major responsibilities for making financial decisions and allocating resources in health care. The ICN emphasizes that financial management is required if resources are to be available due to what seems to be constant factors: finite, and often limited resources, increasing needs for health care and increasing expectations for new services, and an emphasis on efficient use of resources, and rising standards and regulation of quality. It is important to remember that organizational goals are pursued by nurses and others in health care while balancing what is to be achieved with the costs of achieving them. This balancing act calls for financial and **resource management**.

RESOURCE MANAGEMENT

Resource management refers to the management of cash, people, equipment, and buildings so that the mission and goals of the organization are achieved at an expected level of performance. Anyone who works in a health care organization carries some responsibility for the appropriate use and management of resources. Nurse executives and nurse managers have responsibilities for the development and implementation of financial policies and a **budget**, but leadership with respect to resource management can be exhibited by all nurses within a health care organization.

In the early stages of your nursing career you will exhibit novice behaviours in resource management, progressing to advanced beginner, particularly as you experience clinical or other leadership opportunities in an organization. As a beginning nurse you can appreciate the importance of cost-consciousness in health care and learn to balance cost and quality in your use of health care resources. You also can begin to learn about the financial terminology and reports that are used in your workplace and contribute through committees or workplace meetings to the generation of cost-saving ideas and preparation of budgets that contribute to cost-efficient operations in your organization. In working with nurse managers and nurse executives or other organizational leaders, you can contribute to the achievement of goals that enhance patient care and consider the range of resources required to provide services and achieve goals. However, development of the knowledge and skills required for competent, proficient, and expert behaviours with respect to resource management will require information, continuing education, and formal graduate education (Dreisbach, 1994; Pintar, Capuano, & Rosser, 2007; Gould, Goldstone, & Maidwell, 2001).

Human Resource Management

A key aspect of resource management refers to working with people and managing human resources in a way that is cost-effective in achieving the organizational goals. In a large health care organization like a hospital, the major expenditure for the nursing cost centre is the personnel or staffing budget (Carroll, Lacey, & Cox, 2004). Nurses, who provide care on in-patient units on a 24-hours-a-day/7days-a-week basis, normally represent the largest employee group in a hospital. The staffing budget is based on a staffing plan, as discussed in Chapter 8, a plan that is driven in part by the philosophy and model of nursing care used in the organization. The plan considers the numbers and staff mix required to provide care on the unit, but some system of assessing changes in the basic staffing levels, such as patient classification systems or acuity measures, enable staffing levels to be adjusted as required. As the largest component of the budget, it is not surprising that it may be the first one scrutinized in times of budget restraint. In times of economic difficulty, such as the deficit-cutting by governments in the 1990s, great pressure is put on nurse executives and nurse managers to reduce staffing costs. Nurse leaders must use all of their knowledge and skill to make wise decisions and to influence other decision makers in the organization. Several issues arise when some strategies are seen as simple "fixes" for the "problem" of nurse staffing costs (ICN, 2008):

- Staff substitution—replacing qualified nurses with less qualified staff to save money. Examples include substituting licensed practical nurses for registered nurses or unregulated staff for licensed practical nurses. While changing the mix of staff may be appropriate, care must be taken that changes are based on clear principles and a defensible philosophy of nursing care delivery. Otherwise, such an approach can lead to reduced quality of care and result in increased costs, if inappropriate care is provided.

- Reduction in staffing levels—to reduce costs, as opposed to responding to evidence of the need to correct an overstaffing situation, reduces the quality of care. It can result in nurse burnout, errors, and accidents, which ultimately cost more and can cause irreversible damage to patients and the organization.

- **Casualization**—refers to a strategy of reducing staffing costs by hiring a greater percentage of part-time or casual staff or by using agency staff. Use of casual staff can be positive in that it provides flexibility in staffing for those times when unusual events or volumes of activity require additional staff. The cost savings generally relate to the costs of benefits, particularly vacation and sick leave. However, if used to excess casualization can incur higher costs and decreased quality of care, including lack of continuity of care.

The nurse manager must therefore be skilled at examining staffing costs and identifying problems and issues that should be addressed. For example, what are the costs and benefits of using agency or casual nursing staff versus hiring additional full-time staff for a unit that is experiencing higher acuity rates? Value in staffing cannot be measured by dollars alone or by viewing nursing as a series of tasks that any nurse can do, without considering continuity of care, level of experience of nurses on a unit, level of training needed, and other factors. While the manager must be able to use the language of finance and use data to make decisions, the ability to address issues that affect staffing costs depends on leadership skills in communicating with and working with people. For example, seeking benchmarks on absenteeism from similar units in the hospital or peer hospitals is one way a manager can begin to use data to examine an issue. By identifying the absenteeism rate in an exemplary organization, a person can use this as a target to achieve in his or her own organization. However, open discussion and consultation with nursing staff on the unit to examine the issue and seek solutions is essential if the unit as a team is going to achieve a desired target.

Asset Management

Assessment management refers to the assessment, planning, and purchase of equipment or facilities as well as the upgrade or maintenance and care of these. Nurse managers in large organizations must have input into the decisions required in asset management for equipment and facilities needed to provide nursing care, which ICN (2008, p. 33) describes as:

- Assessment of new technologies
- Planning new facilities or upgrading current facilities
- Purchasing or upgrading equipment

- Determining priorities for expenditure
- Determining staffing and training requirements

An asset or equipment inventory is maintained in the organization for items of substantial value, so that information is available on when an asset was purchased, built, or renovated; its cost; and the schedule for maintenance and replacement.

Supplies Management

Supplies include such things as food, drugs, cleaning materials, and one-use products. Many medical supplies are considered consumables as they must be replaced once used, unlike capital equipment, which has a considerable shelf life. Supplies represent a major cost category for health care organizations, particularly acute care hospitals and nursing homes. In large organizations, there are often management information systems for managing the purchase, inventory, and timing of supplies and to analyze changes in costs and quality. Nurse managers oversee substantial volumes of supplies, such as dressings, I/V tubing, and other disposable equipment used by nurses in the delivery of care. They need to analyze financial and inventory control reports to ensure the appropriate use of such materials. In Box 13.1 you will find a description of one example of a project aimed at reducing the cost of nursing care by decreasing supply waste.

Box 13.1

A Budget Awareness Campaign to Reduce Supply Waste

In order to reduce nursing costs, nurse administrators and educators at the Staten Island University Hospital in the United States embarked on a project to make the costs of supplies and their waste visible to employees. An interdisciplinary team of staff RNs and nursing leadership, staff development, and the supply management vice president was formed to direct the project to address supply waste. Councils and staff meetings reviewed supply data and deviations from budgeted supply amounts. Actual supply costs were included in budget information provided by newsletters and formed the basis for discussion at staff meetings. Managers received monthly summaries of unit expenditures to share with staff. Various incentives were considered, such as use of unit savings to purchase key equipment and incorporating supply reductions into employee performance evaluations. The project team considered a wide variety of ideas that came from suggestions, such as finding a convenient spot for items that are frequently used to avoid "stashing" and changing components in sterile kits to reduce the cost by excluding infrequently used items. For example, dressing change kits, IV start kits, and central line catheter insertion kits costs were reduced by changing components, such as including single use tape rather than a full roll of tape.

After the campaign was implemented, expenditures on supplies decreased by $500,000. The project extended to other units, and the ICU Collaborative Council projected an annual savings of $116,000 following a review of supply waste in medical-surgical supplies. As a part of the project, this campaign was incorporated into nurse orientation to the hospital and the nurse manager's regular role changed to include the regular provision of budget information to staff. Monthly tools included details of actual versus budget for salary and supplies; details of charges and expenses to vendors of supplies; a report of supplies by amount and the costs; and unit specific report cards on supply spending. Based on the experience with this campaign, the project team believed that it is better to use volume rather than dollars when evaluating waste because pricing changes affect comparisons.

Source: Johnson, D., Bell, B., Elgendy, J., McDonald, E., West, F., Wenzel, L., Malach, B., & DiStefano, M. (2012). Don't waste green! Launching a budget awareness campaign. *Nursing Management, 43*(8), 51–54.

BUDGETING

Nurses in all positions within an organization, including small ones, usually become aware of the realities of budgets during periods of fiscal restraint. What is most noticeable to the nurse is when resources are constrained to the point that there are shortages of personnel, equipment, and supplies. At those times, nurses are apt to hear more discussion about budgets. A budget is simply a financial plan for income and expenditures, usually for a one-year period. A **fiscal year** refers to the time period for a budget, and it varies from one organization to another. For example, in one province, hospitals may operate on a fiscal year that runs between April 1st in one year and ends March 31st the next year. The dates used relate to the budgeting year of the provincial government that provides the major source of revenue for hospitals as an operating grant. Another organization might use the calendar year January 1st to December 31st as its fiscal year.

There are several kinds of budgets, but the following are the ones commonly referred to in discussions of organizational budgets in health care, and you should understand these different terms.

- **Operating budget** refers to the budget of estimated revenues and expenses for the daily operation of an organization over a period of time, normally a one-year period. It includes the normal operating expenses expected in the daily functioning of the organization and has fairly detailed categories.
- **Capital budget** refers to budgets developed for purchase of items that endure, for example equipment that lasts a number of years, the purchase of major equipment, or the substantial renovation of a building or the construction of a new building(s). Capital costs do not include the costs required to operate or maintain the equipment or new building.
- **Program budget** is a financial plan for a specific area of activity, a planned new activity or service, or a special project. These budgets may be produced when making a decision on whether to add the activity or because they cut across a number of existing departments, or they extend beyond a one-year operating budget but are time-limited.

An organization can have all three kinds of budgets and more, confusing to those who work in the organization. For example, a large organization such as an academic health centre may be engaged in major renovation of its operating rooms and new capital construction projects, such as a parking garage, a family practice building, and a research building. These capital costs are budgeted quite separately from the annual operating budget, and sometimes employees may not understand why they are being asked to conserve supplies because of reduced operating income in a fiscal year at a time when the organization is spending funds on new buildings. Normally, buildings and major equipment are planned years in advance as capital items are purchased to have several years of benefit, and their costs are usually recovered over several years. Therefore, purchase of magnetic resonance imaging (MRI) equipment, which cost millions of dollars, is considered a capital expenditure rather than an operating expense, although the salary costs of the technicians are paid annually and form part of the annual operating budget.

Because of the need to regularly replace equipment in an organization, nurse managers ask direct care nurses annually to submit requests for new or replacement capital equipment. There is normally a lower limit for items to be submitted for this kind of budget, and smaller amounts, for example anything under $10,000, does not require a specific request and justification because it is just part of the regular operating budget. However, if the intensive care nursery requires new isolettes or a post-anaesthetic recovery room requires a large number of intravenous pumps, these requests may be expected to be submitted for consideration in the "small" capital equipment budget.

Budgeting Approaches

The approach to budgeting varies by health care organization and the setting for that organization. In Canada, most health care organizations are publicly funded ones that obtain the majority of their revenue from provincial/territorial governments. The funder or allocator of budgets, such as a regional health authority, therefore sets requirements for the format of a budget that is submitted for approval. One format may be used for internal purposes, for example for submission to a board of directors, and another format is used for submission to an external funder. Typically, a new program that an organization adds to its existing range of services requires a program budget that can be examined and analyzed separately from the overall operating budget, so that explicit decisions are made about funding the new service.

Zero-based budgeting is a budgeting methodology that requires beginning from zero for each cost and building the budget from the ground up. This approach is used in determining the budget for a special purpose or a new program, but has been adopted by many organizations to move away from the traditional **incremental budgeting** approach. In incremental budgeting, most of the change in an operating budget from one year to the next is based on how much the budget should increase based on the assumption that the only change required is a cost-of-living increase. Budgets would be submitted for approval based on a 1, 3, or 5 percent increase and justified based on documented inflation estimates. There are concerns that incremental budgeting leads to bloated budgets as the focus of discussions is about relatively minor adjustments and there may be a failure to scrutinize costs in depth. Incremental budgeting is based on the assumption that the past budget is sufficiently precise in predicting the future budget.

In zero-based budgeting, the intent is to justify every cost and to avoid the tendency for costs to increase each year, without consideration of how new technology, changing procedures, or alternative ways of providing care might be used to lower costs. The downside of this approach is the amount of work required to prepare the budget and analyze alternatives.

Budgeting Process

The process of budgeting varies from one health care organization to another, but in general, three steps are involved: planning and development, obtaining approval, and implementing and controlling the budget.

Budget Preparation

The budgeting process begins in large health care organizations many months before the budget is submitted for approval to a governing body. Input from external and internal stakeholders is required to build an annual operating budget, but major guidance comes from such documents as the mission statement and strategic (or business) plan of the health care organization (ICN, 2008). In Chapter 5 we discussed strategic planning and noted that financial and operational plans are developed that enable accomplishment of strategic plans. Annual operating plans, developed from multi-year strategic plans, identify operational goals and targets for the year. Such plans require input from nursing staff and nurse managers, who oversee the development of a budget. Although a goal may not be accomplished in a one-year time frame, managers who are accountable for a goal must ensure that activities to be undertaken toward the goal during the fiscal year are sufficiently resourced in the annual operating budget to ensure success. In some organizations the budgeting process is overseen by the finance department, a budget committee, or the senior management team. In large organizations, a finance department prepares guidelines, a timeline, and financial expertise to managers (Finkler & McHugh, 2008; Nestman, 1992) as they prepare and develop their budgets. The budgets prepared by each unit or department must adhere to the guidelines or be thoroughly justified, and these are all combined so that the total budget can be reviewed and adjusted if expenditures exceed revenues.

Budgets consist of various types of costs and you will hear these terms used by those who prepare and work with budgets and financial plans. **Fixed costs** refer to those expenses that do not change, no matter what the volume of service is on a nursing or other budget unit. For example, even when there is a slow period, such as a holiday period, in a small clinic practice, the monthly rent or monthly salary of the full-time office manager must be paid. In contrast, **variable costs** refer to those that change as the volume of services change, for example medical supply costs for dressings or syringes that increase as more clients are provided with services. As volumes may vary on a seasonal or other basis, costs are not necessarily incurred evenly across a budget year. Often, costs can be estimated by looking at the previous year's budget, but this does not always work, as costs rise, changes in the environment (for example, a cold or snowy winter affects heating and snow removal), and other fluctuations occur that make cost estimation imperfect. A **responsibility centre** refers to a unit or activity within an organization to which costs can be attributed, and it is therefore referred to as a **cost centre**, for example a neurology unit. In some cases, revenue can be attributed to a responsibility centre and may referred to as a **revenue centre**. A department may be a single responsibility centre or made up of several ones. Both fixed and variable costs can be **direct costs** or **indirect costs**. A direct cost is one that can be attributed to producing a service, for example in providing direct care to a client, while indirect costs support care activity, but are not incurred at the bedside (Dowless, 2007; Wodchis, 1998). Indirect costs are usually allocated to departments based on some formula. For example, housekeeping and maintenance costs can be attributed to departments using a square footage formula or human resource department costs are allocated to direct care departments based on the numbers of employees in the department (Borsa & Anis, 2005). These indirect costs are also referred to as overhead costs. Table 13.3 provides some examples of cost categories and cost items you might find in a small community health centre that provides primary health care services and home care services.

As mentioned earlier, personnel or staffing budgets are usually the largest part of the nursing manager's budget for a unit or department. This component of the operating budget includes the costs of benefits and consideration of the cost effectiveness of some combination of full-time, part-time, casual, and temporary staff. Care must be taken to ensure coverage required for statutory holidays, vacation time, illness, staff orientation and other education events, or other absences. In Canada, most registered nurses and licensed practical nurses who work in hospitals are paid according to a negotiated collective agreement, many of which are multi-year ones, so these major staffing costs are usually known or predictable. Over time, staffing plans must be adjusted, and changes in services and the environment may increase or reduce the staffing needs of an organization. Therefore, the nurse leader must analyze past staffing and forecast future staffing using knowledge of new procedures and developments in health care and the realities of the health care environment (Stichler, 2008). Goddard (2003) identified frequent flaws in staffing and personnel budgeting, and these included failure to understand and define the workloads of specific departments, lack of tools for forecasting workloads in a precise way, and failure to document workload and workflow patterns so that planning for staffing can improve.

Not all budgets that nurses develop are done within large organizations where they may find considerable resources for support and help with budget preparation. Some nurses prepare these as part of a response to a request for proposals (RFPs) from government or related organization for a nursing project, new service, commissioned report, or research on some topic. For example, as highlighted in Chapter 3 on power and politics, the first nurse-led primary health care clinic in Ontario was established by two NPs who had to develop budget proposals for a health care organization that did not yet exist (Heale & Butcher, 2010). They had a vision for a NP-led clinic model that would provide access to primary health care in an underserviced area. Therefore, much in the way that a strategic plan guides budget proposals, this mission and their values guided their proposal development, which included a budget. Heale and Butcher were "very clear that full and comprehensive funding was essential for the success of the NP-led clinical model"

Table 13.3 **Classification of Some Costs in a Community Health Centre**

Cost Category	Cost Centre and Cost Items		
Fixed (expense does not vary with volume)	Indirect (general)	CENTRE BUILDING Rent or mortgage payments Maintenance and security Salaries and benefits Repairs, insurance, hydro Snow removal, landscaping	ADMINISTRATION Adminstrator and support staff Computers Telecommunications Office printing Office staff training Travel costs
	Direct (service)	PRIMARY HEALTH CARE Cleaning equipment Linen supplies Professional consultation	HOME CARE Transportation Vehicle repair and maintenance
Variable (expense varies with volume)	Indirect (general)	PRIMARY HEALTH CARE HOME CARE Cleaning services Travel expenses	HOME CARE Travel expenses

	Direct (service)	PRIMARY HEALTH CARE
		Salaries and benefits
		  Nurse practitioners
		  Physicians
		Medical supplies
		Medications & vaccines
		Diagnostic supplies
			HOME CARE
			Salaries and benefits
			  Registered Nurses
			  Licensed Practical Nurses
			Medical supplies

(p. 25). In the past, some NP positions were not funded with the clerical support and other infrastructure that enabled them to focus fully on clinical practice. Heale and Butcher networked with the professional association and others, reworked unsuccessful proposals, and identified a template used for a family health team model that they could adapt and submit for funding that would achieve "a consistent source of funding" for the envisioned clinic. If you need help with budgeting for a health service or small project and you are not in an organization that can provide administrative or financial expertise, you can explore external sources of help that range from textbooks and articles to consulting with your professional association to hiring an accountant or someone with financial experience in health care. Finding a template that you can use or adapt for your budget proposal is very helpful as it will aid your consideration of the kinds of costs to include, because it may be difficult, if not impossible, to ask for additional funds after approval of your proposed budget.

Obtaining Approval of a Budget

In Canada, most health care organizations have a governing board of directors that reviews and approves of annual budgets prepared by administrators and managers. The board may have a committee that does this review on behalf of the board and makes a recommendation for approval or non-approval followed by a formal vote at a board meeting. The chief executive officer (CEO) and the senior management team answer any questions about the budget and must be prepared to justify items and/or projects, in particular new services or expenditures of any size. Although there was a time when governing boards of health care organizations would approve a **deficit budget** if there was a clear plan to recover and balance the budget in subsequent year(s), approval of a deficit budget is less likely in the current economic environment. The board is apt to send the budget back to the team for revision to ensure that it is balanced. Balance can only be achieved by increasing revenues, more difficult in systems in which government funding is the major source of revenue, or by cutting expenses.

When the budget is not balanced after all of the departmental budgets have been consolidated into one organizational budget, sometimes the senior management team decides where reductions to the proposed budget should be made, for example, by dropping a service that is established or a new service or project that has been proposed and included in the budget for the first time. Cutting an existing service is normally not the approach taken on short notice, as it is presumably a valued service and subject to resistance by those who use the service and who work in that area. New projects or services are responses to a current need or an approach to improving what exists, so this option is also not an attractive one. Difficult decisions must be made by the management team. Depending on the size of the reduction required to balance the budget, all departments may be required to reduce their budgets by a certain percentage, known as "across-the-board" cuts. This approach has frequently been used when a small percentage reduction is required by all departments; however, it is criticized because it penalizes departments that have managed their resources well and have eliminated all of the "fat" from their budget. Other than reducing expenditures or increasing revenues, the only other approach to maintaining service levels while maintaining quality is finding more efficient ways of doing things. Nurse executives and nurse managers in an organization must do their part to prepare balanced budgets and to seek ways to control costs while maintaining and even improving quality of care. Governments or a regional health authority, which are major funders of such organizations as hospitals, expect budgets to be balanced and, depending on the jurisdiction, will insist on balanced operating budgets.

Implementing a Budget and Budget Control

The planned budget must be implemented during the fiscal year, and this step in budgeting involves monitoring performance and controlling costs so that performance is in accordance with the budget plan. Just like the family budget, regular scrutiny of expenditures and activities is required to ensure that costs are under control. If they are not, the family has to take corrective action and get things back on track so as not to incur unwanted debt that will increase costs more in the long run. In an organization, budgetary control is based on the idea that every activity is the responsibility of someone, so budgeting and monitoring relate to a responsibility centre, and the person with that responsibility regularly reviews financial performance in terms of the budget plan (Nestman, 1992). Nurse managers must compare actual performance to the planned or budgeted performance and make adjustments as necessary (Cherry and Jacob, 2008). To do this, managers receive regular reports from financial reporting systems and do a **variance analysis** of the budget categories for their unit (Finkler & McHugh, 2008; ICN, 2008). Nurse managers may be required to submit a **variance report** in which they explain why actual expenses are higher than budget targets for specific costs (Carruth, Carruth, & Noto, 2000). As an example, an unusually high number of patients with cognitive impairment on a unit during a particular month can increase the costs of sitters during that period. In some cases, the monthly report divides the annual amount for an expense into 12 to allocate it evenly throughout the year, even though this linear approach does not always reflect how expenses are incurred. For example, you would expect heating costs to be higher during the winter months, which might explain a negative variance (or seeming overspending) for a particular month, even though the budgeted amount was the same for every month of the year. More **flexible budgets** refer to financial systems that account for reports that are adjusted for expected variations in activities, but these may not be available in an organization or in a project situation that does not have a sophisticated financial system. Flexible budgets can assist the manager in interpreting variance and is most often used for variations in volumes of services. For example, during a major vacation period, the volume of procedures may be expected to be reduced and you could plan for reduced staffing costs during that budget period.

Variances can be explained by many changes that occur during a budget year, from unexpected changes in patient/client or procedure volumes; price changes in drugs, medical equipment, and supplies; or unusual events. An example of the latter took place in 2003 when Toronto experienced the Severe Acute Respiratory Syndrome (SARS) crisis, and hospitals in that city were faced with a crisis management situation involving staff shortages due to quarantine requirements and huge infection control equipment and supply costs (Nagle & Vincent, 2003). Since staffing costs are major ones, nurse managers must address problems that are evident in such indicators as high absenteeism and high staff turnover. Job dissatisfaction will be reflected in high costs for orienting new staff and high levels of replacement staff due to absences. Skilled leadership in human resource management is required to ensure an environment that attracts and retains nurses.

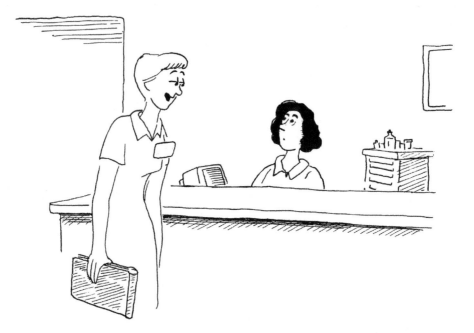

I think we have Mr. Smith's blood sugar balanced.
Now, if we could just balance the unit budget!

Cartoonresource/Shutterstock

BALANCING FINANCIAL PERFORMANCE AND QUALITY IMPROVEMENT

As has been described, nursing leaders at all levels of accountability in health care organizations are involved in budget preparation and monitoring. However, prior to establishing the annual operating budget, decisions are made about strategic goals that involve nurse leaders in decisions that determine what will be included in the budget. Quality improvement is an ongoing challenge for health care organizations and nurse managers lead and participate in design and choice of projects that improve performance while making sense in terms of both benefits and costs.

These was a time when nursing leadership and finance leadership in health care organizations had such differing responsibilities that they had difficulty understanding each other's perspective. However, in enlightened organizations with strong leadership, the two areas come together to address how to improve care in the most efficient way. For that reason, many health care leaders emphasize the importance of a strong relationship between nursing and finance (Brennan, Hinson, & Taylor, 2008; Clarke, 2006; Fifer, 2007; Studer, 2010). Approaches to balancing quality and cost involve an understanding of economic evaluation concepts, the use of outcome data in clinical information systems along with financial data to make decisions, and the idea of a balanced scorecard in health care. Rather than financial performance being divorced from clinical outcomes performance, the two are brought together in planning for and evaluating organizational performance.

Economic Evaluation

Nurse managers might work with health economists to examine alternative projects or approaches when making decisions about nursing care of patients. The basic assumption is that health resources are always limited, so using the various techniques of economic evaluation, decisions are made that provide "the biggest bang for the buck." These techniques are similar in terms of identifying and measuring costs, but they differ in the kind of consequences that result from the alternative approaches or programs being examined (Douglas & Normand, 2005; Drummond et al., 2005). These evaluations are described in Box 13.2.

Box 13.2

Types of Health Economic Evaluation

Cost-minimization Analysis

This kind of analysis is used when two approaches or programs are known to have essentially the same results or outcomes. This relatively simple form of evaluation is done to compare the costs and determine the approach that uses the fewest health care resources. (Some would argue that this technique is not a true economic evaluation.)

Cost-effectiveness Analysis

This kind of analysis can be used when approaches or programs have the same kind of outcome of interest, for example, life-years gained or unwanted pregnancies avoided. Costs for the two approaches can be compared in terms of the effect on the outcome of interest. In this way, two different contraceptives can be compared in terms of their cost in relation to their effectiveness in avoiding unwanted pregnancies.

Cost-utility Analysis

This kind of economic analysis examines outcomes using a generic measure that enables comparison between alternative approaches to a health program. An example of such a measure is the quality-adjusted life-year (QALY), which compares interventions in terms of their impact on quality and quantity of life. The result of the analysis would be described in terms of the cost per quality-adjusted life-year achieved by choosing one program over another. Utility analysis can take both quality and quantity into consideration enabling decisions about treatment or programs on the basis of preferences.

Cost-benefit Analysis

Cost-benefit analysis involves comparing costs and benefits in monetary units. The results of the analysis may be expressed as a ratio of costs to benefits or as a net benefit or net loss sum from choosing one program over another. This kind of analysis can be done when a dollar figure can be arrived at for effects of a program, so it may not be possible with all comparisons of interest. An example of a cost-benefit analysis would be a study that examines two anti-arthritis drugs in terms of disability days avoided that can be measured by their monetary benefit.

Douglas and Normand (2005) believe that economic evaluation can support nurse managers by providing evidence that can either challenge or support resource allocation decisions. They note that, while the effectiveness of the use of specialist nurses in clinics, such as those for cancer care and heart failure, has been demonstrated, only economic evaluation studies that examine cost-effectiveness will provide the evidence required to implement more of these kinds of clinics. They use the example of expanding a clinical nurse specialist (CNS) palliative home care team and illustrate the kinds of costs and outcomes that would be considered in an economic evaluation. For example, costs to be considered include increases in CNS hours, car and fuel costs, and administrative support costs. Outcomes to be considered include improved patient and carer outcomes, satisfaction from early discharge, potentially poorer outcomes, and potentially less team-working and problem solving.

Standardized Clinical Outcomes

In order to measure performance in health care organizations, data are collected on clinical outcomes. These data can be linked to health care structures and inputs, for example staffing data, to examine relationships between inputs and outcomes. Historically, data collected on clients or patients looked at outcomes such as infection or mortality rates. Data on inputs or interventions focused on length of stay and medical procedures, but increasingly, organizations such as hospitals use clinical data to track and measure clinical outcomes as quality indicators (Forster & van Walraven, 2010; The Ottawa Hospital, 2012). Gradually, with more research demonstrating the relationship between nursing inputs and interventions and outcomes, evidence has been established to support the regular collection of data on nursing. In this way, the contribution of nursing to health outcomes becomes more visible than it has been in the past and dispels the notion that nursing is all about the cost of health care, rather than the value added. For example, Goetz, Janney, and Ramsey (2011) describe work toward nursing's clinical and financial goals that resulted in improvements in both cost and quality over a four-year period of more than four million dollars. Savings resulted from reductions in central-line associated blood stream infections, hospital-acquired pressure ulcers, and patient falls.

The development of a nursing minimum data set (NMDS) in Canada was initiated by the Canadian Nurses Association beginning in 1993 (Hannah & White, 2012). This work began with agreement on key nursing data elements. Nursing licensing bodies collect data on individual nurses and nursing workload data became part of national data sets for health care organizations, but information on nursing care provided to patients has been slower to develop (Doran, Mildon & Clarke, 2011).

Gradually, databases are being developed to incorporate nursing-sensitive outcomes, which are those that research studies have linked to nursing care. As discussed in Chapter 11, Quality Improvement, data are needed to establish benchmarks for outcomes and to enable nurse managers to use evidence in decision making about inputs, such as staffing, and patient outcomes. The Health Outcomes for Better Information and Care (HOBIC) program was designed to collect a set of nursing-sensitive outcomes and was implemented in 187 Ontario institutions that included acute care, complex continuing care, home care, and long-term care (Doran, Mildon & Clarke, 2011). Building on this work, the Canadian Health Outcomes for Better Information and Care project, C-HOBIC, collected outcome data in Saskatchewan and Manitoba in such organizations as home care and long-term care. These programs provide information to nurse executives who can obtain outcome reports that they can link to staffing and financial information. In this way nurse leaders can use timely information to understand performance and examine the relationship to workplace structures and policies. Research presented at the end of this chapter by McGillis Hall, Johnson, Hemingway, Pringle, White, and Wodchis (2012) describes the interest by nurse leaders in using such data in their workplace.

Balanced Scorecards and Nursing Report Cards

In health care, organizations have begun to use an approach developed for the business sector in order to examine performance. Use of a **balanced scorecard** refers to collecting and reporting on data from several perspectives—the customer, the core business or internal processes, learning and innovation for improvement, and the financial or shareholder perspective. This approach was adopted in Ontario to produce hospital reports starting in 1998 using four "quadrants": system integration and change, clinical utilization and outcomes, patient satisfaction, and financial performance (Doran, Mildon & Clarke, 2011). Fraser Health, an integrated health network in British Columbia, adopted the balanced scorecard approach in 2006 (Barnardo & Jivanni, 2009).

In 2001, a nursing report was included in *The Hospital Report 2001* (McGillis Hall et al., 2001). The nursing report addressed nursing services, and a range of nursing indicators for each of the overall quadrants was recommended for Ontario's future hospital reports. Some of the clinical outcomes recommended for inclusion were pressure ulcers, patient falls, and failure to rescue. Financial performance and conditions data recommended included such measures as RN, RPN/LPN, and non-professional staff-earned hours per inpatient-weighted case and percentage nursing staff hours utilized for overtime. As has been demonstrated, it is feasible to collect and report on data that provide quality details on nursing care and outcomes. There has been a call for a national report card in nursing in Canada (Doran, Mildon, & Clarke, 2011). Hannah and White (2012) reported that the measures from C-HOBIC were endorsed by the Canadian Nursing Informatics Association (CNIA), and the Canadian Nurses Association sponsored the submission of these for approval as a national standard. They were endorsed as a Canada Approved Standard (CAS) in early 2012, thus receiving approval for use in Canadian health care systems. While there is much more work to be done to provide useful and timely data to those who lead and manage nursing systems, such information systems will support decision making about nursing in health care, facilitate quality improvement, and demonstrate nursing's contribute to care.

RELATED RESEARCH

Nurse Leader Perspectives on Health Outcomes for Better Information and Care (HOBIC) Program

A sample of nurse leaders involved in the Health Outcomes for Better Information and Care (HOBIC) initiative in Ontario health care settings were surveyed to gain an understanding of their experiences with the HOBIC program. Healthcare settings included acute care, long-term care, complex continuing care, and home

(Continued)

care. The descriptive internet survey used open-ended questions to enable in-depth responses. Thirty-seven nurse leaders responded to the survey questions and responses were coded by two members of the study team. Codes were sorted and organized into themes that emerged from the comments of respondents. The codes were reviewed by two team members to ensure agreement on the themes. Four themes were identified in the analysis:

1. benefits to the organization from the HOBIC program,

2. challenges in implementation of the program,

3. management of the challenges, and

4. potential uses of the HOBIC data in the future.

Overall, the participants were very supportive of the program and although it is in the early stages of implementation, respondents saw the benefits, particularly noting the ability to compare data, as a benefit. For example, a long-term care respondent said that they were "better able to track fatigue in our residents" as it was often an early sign of more complex issues. Several respondents thought the information was beginning to influence care planning and delivery by staff nurses as well as nurse mangers, because reports on admission status of patients help focus on their needs and the relationship to staffing levels. A benefit of the program also mentioned was that it was enhancing employee skill in electronic documentation. Implementation of the program was not without its challenges. One of these was the low level of computerization and IT at their site, as well as staff skill levels. In some cases this required double entry, and IT problems were encountered with access to and retrieval of reports. Another challenge at some sites was getting staff nurse engagement in data collection, given the

busy days and especially when it was an additional step in sites that did not have electronic documentation. In some sites, it was a challenge to get the organization to integrate HOBIC into the current systems and get reports that linked back to the unit. In order to overcome implementation changes, leaders used ongoing education and the provision of IT support for staff regarding computer use. Training of the manager group to employ the reports and use set times to discuss and compare data was another way to address the challenges of implementation. One respondent noted that "more proficient users help other." When asked about the future potential of HOBIC data, the majority of respondents was able to identify how it would help them with quality reporting, best practices, policies and protocols, consideration of models of nurse staffing, and discharge planning. One said that "I see a lot of potential to measure outcomes to care, to evaluate the results of staffing changes, etc."

Some of the ways in which the HOBIC initiative has benefitted patients, staff, and organizations were reflected in the results of this study, and it is clear that nurses at all levels of both acute and long-term care saw benefits in having standardized clinical data available. Some of the changes for both individual nurses and organizations are the need to have up-to-date electronic systems and the ability to incorporate nursing data into existing systems to avoid duplication of work. On-going education and support will be needed in these workplaces to assist nurses and their managers to fully benefit from the use of reports to plan and deliver care.

Source: McGillis Hall, L., Johnson, S., Hemingway, A., Pringle, D., White, P., Wodchis, W. (2012). "The potential is unlimited!" Nurse leader perspectives on the integration of HOBIC in Ontario. *Nursing Leadership, 25*(1), 29–42.

Leading Health Care Example

Using a Nursing Balanced Scorecard Approach to Measure and Optimize Nursing Performance

The experience of Bridgepoint Health, a hospital and network, focused on complex chronic care and rehabilitation. Bridgepoint Health developed and implemented a nursing balanced scorecard (NBS) as part of a strategic plan in which the scorecard was a way to "measure and optimize nursing performance." The vision of the strategic plan was "Being Canada's Leader in the Prevention and Management of Complex Disease and Rehabilitation—the New Frontier of Health Care." Priorities were identified by key stakeholders, clinical nurses, nurse educators, and administrators in order to transform nursing professional practice to meet the complex care needs of patients. Priorities included a nursing professional care delivery model, a new clinical skill-mix model, and enhancing the governance structure of nursing. Using a balanced scorecard development process, a team with representation from clinical directors, nursing education, direct care nurses, other health disciplines, business management, and senior nursing staff began to develop a Nursing Balanced Scorecard. They started the planning process with an organizational benchmarking exercise and literature review, and over the planning period developed strategic objectives and indicators in four domains: nursing resource management; nursing internal processes: care delivery and clinical practice; outcomes; and nursing

organizational capabilities. They identified for the scorecard 22 strategic objectives and indicators relating to each objective. For example, under the nursing resource management domain, one strategic objective was to attract and retain the best nursing professionals. Indicators that would be used to monitor achievement of the objective were: nurse retention index, external turnover rate, attrition rate, nurse recruitment index, and nurse satisfaction survey results.

The first quarterly performance report included indicators as either green (progress meeting or exceeding expectations), yellow (progress being made toward target but no changes required yet), and red (progress is below expectations and root-cause analysis and corrective action required to meet performance improvements). Reviewing progress toward targets required explaining variances. For example, progress of some objectives was delayed because there was a major focus on nursing skill-mix change in the six months.

Overall, the NBS was viewed as a valuable way to plan strategic goals in nursing and measure performance. The authors note that data generated from a balanced scorecard helps users and decision makers in the organization understand their progress and evaluate success in achieving goals.

Source: Jeffs, L., Merkley, J., Richardson, S., Eli, J., & McAllister, M. (2011). Using a nursing balanced scorecard approach to measure and optimize nursing performance. *Nursing Leadership, 24*(1), 47–58.

SUMMARY

In this chapter, we have focused on financial leadership in nursing and noted that, as a beginning nurse, you can demonstrate your financial accountability by appropriate use of resources in your workplace. Competency in financial matters can begin early in your career by learning the meaning of financial terms that are used in your workplace, understanding the overall budgeting process, and contributing ideas on better ways of providing nursing care and reducing costs to your unit or organization-wide nursing committees and councils. As you participate in planning exercises and goal setting, you can begin to appreciate the need for nurse executives to provide leadership in transforming a vision into real action that involves real costs. Increasing the value of nursing in the organizations means quality improvements in care while exercising budget monitoring and financial accountability. You will begin to appreciate the knowledge and skill required by managers to manage resources wisely, resources that include people, buildings, equipment, and supplies. Skill in marrying quality improvement with financial performance requires an understanding of how to use the resources and tools available, such as economic evaluation and the use of clinical data on nursing interventions and outcomes, to make decisions. The development of the use of nursing balanced scorecards or nursing report cards is an indication of the many facets of performance that nurse leaders of an organization must consider, and, although financial performance is not the only one, it is a necessary aspect if nursing is to achieve all that it can with the resources available.

Glossary of Terms

Accountability   refers to the obligation of individuals or an organization/government to answer to an authority for the actions and results in carrying out assigned responsibilities.

Balanced scorecard   refers to an approach developed for businesses to look at performance in a comprehensive way using measures related to four aspects: organizational capabilities, internal processes, stakeholders, and financial management over a time period.

Budget   A financial plan that includes expected revenues and expenditures for a specific period of time.

Capital budget   refers to budgets developed for purchase of items that endure, for example, equipment that lasts a number of years, the purchase of major equipment, the substantial renovation of a building, or the construction of a new building(s). The capital costs do not include the costs required to operate or maintain the equipment or new building.

Casualization   refers to changes in the staffing plan that involves hiring a greater percentage of part-time or casual staff or by using agency staff. This approach may be used to reduce staffing costs, but can end up causing more problems than it solves and even increasing costs.

Cost centre   A unit or activity to which costs can be attributed, for example, housekeeping services.

Deficit budget   refers to an operating budget that has more expenses than revenues, a condition known as "being in the red." Either reserve savings must be used or the debt incurred must be repaid in the future. In some jurisdictions, budgets presented for approval must be balanced, and deficit budgets are not allowed. However, because of unexpected expenses or unexpected low revenues, at the end of the fiscal year a budget may turn out to be a deficit one.

Direct costs   Costs that are attributable to the provision of care, such as direct care nursing salaries.

Fiscal year   The 12-month period of the operating budget, which may or may not coincide with the calendar year.

Fixed costs   refers to costs that do not vary with changes in volume of services.

Flexible budget   A budget that is adjusted based on anticipated fluctuations in activities or volumes of services. For example, during seasonal vacation periods, the monthly budget for surgical supplies may be adjusted for the reduced volume of surgery during that period.

Incremental budgeting   refers to building a budget based on a past one by increasing or decreasing amounts based on anticipated but relatively minor changes in revenues and expenditures. The assumption is that the past budget was reasonable and adjustments are made to that base as required.

Indirect costs   refers to costs that support direct care but do not directly involve care to patients, for example, human resources office or housekeeping. These are sometimes referred to as overhead costs.

Operating budget   refers to the budget of estimated revenues and expenses for the daily operation of an organization over a period of time, normally a one-year period. It includes the normal operating expenses expected in the daily functioning of the organization and is fairly detailed in terms of categories.

Program budget   is a financial plan for a specific area of activity, a planned new activity or service, or a special project. These budgets may be produced to make a decision about adding the activity, because they cut across a number of existing departments, or they extend beyond a one-year operating budget and are time-limited.

Resource management   refers to management of the full range of resources within an organization, including money, people, buildings, equipment, and so on.

Responsibility centre   refers to a unit or activity within an organization to which costs can be attributed, for example, a primary health care team in a community centre with many programs.

Revenue centre   refers to a unit or activity within an organization to which income can be attributed, for example a gift shop in a hospital.

Staffing budget/Personnel budget   refers to the portion of the operating budget that provides for salaries, wages, and benefits and is typically the largest portion of a health care organization's budget. It may also be referred to as a labour budget in some organizations.

Variable costs   Costs that change as volume of services increase or decrease.

Variance analysis   An examination that compares actual to budget to determine any variation between what was planned and what actually occurred during a specific period of time, along with an explanation of any substantial variation between the two.

Variance report   refers to reports than an organization may require of managers on a regular basis following variance analysis that explain the reasons for a variance and, in some cases, a plan to address any shortfall or other corrective action.

Zero-based budgeting   refers to a budgeting methodology that builds expenses in a budget from zero every time the budget is prepared. In this approach, every item is justified every year.

CASE

Tim Levinson is a newly appointed nurse manager for a busy medical unit in an acute care hospital. Shortly after he begins his work, the nurse to whom he reports, the director of surgical services, tells him that his unit staffing budget had a negative variance in the past three monthly budget reports and he needs to get the budget "under control."

Questions

1. What kinds of factors do you think Tim needs to consider in examining why the budget is overspent?

2. What kinds of information or reports that do you think Tim will need to determine where the problem(s) are?

Tim quickly discovers that a large number of agency nurses were used in the previous three months to cover the costs of covering for staff absences. He also learns that overtime costs for regular staff have increased in the past three months.

3. What further information do you think that Tim requires and how do you think he can obtain it?

4. How do you think Tim should proceed in the short term? In the long term?

5. What kinds of data or information do you think Tim needs in assessing the consequences of overtime and high agency nurse staffing? Where do you think he could find it?

6. How could he use this information in making the case that there is a need to reconsider the staffing plan for the unit?

Critical Thinking Questions and Activities

1. Think about your current workplace and the supplies that are used on a daily basis by nursing staff in providing care. Can you identify any ways in which supply costs might be reduced?

2. In your current health care organization, see if you can find a copy of the operating budget of the organization. This may be available in a format that shows the major cost categories and dollar figures for the organization overall that has been prepared for the board of directors or an annual meeting. See if you can identify the cost categories that would be influenced in a major way by nursing services.

3. Ask a nurse manager if you could learn more about the unit budget for which he or she is responsible. Ask if you can view the unit's budget and interview the manager to ask about the process of budgeting and major challenges in managing the budget.

4. Reflect on the costs of providing care in your workplace. Do you think that the people you work with are aware of those costs? Does your workplace provide any information about reducing costs or waste? If not, how do you think they could increase awareness and secure cooperation?

5. Does your workplace provide any clinical information on nursing outcomes? Are there any goals with regard to improving nursing outcomes? If not, do you think there is an area in which nursing performance could improve? What cost savings for the nursing unit and/or the health system might you see if there was an improvement in this area? What kind of data would you need to be collected to find out if there was an improvement?

Self-Quiz

You are a nurse educator in a community hospital, and a nurse manager has asked you to plan a workshop for the nursing staff on her unit on the topic of health assessment. She expects you to prepare a budget so that she knows what to include in her annual budget in the coming year. The following questions relate to this request.

1. The budget you prepare for the nurse manager would best be described as a/an:
   a. Capital budget
   b. Operating budget
   c. Program budget
   d. Staffing budget

2. You plan a one-day (8-hour) workshop that you will offer three times and you will plan to release 20 nurses in total to attend the workshop. The expenditures for coverage for these nurses would increase which of the following?
   a. Flexible budget
   b. Cost-effectiveness
   c. Productivity
   d. Personnel costs

3. The coverage costs that would be attributed to the manager's budget to conduct the workshop would be considered:
   a. Fixed, direct
   b. Variable, direct
   c. Fixed, indirect
   d. Variable, indirect

4. You want to acquire satellite transmission equipment in the nursing education centre to use as part of the workshops that your centre conducts on a yearly basis. You would expect that your manager would tell you that this request would be part of a:
   a. Strategic planning exercise
   b. Balanced nursing scorecard
   c. Operating budget
   d. Capital budget

Useful Websites

Academy of Canadian Executive Nurses
http://acen.ca/

Accreditation Canada
www.accreditation.ca

Canadian Foundation for Healthcare Improvement
www.cfhi-fcass.ca/AboutUs.aspx

Canadian Health Leadership Network
www.chlnet.ca/

Canadian Institute for Health Information Health System Performance
www.cihi.ca/CIHI-ext-portal/internet/EN/Theme/health+system+performance/cihi010646

Nursing Leadership Network of Ontario
www.nln.on.ca/

References

Barnardo, C., & Jivanni, A. (2009). Evaluating the Fraser Health balanced scorecard—A formative evaluation. *Healthcare Management Forum, 22*(2), 49–60.

Borsa, J., & Anis, A. (2005). The cost of hospital care in Canada: A comparison of two alternatives. *Healthcare Management Forum, 18*(1), 19–27.

Brennan, T., Hinson, N., & Taylor, M. (2008). Nursing and finance. Making the connection. *Healthcare Financial Management, 62*(1), 90–94.

Carroll, C.A., Lacey, S.R., & Cox, K.S. (2004). Comparing variations in labor costs for two vs. one full-time nurse manager. *Nursing Economic$, 22*(5), 254–257.

Carruth, A.K., Carruth, P.J., & Noto, E.C. (2000). Nurse managers flex their budgetary might. *Nursing Management, 31*(2), 16–17.

Cherry, B., & Jacob, S.R. (2008). *Contemporary nursing. Issues, trends, & management.* 4th ed. St. Louis, Missouri: Mosby.

Clarke, R.L. (2006). Finance and nursing. The business of caring. *Healthcare Financial Management, 60*(1), 50–56.

Dohmann, E.L., & Hahn, J.A. (2011). Achieving accountability. It's all about you! *Nursing Management, 42*(11), 39–42.

Doran, D., Mildon, B., & Clarke, S. (2011). Towards a national report card in nursing: A knowledge synthesis. *Nursing Leadership, 24*(2), 38–57.

Douglas, H., & Normand, C. (2005). Economic evaluation: what does a nurse manager need to know? *Journal of Nursing Management, 13,* 419–427.

Dowless, R.M. (2007). Your guide to costing methods and terminology. *Nursing Management, 38*(4), 52–57.

Dreisbach, A.M. (1994). A structured approach to expert financial management: A financial development plan for nurse managers. *Nursing Economic$, 12*(3), 131–139.

Drummond, M.F., Sculpher, M.J., Torrance, G.W., O'Brien, B.J., & Stoddart, G.L. (2005) *Methods for the economic evaluation of health care programmes.* 3rd ed. Oxford: Oxford University Press.

Fifer, J.J. (2007). Bridging the gap between nursing and finance. *Healthcare Financial Management, 61*(4), 28.

Finkler, S.A., & McHugh, M.L. (2008). *Budgeting concepts for nurse managers.* 4th ed. St. Louis, Missouri: Saunders.

Fooks, C., & Maslove, L. (2004). *Rhetoric, fallacy or dream? Examining the accountability of Canadian health care to citizens.* Ottawa: Canadian Policy Research Networks.

Forster, A.J., & van Walraven, C. (2010). The use of quality indicators to promote accountability in health care: the good, the bad, and the ugly. *Open Medicine, 6*(2), 75–79.

Goddard, N.L. (2003). The five most common flaws in health care staffing and personnel budgeting. *Nurse Leader, 1*(5), 44–48.

Goetz, K., Janney, M., & Ramsey, K. (2011). When nursing takes ownership of financial outcomes: Achieving exceptional financial performance through leadership, strategy and execution. *Nursing Economic$, 29*(4), 173–182.

Gould, D., Kelly, D., Goldstone, L., & Maidwell, A. (2001). The changing training needs of clinical nurse managers: exploring issues for continuing professional development. *Journal of Advanced Nursing, 34*(1), 7–17.

Hannah, K., & White, P.A. (2012). C-HOBIC: Standardized clinical outcomes to support evidence-informed nursing care. *Nursing Leadership, 25*(1), 43–46.

Heale, R., & Butcher, M. (2010). Canada's first nurse practitioner-led clinic: A case study in healthcare innovation. *Nursing Leadership 23*(3), 21–29.

International Council of Nurses. (2008). *Financial management for nurses.* Geneva: ICN.

Jeffs, L., Merkley, J., Richardson, S., Eli, J., & McAllister, M. (2011). Using a nursing balanced scorecard approach to measure and optimize nursing performance. *Nursing Leadership, 24*(1), 47–58.

Johnson, D., Bell, B., Elgendy, J., McDonald, E., West, F., Wenzel, L., Malach, B., & DiStefano, M. (2012). Don't waste green! Launching a budget awareness campaign. *Nursing Management, 43*(8) 51–54.

McGillis Hall, L., Doran, D., Lascenger, H.S., Mallette, C., O'Brien-Pallas, L.L., & Pedersen, C. (2001). *Hospital Report 2001: Preliminary studies, volume 2: Exploring nursing, women's health, population health.* Toronto: HSPRN. Retrieved June 26, 2013, from www.hsprn.ca/reports/2001/nursing_2001.html

McGillis Hall, L., Johnson, S., Hemingway, A., Pringle, D., White, P., Wodchis, W. (2012). "The potential is unlimited!" Nurse leader perspectives on the integration of HOBIC in Ontario. *Nursing Leadership, 25*(1), 29–42.

Nagle, L.M., & Vincent, L. (2003). A SARS postcard—reflections of two health-care leaders. *Nursing Leadership, 16*(2), 24–26.

Nestman, L.J. (1992). *Management control and funding systems: For Canadian health service executives.* Ottawa: Canadian College of Health Service Executives.

The Ottawa Hospital. (April 1, 2012). *2012/13 Quality improvement plan (short form).* Ottawa: The Ottawa Hospital. Downloaded from www.ottawahospital.on.ca/wps/portal/Base/TheHospital/QualityAndSafety/Planning/QualityImprovementPlan

Pintar, K.A., Capuano, T.A., & Rosser, G.D. (2007). Developing clinical leadership capability. *The Journal of Continuing Education in Nursing, 38*(3), 115–121.

Porter-O'Grady, T., & Malloch, K. (2013). *Leadership in nursing practice. Changing the landscape of health care.* Burlington, MA: Jones & Bartlett.

Stichler, J.F. (2008). The bottom line. Financial management skills for nurse leaders. *Nursing for Women's Health, 12*(2), 157–162.

Studer, Q. (2010). Do your nurses speak finance? *Healthcare Financial Management. 64*(6), 80–84.

Wodchis, W. P. (1998). Applying activity-based costing in long term care. *Healthcare Management Forum, 11*(4), 25–32.

Chapter 14
Ethical Leadership and the Context for Ethical Practice in Health Care Organizations

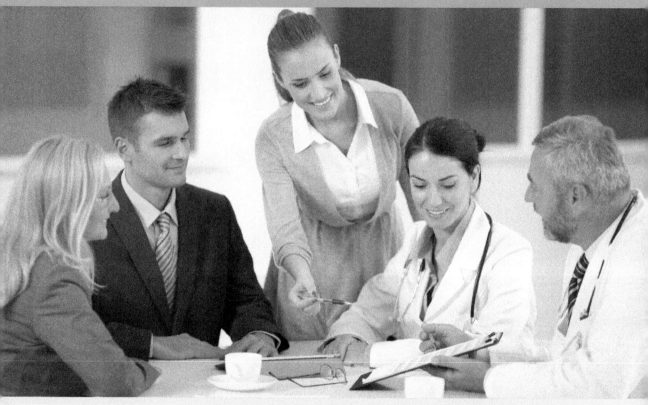

svetikd/Getty Images

Learning Objectives

After reading, studying, and reflecting on this chapter's content, you will be able to:

1. Discuss the concepts of moral agency, moral distress, and moral climate
2. Discuss the concept of character and the characteristics of ethical leadership
3. Describe qualities of a workplace that would promote a positive ethical climate
4. Discuss ways in which nursing leaders can promote ethical practice in the workplace
5. Identify resources for ethics in the workplace and discuss their use in supporting ethical practice

INTRODUCTION

In your nursing classroom and clinical courses, you learn about the ethical aspects of nursing practice and focus on the kinds of issues that may arise in different clinical settings. For example, consent to treatment may be an issue in areas where nurses work with individuals whose cognitive capacity is in question, such as pediatrics, neurology, psychiatry, and geriatrics. Your nursing courses introduce you to knowledge, tools, and skills that you use to address ethical concerns. For example, you learn about nursing codes of ethics and ethical principles such as autonomy and beneficence that are considerations in analyzing moral situations. (Please note that we use the terms "ethical" and "moral" interchangeably in this chapter.) The focus of these courses is usually on the ethical responsibilities of the individual nurse in relation to patients and their families, obligations to individuals, and the duty of care. The focus on decisions at the individual level is a micro-level one, while a focus on health policy at the government level would involve macro-level decisions (Rodney, et al., 2013). In this chapter we focus on the middle or meso-level, where decisions are made within the context of health care organizations. We do not address specific ethical or legal issues related to clinical situations, but rather how nurses experience these issues in daily practice, how organizations can be structured to address the ethical aspects of health care, and the ethical aspects of leadership roles in nursing.

We begin the chapter with a focus on the ethical aspects of practice in the workplace and discuss what is known about the experiences of nurses in this regard. We discuss key concepts in ethical practice, such as the moral climate and moral culture of a workplace. As all nurses have opportunities and experiences in leadership, we discuss the concepts of ethical leadership and ethical leaders. In particular, we discuss ethical leadership in nursing and how formal leaders can facilitate ethical practice in the workplace. We discuss standards for health care organizations with respect to ethics, issues in organizational ethics, and resources for nurses in the workplace.

ETHICS IN THE NURSING WORKPLACE

The expectations for ethical practice in nursing are identified in nursing codes of ethics or ethical guidelines, be they international (International Council of Nurses, 2012), national (American Nurses Association, 2009; Canadian Nurses Association, 2008), or jurisdictional. For example, in Canada, some provincial nursing regulatory bodies have a code or guidelines on ethics for nurses who are registered or licensed to practise in that province (College of Nurses of Ontario, 2009; L'Ordre des infirmières et infirmiers du Québec, 2012). Although these codes and guidelines set the norms or standards for ethical behaviour, to what extent do nurses believe they meet these standards in their daily practice? Although there has been evidence from many countries that nurses may experience moral distress because of workplace constraints on their practice, concerns about this problem were heightened in Canada during the healthcare cutbacks of the 1990s (Baumann et al., 2001; Cummings & Estabrooks, 2003). The cutbacks led to loss of nursing positions and increased workloads while decreasing supports in the workplace. As a result, a number of studies have been done over the past 15 years and we have learned more about the experiences of nurses, their perceptions of ethical issues in their work settings, and contextual factors that affect their ability to practise in accordance with their ethical beliefs (Gaudine, et al. 2011a; Storch, et al., 2002). Several key concepts have emerged from theory and research about ethical nursing practice, and these ideas are discussed next.

Moral Agency

Moral agency refers to "the capacity or power of a nurse to direct his or her motives and actions to some ethical end" (CNA, 2008, p. 26). In essence, the moral agency of a nurse refers to doing what is right through choice and deliberate action. As Rodney, Buckley, Street, Serrano, and Martin (2013) note, one difficulty with the traditional notion of moral agency is that it assumes all those involved in a situation are independent and in a similar situation. They point out that, in the health care environment, there are often power imbalances that constrain nurses from acting as moral agents. In some settings, nurses become socialized into thinking and feeling constrained to the point that they do not act as autonomous moral agents. Such situations are serious and must be corrected through nursing leadership in action.

Moral Distress

Andrew Jameton (1984) is a philosopher who explored the ethical dilemmas of nurses in their practice, and he defined **moral distress** as occurring "when one knows the right thing to do, but institutional constraints make it nearly impossible to pursue the right course of action" (p. 6). Wilkinson (1987/88) developed a moral distress model based on her study of 24 nurses and described the "psychological disequilibrium and negative feelings state" (p. 16) of nurses who did not act in accordance with their moral decisions due to external or internal constraints. External constraints were most often physicians, law, nursing administration, and hospital administration/policy. Internal constraints referred to such things as fear of job loss, self-doubt, a sense of futility based on previous experience, and internalized socialization of nurses to carry out orders. Corley (2002) proposed a theory of moral distress that addressed the internal psychological effects on nurses and nurses' external context, that is, institutional constraints. The psychological effects on nurses range from anger and frustration to sadness, anxiety, and guilt. Webster and Baylis (2000) describe **moral residue** as a lingering sense of having compromised one's own values. Nurses may carry this sense of guilt and of having betrayed themselves long after an experience of moral distress.

Most of the research on moral distress among nurses has focused on nurses in acute care hospitals, although there have been some studies in long-term care (Green & Jeffers, 2006) or some that included nurses from such settings (Austin, Bergum, & Goldberg, 2003). In a meta-synthesis of studies of the experience of moral distress of nurses in hospital settings, Rittenmeyer and Huffman (2009) included 39 studies that met the review criteria. Their key findings or syntheses are presented in Box 14.1

Similar experiences of moral distress seem to occur among nurses no matter what the work setting. In their hermeneutic phenomenological study of Canadian nurses in mental health-care settings, Austin, Bergum, and Goldberg (2003) describe the anguish of nurses in long-term care and acute care settings who feel overworked and too busy to sit with a

Syntheses of Key Findings on Research of Moral Distress Experienced by Professional Nurses Working in Hospital Environments

1. **Human Reactivity:** Nurses who experience moral distress respond with a myriad of biological, psychological and stress reactions.

2. **Institutional Culpability:** Moral distress is experienced when nurses feel the need to advocate for patients' well-being, while coping with institutional constraints.

3. **Patient Pain and Suffering:** The perception of patient pain and suffering as

a result of medical decisions, of which the nurse has little power to influence, contribute to the experience.

4. **Unequal Power Hierarchies:** Unequal power structures, prevalent in institutions, exacerbate the problem.

Source: From Syntheses of Key Findings on Research of Moral Distress Experienced by Professional Nurses Working in Hospital Environments, *JBI Systematic Reviews*. Reprinted by permission.

patient who is dying or address someone who is screaming due to "mental pain." One nurse describes the frustration of seeing colleagues "give up" and feeling alone and "disconnected" (p. 181).

Moral Climate

Ethical or **moral climate** refers to the current values (both explicit and implicit) that influence a workplace and the professional practice within that workplace (CNA, 2008; Rodney, Buckley et al., 2013). For example, a work setting that values the dignity and privacy of patients has a structural configuration, equipment, supplies, and policies that enable staff to practise in a way that promotes these values. There are locations in the setting for private discussion with patients and families about personal issues, patient gowns and curtains are in working order, and staff members do not discuss patients in public areas. Values in the broad health care system can also influence moral climate, for example, when an emphasis on cost savings or business efficiency prevails and leads to decisions that fail to take patient safety into consideration. Moral culture is a similar concept, but refers to the part of an organization's culture that can influence moral reasoning and decision making within the organization. The formal and informal systems in an organization that influence moral decision making include peer and leadership behaviour, ethical norms, codes of conduct/practice, and reward systems (Brown & Treviño, 2006). For example, in the culture of a hospital, nurses may receive positive comments and congratulations for ensuring patients are discharged by 10:00 hours without regard to the quality of discharge planning and readiness of patients to return home.

Moral distress among nurses has been shown to be associated with the ethical climate of a workplace. Pauly, Varcoe, Storch, and Newton (2009) studied registered nurses working in acute care hospitals in British Columbia using a survey method that involved the measurement of moral distress intensity and frequency as well as hospital ethical climate. A random sample of 1,700 nurses yielded a total of 374 returned surveys (22 percent). Moral distress intensity scores could range between 0 and 6, and moral distress frequency between none (0) and very frequently (6). The items with the highest moral distress intensity scores (greater than 4) were:

- working with perceived unsafe RN staffing,
- being required to work with patients when the nurse did not feel competent to do so,
- working with RNs who were perceived to not be as competent as the patients required,
- working with doctors who were perceived to not be as competent as the patients required, and
- assisting a physician who was viewed as providing incompetent care.

Although moral distress was not a frequent occurrence among respondents, it tended to be intense when it did occur.

Pauly and colleagues (2009) measured hospital ethics climate with a scale that ranged from 1 (almost never true) to 5 (almost always true) and that addressed five factors: peers, patients, managers, hospital, and physicians. A high total score indicated a positive ethical climate. The researchers found a significant, negative correlation between the hospital's ethical climate and nurses' levels of moral distress—higher levels of hospital's ethical climate were associated with lower levels of nurses' moral distress. All the five factors in the hospital ethics climate scale correlated with nurses' moral distress, indicating that there are different contributing factors for a hospital's ethical climate. While many authors have focused on institutional constraints as a source of moral distress, Pauly et al.'s research findings highlight five sources. They conclude that further study and consideration of the relationship of moral distress and ethical climate is needed so that improvements in care can result from consideration of multiple strategies. For example, improvements in relationships with peers, managers, physicians, and others might enhance the ethical climate in a workplace. As Storch (2010) notes: "Although nurses share responsibility for working together to enhance the quality of their work environment, they cannot do so alone. Health agencies are complex organizations that involve many players and many policies that may at times be at odds with good nursing practice and nursing ethics" (p. 20).

Moral Community

Moral community, in the context of a workplace, involves clear and shared values that guide practice and fosters a safe climate for all participants to be heard (CNA, 2008). Discussion of ethical issues, problems, and values is encouraged and supported. Rodney, Buckley et al., (2013) refer to the period of the 1990s in Canada as having had a profound impact on the moral climate for nursing practice. Reductions in staff and nursing leaders within health care organizations along with rapid changes with little or no input from nurses led to burnout and job dissatisfaction. Rodney, Buckley et al. believe that workplaces where nurses have been devalued, disenfranchised, and demoralized must be rebuilt and values-based change is required if good nursing care is to prevail: "A minimal requirement for improving the moral climate for nursing practice and fostering the development of nursing as a moral community is to turn the negative characteristics around and strengthen the positive characteristics" (p. 198).

They indicate that a beginning would involve assisting nurses to find their moral voices, to help them use the language of ethics, and to engage in ethics education for nurses and all those who work in health care. The Leading Health Care Example in this chapter describes one approach to building moral community in a range of workplace settings.

Leading Health Care Example

Exploring Ethics in Practice: Creating Moral Community in Healthcare One Place at a Time.

Scott, Marck, and Barton (2011) describe an approach that they have used with nurses in practice to address the ethical issues that arise on a daily basis. The use of ethics in practice sessions (EIP) was developed in an acute care hospital in Alberta, but was subsequently adapted for community-based nursing in a rural home care practice setting and a rural public health nursing office in Alberta. These sessions are viewed as a way to build moral community as they provide a safe place for nurses, both practitioners and managers, to explore ethical issues using relevant research and the support of colleagues.

A group of nurses undertaking an EIP session drew on recent experiences to select one or more topics for discussion at the session. The group also identified colleagues who may be willing to present and discuss a topic, and the presenter could partner with a colleague from within the setting or from outside the setting. Managers provided support to the presenters who examined current policies and related literature and also developed one

or more case studies to use in the presentation. The collected material, along with key questions, were provided to those who attended the EIP session, which lasted about 45 minutes—a 15-minute presentation followed by a 30-minute discussion. Topics addressed in these sessions have ranged from handling mistakes in practice, to triage in the emergency room, to small town practice. In their article, the authors describe an initial EIP discussion among rural public health nurses, who shared their stories and began to identify ethical concerns that they shared. A key one for these nurses was the blurring of boundaries between professional and personal lives and how to deal with situations in an ethical way when nurses lived in the community with their clients. An experienced public health nurse co-led the presentation that involved describing the problem identified by staff, summarizing relevant articles, and presented the case of an influenza outbreak that was used as a meaningful one for this group of nurses to discuss ethical aspects of boundary concerns. The case gave rise to a range of ethical concerns that nurses shared with each other in relation to the implementation of the H1N1 vaccine. The sharing of these stories

(Continued)

was one way in which nurses learned about ethics and the authors note that such narratives can increase understanding of the ethical nature of practice experiences. The authors believe that the telling of stories is an important aspect of reflective practice that enables nurses to think deeply about ethics in practice. The nurses in the group valued the ability to discuss ethical concerns and listened respectfully to colleagues and how they handled boundary issues and why they did so. They were able to think about and discuss future situations and how they might act in the future as individuals and as part of a larger system of health care, something the authors refer to as "moral imagination."

Nurses who participated in the EIPs evaluated the sessions very positively. They learned from hearing about different approaches and thought that they would be able to incorporate some of what they heard into future practice situations. The authors emphasize the importance of participants identifying the issues for discussion and have found that such sessions can foster the growth of a "moral community" where moral imagination can develop in a safe, trusting environment.

Source: Scott, S. L., Marck, P., Barton, S. (2011). Exploring ethics in practice: Creating moral community in healthcare one place at a time. *Nursing Research, 24*(4), 78–87.

ETHICAL LEADERSHIP

In Chapter 1 we described ethical leadership in terms of appropriate conduct or conduct consistent with ethical norms for personal behaviour and interpersonal relationships. Ethical leadership also involves promoting such conduct among followers. Scholars of leadership and organizational science became more interested in ethical leadership following major business scandals in the United States (Brown & Treviño, 2006; Reed, 2012). Questionable business practices and financial scandals affecting Canadian health care have been reported in the press and have ranged from alleged excessive expense accounts of health care executives ("Alberta Health expense scandal," 2012) to alleged fraud in the building of a superhospital in Montreal (McArthur & Montero, 2012) and out-of-control spending and the awarding of untendered contracts for the development of electronic health records in Ontario by eHealth Ontario ("EHealth scandal a $1B waste," 2009). Despite high profile scandals in the media, several U.S. studies of employees in organizations rate ethical leadership quite highly (Brown & Treviño, 2006).

Brown and Treviño reviewed the literature on ethical leadership to address the question: What is ethical leadership? They identified the ways in which ethical leadership was similar to and different from the theories of authentic leadership, spiritual leadership, and transformational leadership (discussed in Chapter 1 of this text). All three types were similar to ethical leadership in terms of an emphasis on altruism (concern for others), integrity, and role modelling. However, authentic leaders are characterized by authenticity and self-awareness, whereas ethical leaders focus on moral management and awareness of others. Spiritual leaders focus on hope and faith as well as work as vocation more than the moral management approach.

Transformational leaders focus on vision and values whereas ethical leadership emphasizes ethical standards (Brown & Trevino, 2006).

There is considerable overlap between values-focused theories of leadership with respect to the ethical character and behaviour of leaders, with some differences in the overall approach to leadership. The idea of ethical leadership includes a more explicit focus on influencing others by establishing explicit ethical standards and holding followers accountable through reward and discipline, a style considered more transactional than transformational. This moral management style is similar to the approach used by regulatory bodies that set standards and can apply sanctions if there are violations of these standards. Transformational leadership style involves more personal qualities in a leader who is inspirational, charismatic, or intellectually stimulating and uses idealized influence (as discussed in Chapter 1).

Ethical Leaders

How do ethical leaders develop and how does one recognize ethical leadership in their work setting? According to Brown and Treviño (2006), there are influences in the development of ethical leaders: an ethical role model that a leader has worked with closely during his or her career, working in a positive ethical climate or culture that supports and promotes ethical behaviour and practices, and facing and dealing with morally intense situations in a workplace. Morally intense situations are those that have potential for great harm, and these are the situations that are apt to draw attention to the behaviour of a leader. If the leader handles these events in an ethical manner, he or she will be judged by others as an ethical leader. Ethical leadership theory proposes that ethical leaders influence the conduct of followers and the ethical decision making of these employees through role modelling and communicating the importance of ethical standards. Because followers will be held accountable for decisions, they will be more apt to consider the ethical implications of their decisions, leading to more ethical decisions.

A number of organizational scholars have focused on the role of **character** in ethical leadership, a focus that is reminiscent of the discussion in Chapter 1 of Great Man theories or trait theories of leadership (Hannah & Avolio, 2011a, 2011b; Quick & Wright, 2011; Wright & Quick, 2011). It is interesting to note that the founding editor of *Nursing Ethics* summarized a decade of nursing ethics (2000 to 2010), as reflected in that journal, and noted that "Virtue ethics is now definitely the theory of choice" (Tscudin, 2010, p. 130). The return to the notion of character as critical in leadership in organizations is relatively recent and is likely a reflection of concerns about the lack of ethical leadership evident in media reporting of high-profile scandals. Wright and Quick refer to character as morally based values, noting that character-based leadership is focused on qualities aimed at the betterment of society, as well as personal qualities aimed at the improvement of individuals. Values-based leadership has a wider focus in than character-based leadership, because moral values are only a subset of a wider range of values, for example, competence, pleasure, comfort, and so on. According to Wright and Quick:

> ... a character-based leader is best viewed as an agent for moral change ... one with
> the requisite self-control (moral discipline) to selflessly act on their own volition

(moral autonomy) to inspire, sustain and transform the attitudes and beliefs of both themselves and their followers. Best viewed as providing an overarching moral compass, the character-based leader has the perspective to continuously strive to move their team or organization beyond narrow, self-interest pursuits toward the attainment of common good goals (moral attachment). (p. 976)

There is agreement among some scholars about the concept of character, for example, that character refers to a moral component that is distinct from values (which have a broader range than moral matters) and from personality (which may include non-moral traits such as creativity) (Hannah & Avolio, 2011b). They also agree that character is something that can be developed and that it resides within the leader, is affected by context, and that some strengths of character (for example, courage) may fit specific contexts (for example, bravery in a firefighter). According to Hannah and Avolio (2011b), ethical behaviour and leader character might be expanded beyond the normal considerations, so that similar to performance on a continuum, behaviour may range from unethical to ethical to virtuous, and character may range from low to high to **ethos**. Ethos is described as "… an inner strength driving virtue … a distinct class of character—a class that when possessed by an individual will provide the inner strength or resources to step up and perform extra-ethical, virtuous action" (p. 991). To illustrate virtue, they cite the example of extreme dedication in a nurse to a patient when required by the context. The Canadian experience of nurses who cared for patients with Severe Acute Respiratory Syndrome (SARS) when there was great uncertainty about the illness illustrates virtue (see Campbell, 2006). Hannah and Avolio also believe leaders operating under extreme contexts (high moral intensity) require high levels of character, individuals are influenced by group members, and groups develop collective norms.

ETHICAL LEADERSHIP IN NURSING

All nurses are expected to practise in accordance with the ethical standards and guidelines that are explicitly set out by the regulatory body to which the nurse is accountable. For example, one might expect registered nurses in Prince Edward Island to adhere to the *Code of Ethics for Registered Nurses* of the Canadian Nurses Association (CNA) (2008), as the Association of Registered Nurses of Prince Edward Island (2011) has adopted that code in their *Standards for Nursing Practice*. However, although a code provides guidance, it cannot address every situation, and the code authors recognize that "practice environments have a significant influence on nurses' ability to be successful in upholding the ethics of their practice" (CNA, 2008, p. 4). They also identify other key influences on ethical practice: other health-care practitioners, organizations, and government policy-makers. All nurses are encouraged to work with nursing colleagues and others to create moral communities that promote ethical care (CNA, 2008). As nurse managers and nurse executives are in key positions to influence the practice environment, leadership in ethics is expected of those who occupy such administrative positions (American Nurses Association, 2009; CNA, 2010).

We have much evidence from research in nursing that nurses experience moral distress due to external constraints (Corley, 2002; Pauly et al., 2009; Rittenmeyer &

Box 14.2

Currents Affecting Navigation

Currents Constraining Navigation
Privileging of biomedicine
Corporate ethos

Currents Facilitating Navigation
Supportive colleagues
Professional guidelines and standards
Education in ethics

Source: Navigating Towards a Moral Horizon: A Multisite Qualitative Study of Ethical Practice in Nursing, *Canadian Journal of Nursing Research, 34*(3), 75–102. Reprinted by permission of McGill University.

Huffman, 2009). To a somewhat lesser extent, researchers have identified what helps or does not help nurses in practising ethically and what nurse leaders can do to promote an environment that supports ethical nursing practice. An example is a qualitative study using focus groups that examined the meaning of ethics for nurses providing direct care (Rodney, Varcoe et al., 2002). In total, 19 focus groups were conducted involving 87 nurses from a variety of settings. The researchers used the metaphor of navigation on the water to describe their finding that nurses sought to reach the "good" in harmony with patients, families, and teams, which was not always easy: "they were navigating towards a moral horizon, but their course was often not smooth or certain" (p. 80). The nurse participants in the study described how their practice was helped or hindered in moving toward a moral horizon. Factors that constrained them included a culture that emphasized biomedicine over supportive time with patients and workplace efficiency over patient well-being. Several factors helped nurses with ethical practice: nursing colleagues and practitioners from other disciplines who were supportive, guidelines and policies that improved practice, and ethics education. The "currents" that affected navigation toward the moral horizon are listed in Box 14.2

Based on the study, Storch et al. (2002) identified the findings that were of particular relevance to nursing leaders. They noted three areas of concern to practising nurses that called for moral leadership:

- The climate and policies of organizations—nurses need to be able to raise ethical questions and not feel that they are silenced. In addition, policies that are lacking, too restrictive, or problematic for nurses in ethical situations need to be addressed.

- Allocation of resources was a concern, either because resources were wasted at times in maintaining life support when treatment seemed futile, or workload and understaffing prevented time to listen to patients or to reflect on ethical practice.

- Power inequities in the health care system created conflicts between loyalty to patients or to senior nurses and physicians. The imbalance in health care hierarchy might mean that nurses were excluded from decision making or were unable to get morally distressing situations addressed.

Addressing these concerns in a health care organization requires moral leadership among nurse leaders. Nurses in this study mentioned that nurse leaders, such as nurse managers, did not always provide support for nurses to address issues, raise questions, or advocate for clients, although there were some exceptions cited. Some nurses considered their managers as having little power themselves, but for the most part, these leaders seemed unwilling to take action. The researchers emphasized the need for nurse leaders to support nurses, act as moral agents, and make the point that these leaders might begin by self-reflection on what is preventing them from doing so. Then, they must help nursing staff identify the ethical issues, and in naming them, begin to address them. They need to find their moral courage and become a "moral compass" for nurses with whom they work (Storch et al., p. 12).

The sense that nurse managers as a group face challenges when addressing ethical issues was evident in a study by Gaudine and Beaton (2002) of nurse managers from seven hospitals. This qualitative study involved interviews with 15 managers. Four themes of ethical conflict between these managers and their organization emerged. These themes were:

1. voicelessness,

2. "where to spend the money,"

3. rights of the individual versus the organization's needs, and

4. unjust practices by senior management or the organization.

These nurse managers experienced what could be considered moral distress and the researchers noted that:

> it is difficult to convey the extent of the frustration, stress, pain, and powerlessness expressed in the interviews. The nurse managers shared the concern of their staff nurses when quality care could not be delivered, and they perceived themselves as the person responsible for improving patient care and for alleviating staff concerns." (p. 28)

These findings have implications for hospitals and other kinds of health care organizations that need to attract and retain strong and effective leadership in nursing and retain strong and competent nursing staff.

Gaudine and Thorne (2009) examined the relationship between ethical conflict (as measured by perceptions of ethical value congruence with the hospital and shared ethical priorities) and adverse outcomes (using measures of stress, organizational commitment, absenteeism, intention, and turnover). In a sample of 126 nurses from one hospital, they found a relationship between perceptions of ethical disagreement and negative outcomes, underscoring the importance of organizations working to reduce ethical conflict in the workplace. In a subsequent analysis with a sample of 410 nurses in four hospitals, Gaudine and Thorne (2012) found three areas of nurses' ethical conflict with their organizations:

1. patient care values,

2. value of nurses, and

3. staffing policy values.

In this longitudinal study of outcomes, they found that all of these areas were associated with stress, that patient care values conflict was associated with turnover when measured over one year, that conflicts around staffing policy values affected turnover intention, and that patient care values conflict predicted absenteeism. Nurses and nurse managers are not the only groups to identify conflicts with the organization in which they work. In a qualitative study of nurses and physicians in four hospitals, shared conflicts experienced by these two groups included lack of respect for professionals, insufficient resources affecting patient care and work life, clashes with organizational policies, administration turning a "blind eye" to problems, and lack of transparency or openness in the organization (Gaudine, LeFort, Lamb, & Thorne, 2011b).

There have been some encouraging examples and models for supporting nurses to "name" and address ethical issues that affect their daily practice. Storch, Rodney, Varcoe, et al. (2009) embarked on research to address how the ethical climate of the workplace can be improved for nurses in a three-year endeavour entitled, *Leadership for Ethical Policy and Practice (LEPP)*. A description of this work is provided in the Related Research box at the end of this chapter. The next section also addresses some of the resources that nurses have reported as useful with respect to ethics in practice (Gaudine & Beaton, 2002; Rodney, Varcoe et al., 2002; Shirey, 2005).

ETHICS IN HEALTH ORGANIZATIONS

What is required of health care organizations with respect to ethics? If nurses and nurse managers are encountering ethical problems that do not seem to get resolved, what standards are in place that promote ethics and direct an organization with respect to ethical matters? Although nurses in Canada have reported moral distress and ethical concerns in practice, this seemed to be particularly intense during the aftermath of cutbacks and workload increases in the 1990s (Gaudine & Thorne, 2000; Rodney, Varcoe et al., 2002). Since that period, there seems to have been greater attention given to ethics within organizations. According to Gibson (2012), there has been a "dramatic increase in attention paid to ethics in Canadian health institutions" in the past 10 years (p. 37).

At the national level, there have been some steps taken to promote ethics within Canadian health care organizations. Accreditation Canada (2010) developed new standards that were introduced in 2008, and health care organizations that pursue the voluntary program of accreditation examine their own organization in terms of those standards, prior to a site visit by external reviewers. Although the program is voluntary, the majority of hospitals and increasing numbers of institutional and community-based services that employ nurses are undergoing accreditation. The revised program, called Qmentum that was introduced in 2008, has a greater focus than the earlier one had on quality improvement and patient safety (Accreditation Canada, 2009). Standard 5 under the section on "Effective Organization" requires the organization's leaders make decisions consistent with the stated values and ethics that they have defined. These standards also indicate that the leaders "develop and implement an ethics framework" (Accreditation Canada, 2010, p. 7). The ethics framework defines the formal process for managing ethical issues, and includes a process for reviewing the ethics of research conducted in the organization. The organization's leaders must identify who monitors the ethics framework and the processes for ethics, and they must also develop and improve the ethics knowledge of all the players—board of governors, leaders, staff members, and service providers. In 2009, Accreditation Canada held a national conference on Ethics in Health Care "showcasing the tools and strategies organizations need to deal with sensitive ethical issues that arise in health care" (p. 6).

Accreditation Canada mentions several kinds of issues that might be addressed by an ethics framework that a health care organization develops and adopts. One guideline reads: "The ethics framework may address issues related to organizational ethics, research ethics, clinical ethics, and bioethics, as applicable" (Accreditation Canada, 2010, p. 7). **Organizational ethics** are typically distinguished from **clinical ethics** in that clinical ethics focuses on issues that arise for patients and providers in the provision of health care. An ethical situation that recurs may give rise to an organizational policy, for example, a policy on how decisions about resuscitation should be made and documented. However, organizational ethics generally refers to administrative and management ethical issues, including standards of business practice, the treatment of employees, resource allocation and management, and leadership practices that promote a positive moral climate within the organizations (Gibson, 2012; Keatings & Smith, 2010; Suhonen, Stolt, Virtanen & Leino-Kilpi, 2011). **Research ethics** refers to the policies on ethical review and monitoring of health care studies that are conducted within a health care organization. Some system of review of research proposals is established by organizations to ensure that such issues as consent, consideration of benefits and burdens, and scientific merit are addressed before approval to proceed with research is provided by an organization.

Ethical Resources in the Workplace

Health care organizations are apt to vary in what might be available in the workplace with respect to ethics resources. At a minimum, a health care organization or regional health service will have some statement of vision, mission, and values that can provide broad ethical direction for the services provided by that organization (Accreditation Canada, 2010). As an example, Box 14.3 contains this kind of statement from the Horizon Health Network in New Brunswick, which is a regional health care organization composed of hospitals, health centres, home care, public health, and other services in the province. As you can see, value statements typically contain a mixture of ethical and other kinds of values.

Box 14.3

Horizon Health Network Strategic Directions

Our Vision:	Leading for a Healthy Tomorrow
Our Mission:	Care for People, Educate, Innovate and Foster Research
Our Values:	Compassion, Respect, Integrity, Collaboration, Excellence, Sustainability, Innovation

Source: Reprinted by permission of Horizon Health.

Some of the other ethics resources that may provide useful guidance in health care organizations are discussed next.

Ethical Guidelines and Codes of Ethics

Some organizations may adopt a Code of Conduct or a Patient Bill of Rights that provide patients/clients and employees with statements about ethical conduct and standards that are expected in the organization. For example, hospitals with a religious sponsor may adhere to a specific code, such as the Health Ethics Guide of the Catholic Health Alliance of Canada (2012). However, in most health care organizations, practice is guided by the codes of ethics of the various health professions, because members of regulated health professions are accountable to their regulatory bodies, whether it is nursing, medicine, or physiotherapy, and to the standards set by the profession in the province or territory. For that reason, as a nurse, you should have a copy of your ethical guidelines or code of ethics that provides guidance for your practice. A copy might be available in your workplace, but these kinds of documents are easily accessed on nursing websites. Some national and provincial or territorial websites might provide additional ethical resources that are useful for the workplace. The section on Useful Websites will provide some sources for nurses in every part of the country; for example, there is a Canadian website on nursing ethics: www.nursingethics.ca/.

Ethics Committees

In some health care settings, there are ethics committees that have one or more functions related to ethical matters, but you are most apt to find these in large, acute care hospitals. In a 2008 survey of Canadian acute care hospitals with 100 beds or more, 126 responses were received for a response rate of 51% (Gaudine, Thorne, LeFort & Lamb, 2010). Approximately 85% of respondents reported having such a committee, with more than half of them established in the previous 10 years. These committees were advisory in nature, rather than making decisions about ethics, and the most common functions were education for committee members and health professionals (over 84%), counselling and support to health professionals (approximately 80%), and advising administration on organizational ethics issues (68%).

Ethics committees are typically interdisciplinary, with representation from such groups as nursing, medicine, and other health professionals, administration, law, ethics, clergy, board members, and so on. In addition to planning and organizing ethics education for the organization, some ethics committees provide consultation to health professionals and or patients and families with respect to clinical ethical issues in the hospital. Based on a case study of four Canadian hospitals, however, one might expect considerable variation in how hospitals handle ethics consultation. For example, in two settings in that study, a subset of the ethics committee offer consultations: one setting used an administrative-led ad hoc group, and one used a clinical ethicist who later reported briefly on consultations at ethics committee meetings (Gaudine, et al., 2011b).

There is some evidence that health professionals do not consult ethics committees when they are dealing with an ethical issue. In a qualitative study involving 34 nurses, 10 nurse managers, and 31 physicians from four hospitals, barriers to and facilitators to using the committees by these professionals were identified (Gaudine, et al., 2011a). A common barrier was lack of knowledge about the committee and how it could be used, but some fear of the reaction of others was also identified, notably nurses' concern about the chain of command. Physicians identified lack of expertise among committee members in medicine or ethics as a reason for not consulting ethics committees. Facilitators to using these committees included support within the unit and hospital by someone (a manager, ethicist, or patient advocate) and ethics education.

Ethics Education

Ethics education in health care organizations consists of a variety of approaches to raise ethical awareness and understanding among all those who work in or volunteer in those settings. As mentioned earlier, these endeavours are often the responsibility of an ethics committee, especially in large organizations, and may take many forms: a specific portion of orientation programs for new employees; luncheon seminars or discussion groups focused on an ethics scenario or ethics topic; ethics rounds wherein a real case situation is presented and discussed by those who were involved; and ethics workshops and conferences hosted by an organization or for which some employees are funded to attend. Nurses welcome activities designed to support learning about ethics (Storch, et al., 2009). The Ethics in Practice sessions discussed in the Leading Health Care Example in this chapter incorporated ethics education, but rather than something planned for a whole organization by an ethics committee, a group of nurses in a work setting choose the issue of greatest relevance to their practice for study and discussion (Scott, Marck, & Barton, 2011). In these sessions, the nurse leader identified relevant articles for the group participants to read. This activity is similar to the practice of ethics journal clubs in which nurses meet as a group on a regular basis to discuss a journal article on ethics.

Clinical Ethicists/Clinical Ethics Services

Clinical ethicist or bioethicist roles have developed since about the 1980s and these kinds of positions are most often found in large teaching hospitals. The ethicist is an individual with graduate preparation in philosophy, ethics, bioethics, or health care ethics, and typically, part of the preparation for the role is a placement or internship in a health care setting dealing with clinical or health care ethics consultation (Canadian Bioethics Society, 2008; Keatings & Smith, 2010). Health professionals from a variety of backgrounds pursue studies and a career in this kind of role, so you may meet clinical ethicists with a background in nursing or medicine. The role usually involves working with health care professionals, patients, and families to address issues and provide support for decision making in difficult situations. An ethicist employed by a health care organization provides ethics consultations, but also may be expected to plan and organize an ethics program or service that provides not only consultation, but also ethics education and advice on the ethical aspects of organizational policies and processes. For example, the Hospital for Sick Children (2013) in Toronto has a Department of Bioethics that "offers a consultation service for patients, families, and staff. This service is available to all patients, families, and health care practitioners who want help making difficult ethical decisions" (Hospital for Sick Children, 2013).

Leadership for Ethical Policy and Practice (LEPP): Participatory Action Project (2009)

At several sites in British Columbia a three-year research study that focused on how nurses could improve the ethical climate in health care was conducted. The researchers planned this study based on the belief that "researchers, policy makers, administrators and health-care providers, through participatory democratic processes informed by ethical perspectives, can make critical changes to health care oriented to the good of patients" (Storch et al., 2009, p. 71). The project, Leadership for Ethical Policy and Practice (LEPP), was designed to involve nurses in direct practice, supported by formal nurse leaders, in developing and trying out strategies in daily work that promoted a positive ethical climate in the workplace. The overall project had a lead team, an operations team, an advisory group, and site project teams. Six site project teams were involved in the project, and they ranged from one part of a large health facility to an entire small hospital. The teams varied by site and were composed of direct care nurses and other health care providers with the support of the chief nursing officer (CNO) or equivalent.

The methodology for the study was participatory action research (PAR) as it is suited to looking at change and learning as the study unfolds. With PAR, participants are involved in determining the purposes, actions, data collection, and analysis of the study as the project proceeded, and therefore sites in this study were able to tailor the project to their situations. The site team participants met on a regular basis to share and discuss ethical concerns and problems in practice and to problem-solve solutions in their workplace. There were differences in site projects, but the overall study was overseen by the lead team and the operation team. All teams came together for an annual conference at which participants shared experiences and evaluated the progress of the study.

The authors identified what had been learned during the PAR study. Nurses at the different sites varied in their approach to addressing practice issues using an "ethics lens" and used strategies that fit with their unique situations. Strategies included ethics debriefings, integration of the ethics work with ongoing site projects, such as patient safety, or focused on interdisciplinary collaboration to resolve ethical challenges. Some site teams pursued and obtained research funding for their projects. Overall study findings identified by the authors included the following:

- the importance of nurses' addressing their own issues in a practice setting
- nurses in formal leadership roles are key in supporting an ethical climate
- direct or indirect support of decision makers, Chief Nursing Officers (CNO), gave many nurses a sense of hope and connection to other nurses
- nurses valued the ethics lens, and PAR methods often provided them with new ideas about helpful actions

The authors acknowledge that PAR projects take considerable time and persistence to bring about changes and recognize the challenge of sustaining such projects. On the plus side, however, they note that there was considerable spillover from the projects and that knowledge transfer took place to other nursing groups and locations during the project.

Source: Storch, J., Rodney, P., Varcoe, C., Pauly, B., Starzomski, R., Stevenson, L., Best, L., Mass, H., Fulton, T. R., Mildon, B., Bees, F., Chisolfm, A., MacDonald-Rencz, S., McCutcheon, A. S., Shamian, J., Thomspon, C., Makaroff, K. S., & Newton, L. (2009). Leadership for ethical policy and practice (LEPP): Participatory action project. Nursing Leadership, 22 (3), 68–80.

SUMMARY

Your nursing career can lead you to work in a variety of health care organizations and settings, and you may notice differences in the moral climate and culture of these workplaces. Ethical reflection throughout your career will enable you to identify when and where you have enacted your moral agency and when you have experienced moral distress. The ability to recognize ethical issues and reflect on why you may feel constraints that prevent doing what you feel is the right thing to do are skills and practices that will serve you well. They will help you find your moral voice. Sometimes, just being able to "name" a problem or issue helps you consider what resources to draw on and how to seek a resolution in an effective way. In this chapter, you have been introduced to the idea of ethical leadership and character in ethical leaders. You will recognize such leadership in others and in yourself as you reflect on your practice. You will also play a role in building a moral community in your workplace as you seek to contribute to and promote a positive moral climate.

Glossary of Terms

Character   refers to a multidimensional concept that includes moral discipline (personal needs are subordinated to the greater social good), moral attachment (commitment to something greater than yourself), and moral autonomy (discretion and judgment to freely act in a moral way) (Wright & Quick, 2011). Character implies habitual qualities to act in a moral way.

Clinical ethics   refers to the standards that apply to clinical situations and issues in health care; these typically involve the practice of health care professionals and their concerns about care of patients/clients.

Ethos   as described by Hannah and Avolio (2011b, p. 991), refers to "... an inner strength driving virtue ... a distinct class of character—a class that when possessed by an individual will provide the inner strength or resources to step up and perform extra-ethical, virtuous action."

Moral agent/agency   refers to the ability to deliberate, choose, express, and act upon moral responsibilities. Nurses enact their moral agency when they reflect on and act in an ethical manner as they engage in professional practice.

Moral community   refers to clear and shared values within a workplace that enable ethical action and discussion of ethical values and issues.

Moral distress   refers to the negative feelings, such as anger and guilt, that are experienced when an individual acts contrary to his or her moral choice because of internal and/or external constraints.

Moral/Ethical climate   refers to the prevailing values that influence a workplace or the health care system in general and that have an effect on professional practice within it.

Moral/Ethical culture   refers to formal and informal systems in an organization that support either ethical or unethical behaviour. Examples include codes, ethical norms, leadership, policies, reward systems.

Moral residue   refers to the lingering guilt or feelings that persist with unresolved moral distress or from acting in a way that is inconsistent with moral values due to choice or external constraints.

Organizational ethics   refers to the ethical issues and standards related to administration and management within an organization and how these influence organizational life; often this refers to the business aspect of a health care organization, human resource practices and the ethical aspects of decisions.

Research ethics refers to ethical standards for the conduct of research. Organizations establish some system for review of research proposals to ensure that they meet ethical standards and that ongoing monitoring is carried out, as required.

CASE

Danielle works on a medical unit that increasingly has patients who are drug users and who are hospitalized for treatment of other medical conditions. The nurses on the unit find that these patients are challenging to care for—their behaviour is sometimes aggressive and they frequently leave the unit. The nurses sometimes suspect they are seeking drugs and even using their IV lines for drug use. Danielle is concerned that the disapproval and dislike of these patients by colleagues might lead to care that is inadequate, and she sees this as an ethical issue. Some nurses complain to the nurse manager and to physicians and tell them that such patients should be treated on a psychiatric unit rather than a medical one.

Questions

1. Do you agree with Danielle that this situation raises ethical issues? If so, how would you describe these?

2. What role do you think Danielle could play in addressing this issue? What role do you think the nurse manager has regarding this issue?

3. What resources in the organization might contribute to addressing ethical issues in this situation?

4. How might such situations affect the ethical climate?

5. What do you think of the suggestion that these patients should be treated on psychiatric units?

Critical Thinking Questions and Activities

1. Reflect on a clinical experience in which you felt constrained to do what you thought was the "right thing" in providing care. What was it that caused you to feel constrained? Was there some aspect of the moral culture that influenced you?

2. Identify a formal or informal leader in your organization who you think is an ethical leader. Does this person demonstrate qualities that you think illustrate character? How has this person behaved that led you to identify him or her as an ethical leader?

3. Look for the formal values espoused in the organization in which you work. How many of these values do you consider to be ethical ones? Can you imagine a situation in which espoused values might conflict with each other? Have you seen evidence of one or more of these values

in the way the organization functions or makes decisions?

4. Investigate the ethical resources available in your health care organization. Informally survey your colleagues to see if they have used any of these resources to address an ethical issue.

5. Do you have a moral community in your work setting? If you think you do, identify what it is that makes you think you do. If you think you do not, what do you think you could do to promote building a moral community?

Self-Quiz

A registered nurse who is a staff nurse in a long-term care setting leaves work following the night shift after a patient died during the shift. The night shift was short-handed, and despite the nurse asking for a replacement nurse, the facility did not provide one. The nurse is feeling sad and guilty because her usual rounds were interrupted due to another resident's seizures that took everyone's attention, and she only discovered the death of her elderly patient when she resumed her rounds later. The following questions relate to this situation.

1. The feelings the nurse is experiencing are characteristic of:
   a. Institutional culpability
   b. Power imbalance
   c. Moral distress
   d. Ethical character

2. If the health care setting continues to emphasize controlling staffing costs, which causes nurses to feel as though the care of patients is compromised, it is likely to have a negative effect on:
   a. Transformational leadership
   b. Idealized influence
   c. Ethical disengagement
   d. Moral climate

3. A nurse manager who addressed this issue by drawing on the nursing code of ethics and standards to argue for improved staffing would be exhibiting which kind of leadership?
   a. Ethical
   b. Authentic
   c. Transactional
   d. Transformational

4. In health care settings, ethical issues related to staffing and human resources are considered to be matters of:
   a. Research ethics
   b. Clinical ethics
   c. Bioethics
   d. Organizational ethics

Useful Websites

Accreditation Canada
www.accreditation.ca/en/

Canadian Bioethics Society
www.bioethics.ca/

Canadian Nurses Association on Nursing Ethics
www.cna-aiic.ca/en/improve-your-workplace/nursing-ethics/

Catholic Health Alliance of Canada
Health Ethics Guide
www.chac.ca/resources/ethics/ethicsguide_e.
php

International Council of Nurses
www.icn.ch/about-icn/about-icn/

Nursing Ethics.ca
www.nursingethics.ca/

References

Accreditation Canada. (2009). *Annual report 2009. Driving quality health services.* Ottawa: Accreditation Canada. Retrieved from http://www.accreditation.ca

Accreditation Canada. (2010). Qmentum Program. *Effective organization. Standards.* Ottawa: Author.

Alberta Health expense scandal claims former CEO. (2012, August 3). CBC News. Retrieved from www.cbc.ca/news/health/story/2012/08/02edmonton-weatherill-resigns-merali.html

American Nurses Association. (2009). *Nursing administration. Scope and standards of practice.* Silver Spring, Maryland: Author.

Association of Registered Nurses of Prince Edward Island. (2011). *Standards for nursing practice.* Charlottetown, PEI: Author.

Austin, W., Bergum, V., & Goldberg, L. (2003). Unable to answer the call of our patients: mental health nurses' experience of moral distress. *Nursing Inquiry, 10*(3), 177–183.

Baumann, A., Giovannetti, P., O'Brien-Pallas, L., Mallette, C., Deber, R., Blythe, J., Hibberd, J., & DiCenso, A. (2001). Healthcare restructuring: The impact of job change. *Canadian Journal of Nursing Leadership, 14*(1), 14–20.

Brown, M.E., & Treviño, L.K. (2006). Ethical leadership: A review and future directions. *The Leadership Quarterly, 17*(6), 595–616.

Campbell, A. (December, 2006). *Spring of fear. The SARS commission final report.* Available from www.archives.gov.on.ca/en/e_records/sars/report/v3.html

Canadian Bioethics Society. (May, 2008). *The development of a model job/role descriptions.* Report to the CBS from the Task Force on Working Conditions for Bioethicists. Retrieved January 10, 2013, from www.bioethics.ca/

Canadian Nurses Association. (2008). *Code of ethics for registered nurses.* Ottawa: CNA.

Canadian Nurses Association. (January, 2010). *Ethics in practice for registered nurses. Ethics, relationships and quality practice environments.* Ottawa: CNA.

Catholic Health Alliance of Canada. (2012). *Health ethics guide.* 3rd ed. Available from www.chac.ca/resoures/ethics/ethicsguide_e.php

College of Nurses of Ontario. (2009). *Ethics. Practice standard.* Available from: www.cno.org

Corley, M. (2002). Nurse moral distress: a proposed theory and research agenda. *Nursing Ethics, 9*(6), 636–650.

Cummings, G., & Estabrooks, C.A. (2003). The effects of hospital restructuring that included layoffs on individual nurses who remained employed: A systematic review of impact. *International Journal of Sociology and Social Policy, 23*(8/9), 8–53.

EHealth scandal a $1B waste: auditor. (2007, October 7). CBC News. Retrieved from www.cbc.ca/news/canada/toronto/story/2009/10/07/ehealth-auditor.html

Gaudine, A.P., & Beaton, M.R. (2002). Employed to go against one's values: Nurse managers' accounts of ethical conflict within their organizations. *Canadian Journal of Nursing Research, 34*(2), 17–34.

Gaudine, A., Lamb, M., LeFort, S., & Thorne, L. (2011a). Barriers and facilitators to consulting hospital clinical ethics committees. *Nursing Ethics, 18*(6), 767–780.

Gaudine, A., Lamb, M., LeFort, S., & Thorne, L. (2011b). The functioning of hospital ethics committees: A multiple-case study of four Canadian committees. *HEC Forum, 23,* 225–238.

Gaudine, A., LeFort, S., Lamb, M., & Thorne, L. (2011a). Clinical ethical conflicts of nurses and physicians. *Nursing Ethics, 18*(1), 9–19.

Gaudine, A., LeFort, S., Lamb, M., & Thorne, L. (2011b) Ethical conflicts with hospitals: The perspective of nurses and physicians. *Nursing Ethics, 18*(6), 756–766.

Gaudine, A., & Thorne, L. (2000). Ethical conflict in professionals. Nurses' accounts of ethical conflict with organizations. *Research in Ethical Issues in Organizations, 2,* 41–58.

Gaudine, A., & Thorne, L. (2009). The association between ethical conflict and adverse outcomes. *Journal of Business Ethics, 92*(2), 269–276.

Gaudine, A., & Thorne, L. (2012). Nurses' ethical conflict with hospitals: A longitudinal study of outcomes. *Nursing Ethics, 19*(6), 727–237.

Gaudine, A., Thorne, L., LeFort, S., & Lamb, M. (2010). Evolution of hospital clinical ethics committees in Canada. *Journal of Medical Ethics, 36,* 132–137.

Gibson, J.L. (2012). Reflections on healthcare leadership ethics. Organizational ethics: No longer the elephant in the room. *Healthcare Management Forum, 25,* 37–39.

Green, A., & Jeffers, B. (2006). Exploring moral distress in the long-term care setting. *Perspectives, 30*(4), 5–9.

Hannah, S.T., & Avolio, B.J. (2011a). The locus of leader character. *The Leadership Quarterly, 22*(5), 979–983.

Hannah, S.T., & Avolio, B.J. (2011b). Leader character, ethos, and virtue: Individual and collective considerations. *The Leadership Quarterly, 22*(5), 989–994.

Horizon Health Network. (2013). *Strategic directions.* Retrieved January 13, 2013, from www.horizonnb.ca/home/about-us/strategic-directionsaspx.

Hospital for Sick Children. (2013). *Department of Bioethics. Who we are.* www.sickkids.ca/bioethics/index.html

International Council of Nurses. (2012). *The ICN code of ethics for nurses.* Geneva: ICN.

Jameton, A. (1984). *Nursing practice: The ethical issues.* Englewood Cliffs, NJ: Prentice Hall.

Keatings, M., & Smith, O. (2010). *Ethical and legal issues in Canadian nursing.* 3rd ed. Toronto: Mosby.

McArthur, G., & Montero, D. (2012, December 22). Meet Arthur T. Porter, the man at the centre of one of Canada's biggest health-care scandals. *The Globe and Mail.* Retrieved from www.theglobeandmail.com

L'Ordre des infirmières et infirmiers du Québec. (2012). *Code de déontologie des infirmières et infirmiers.* Available from www.oiiq.org/lordre/qui-sommes-nous/lois-et-reglements

Pauly, B., Varcoe, C., Storch, J., & Newton, L. (2009). Registered nurses' perceptions of moral distress and ethical climate. *Nursing Ethics, 16*(5), 561–573.

Quick, J.C., & Wright, T.A. (2011). Character-based leadership, context and consequences. *The Leadership Quarterly, 22,* 984–988.

Reed, G.E. (2012). Leading questions. Leadership, ethics, and administrative evil. *Leadership, 8*(2), 187–198.

Rittenmeyer, L., & Huffman, D. (2009). How professional nurses working in hospital environments experience moral distress: A systematic review. *JBI Library of Systematic Reviews 7*(28), 1233–1290.

Rodney, P., Buckley, B., Street, A., Serrano, E., & Martin, L.A. (2013). The moral climate of nursing practice: Inquiry and action. In J.L. Storch, P. Rodney & R. Starzomski (Eds.) *Toward a moral horizon. Nursing ethics for leadership and practice.* 2nd ed. (pp. 188–214). Toronto: Pearson.

Rodney, P., Harrigan, M., Jiwani, B., Burgess, M., & Phillips, J.C. (2013). A further landscape: Ethics in health care organizations and health/health care policy. In J.L. Storch, P. Rodney & R. Starzomski (Eds.) *Toward a moral horizon. Nursing ethics for leadership and practice.* 2nd ed. (pp. 358–383). Toronto: Pearson.

Rodney, P., Varcoe, C., Storch, J.L., McPherson, G., Mahoney, K., Brown, H., Pauly, B., Hartrick, G., & Starzomski, R. (2002).

Canadian Journal of Nursing Research, 34(3), 75–102.

Scott, S.L., Marck, P., & Barton, S. (2011). Exploring ethics in practice: Creating moral community in healthcare one place at a time. *Nursing Research, 24*(4), 78–87.

Shirey, M.R. (2005). Ethical climate in nursing practice. The leader's role. *JONA'S Healthcare Law, Ethics, and Regulation, 7*(2), 59–67.

Storch, J.L. (2010). Comment on Pattison and Wainwright: 'Is the 2008 NMC code ethical?' *Nursing Ethics, 17*(1), 19–21.

Storch, J.L., Rodney, P., Pauly, B., Brown, H., & Starzomski, R. (2002). Listening to nurses' moral voices: Building a quality health care environment. *Canadian Journal of Nursing Leadership, 15*(4), 7–16.

Storch, J., Rodney, P., Pauly, B., Fulton, T.R., Stevenson, L., Newton, L., & Makaroff, K.S. (2009). Enhancing ethical climates in nursing work environment. *Canadian Nurse, 10*(3), 20–25.

Storch, J., Rodney, P., Varcoe, C., Pauly, B., Starzomski, R., Stevenson, L., Best, L., Mass, H., Fulton, T.R., Mildon, B., Bees, F., Chisolfm, A., MacDonald-Rencz, S., McCutcheon, A.S., Shamian, J., Thomspon, C., Makaroff, K.S., & Newton, L. (2009). Leadership for ethical policy and practice (LEPP): Participatory action project. *Nursing Leadership, 22*(3), 68–80.

Suhonen, R., Stolt, M., Virtanen, H., & Leino-Kilpi, H. (2011). Organizational ethics: A literature review. *Nursing Ethics, 18*(3), 285–303.

Tschudin, V. (2010). Nursing ethics: The last decade. *Nursing Ethics, 17*(1), 127–131.

Webster, G., & Baylis, F. (2000). Moral residue. In S. Rubin & L. Zoloth (Eds.), *Margin of error: The ethics of mistakes in the practice of medicine* (pp. 217–230). Hagerstown, MD: University Publishing.

Wilkinson, J.M. (1987/88). Moral distress in nursing practice: Experience and effect. *Nursing Forum, 23*(1), 16–29.

Wright, T.A., & Quick, J.C. (2011). The role of character in ethical leadership research. *The Leadership Quarterly, 22*, 975–978.

Appendix– Answer Key

Chapter 1
1) c   2) c   3) a   4) d

Chapter 2
1) d   2) c   3) c   4) a

Chapter 3
1) a   2) b   3) d   4) c

Chapter 4
1) b   2) a   3) d   4) b

Chapter 5
1) c   2) d   3) a   4) d

Chapter 6
1) d   2) d   3) d   4) a

Chapter 7
1) d   2) b   3) a   4) c   5) b   6) c

Chapter 8
1) a   2) b   3) d   4) c

Chapter 9
1) d   2) a   3) c   4) b

Chapter 10
1) a   2) c   3) c   4) c   5) c

Chapter 11
1) d   2) a   3) c   4) a

Chapter 12
1) c   2) a   3) c   4) d

Chapter 13
1) c   2) d   3) a   4) d

Chapter 14
1) c   2) d   3) a   4) d

Index

Note: *f* denotes a figure and *t* denotes a table.